AF717510

Theater Ballistic Missile Defense

Theater Ballistic Missile Defense

Edited by
Ben-Zion Naveh (Editor)
WALES Ltd., Ramat-Gan, Israel
Azriel Lorber (Associate Editor)
WALES Ltd., Ramat-Gan, Israel

Volume 192
PROGRESS IN
ASTRONAUTICS AND AERONAUTICS

Paul Zarchan, Editor-in-Chief
MIT Lincoln Laboratory
Lexington, Massachusetts

Published by the
American Institute of Aeronautics and Astronautics, Inc.
1801 Alexander Bell Drive, Reston, Virginia 20191-4344

Copyright © 2001 by the American Institute of Aeronautics and Astronautics, Inc. Printed in the United States of America. All rights reserved. Reproduction or translation of any part of this work beyond that permitted by Sections 107 and 108 of the U.S. Copyright Law without the permission of the copyright owner is unlawful. The code following this statement indicates the copyright owner's consent that copies of articles in this volume may be made for personal or internal use, on condition that the copier pay the per-copy fee ($2.00) plus the per-page fee ($0.50) through the Copyright Clearance Center, Inc., 222 Rosewood Drive, Danvers, Massachusetts 01923. This consent does not extend to other kinds of copying, for which permission requests should be addressed to the publisher. Users should employ the following code when reporting copying from this volume to the Copyright Clearance Center:

1-56347-385-2 $2.00 + .50

Data and information appearing in this book are for informational purposes only. AIAA is not responsible for any injury or damage resulting from use or reliance, nor does AIAA warrant that use or reliance will be free from privately owned rights.

ISBN 1-56347-385-2

This book is dedicated to the memory of the late Brig. Gen. (Ret.) Michael Cohen, head of Materiél Directorate at the Israeli Air Force, founder of WALES Ltd., and recipient of the David R. Israel Award for Meritorious Achievement for his work on the Israeli BMD architecture

Progress in Astronautics and Aeronautics

Editor-in-Chief
Paul Zarchan
MIT Lincoln Laboratory

Editorial Board

John Binder
MathWorks, Inc.

Richard Lind
NASA Dryden Flight Research Center

Lt. Col. Steven A. Brandt
U.S. Air Force Academy

Richard M. Lloyd
Raytheon Electronics Company

Fred DeJarnette
North Carolina State University

Ahmed K. Noor
NASA Langley Research Center

Leroy S. Fletcher
Texas A&M University

Albert C. Piccirillo
ANSER, Inc.

Michael D. Griffin
Orbital Sciences Corporation

Vigor Yang
Pennsylvania State University

Phillip D. Hattis
Charles Stark Draper Laboratory, Inc.

Ben T. Zinn
Georgia Institute of Technology

Foreword

While writing this foreword, I was informed of the spectacular success of the Arrow system as it intercepted a Black Sparrow missile simulation of a SCUD ballistic missile.

I was deeply involved with both the Arrow and Black Sparrow projects from their inception and saw them through advanced stages of funding and development. I was at the center of the early crises, including budgetary difficulties and failed prototypes. Because of my close personal involvement with this project, I was deeply satisfied with its latest success. Yet we must remember to constantly examine our assumptions and focus on future challenges and ways to cope with them, while striving to obtain timely answers in advance and not after the fact. After all, we had the technological capabilities to develop the Arrow system even before the Gulf War, yet we did not prepare ourselves sufficiently for the crisis of 1991. Our assessment of the risks involved in the acquisition of ground-to-ground tactical missiles by the countries of the region was inadequate.

The general trend of thought during the 1970s and 1980s downplayed the importance of defense systems against tactical ballistic missiles carrying conventional warheads. Since the accuracy of the tactical missiles left much to be desired, many concluded that they did not constitute a material threat to military forces or strategic assets. In addition, it was argued that deterrence measures, such as the threat of a significant offensive response, were sufficient to prevent attacks against civilian targets and population centers. Furthermore, it was assumed that hostile countries would not dare to fire missiles armed with chemical or biological warheads at civilian targets.

Indeed, a survey of the brief history of the use of ballistic missiles in various conflicts should have contradicted these assumptions and conclusions. However faced with shrinking budgets and immediate requirements, there was an understandable tendency to postpone long-term needs. Thus, immediate security threats received full attention and support, while uncertain threats, such as the deployment of ballistic missiles, became a secondary budgetary priority.

Ballistic missiles were first used in the Second World War when the Germans developed the extraordinary V-2, a tactical ballistic missile. The V-2 was further developed by the Soviet Union and eventually turned into the ubiquitous SCUD. The V-2 was initially intended for use against large population centers. The British failed in attempts to develop a defense against it. They tried to locate the launchers on the French coast and destroy them by aerial attack but these were well dispersed and, by their very nature, difficult to identify.

The Normandy invasion pushed the launching sites further back and out of Britain's range (although the attacks against Antwerp continued, with more missiles hitting that city than London). This prevented the V-2 from becoming a successful and effective weapon against the British population. Otherwise, the Second World War might have proceeded differently.

During the Iran–Iraq War, in the 1980s, both sides fired ballistic missiles against each other's population centers. Tehran suffered great losses as a result, although the Iraqi warheads were conventional. The city's inhabitants clearly demonstrated concern and fear as they evacuated the city in droves. It is argued that the effect of missile attacks was one of the reasons for the war's conclusion. Moreover, this experience probably contributed to Iran's decision to launch an intensive program of acquisition and development of ballistic missiles.

On a different note, the Syrian military leadership claimed that the uncontested superiority of the Israeli Air Force was the decisive factor in the 1982 Lebanon war. The Syrians' declared conclusion was that while the Lebanon War was fought using ground-to-air missiles, the next war would be characterized by ground-to-ground missiles. (In 1982, the Syrian air defense, based on ground-to-air missiles, suffered a defeat in the Bekka Valley.) As such, the Syrians intensified their efforts to aquire additional SS-21 and SCUD-B ballistic missiles. They later developed an indigenous capability to produce ballistic missiles while also acquiring longer range missiles, such as the SCUD-C and the SCUD-D.

These facts notwithstanding, the assessment of Israel's defense establishment until the 1991 Gulf War held that there was no justification to develop an antiballistic missile defense system. It is important to note that this assessment was not the result of faulty intelligence. There was no lack of data regarding the armaments of the region.

Undoubtedly, the Gulf War significantly shifted the appraisal of the situation. On the one hand, it encouraged the countries of the region to intensify their efforts to acquire ballistic missiles. After all, even a superpower such as the United States, armed with commanding satellite systems and the most advanced reconnaissance capabilities and attack aircraft, failed to stop the launches until the end of the war. At the same time, countries faced with the threat of a ballistic missile attack were encouraged to develop antiballistic missile defense systems as a result.

The ground-to-ground ballistic missile has introduced a new dimension to conventional warfare. It is no longer necessary to share a border in order to mount an attack against an enemy country. Consequently, military doctrines are undergoing change since up until now ground forces constituted the decisive force in warfare. Absent a common border, decisions on the ground are rendered obsolete, making it very difficult to achieve a decisive victory in a conventional war. As a result, several countries have developed chemical warheads to obtain a military advantage by means of non-conventional weapons. This development heightened the need for antiballistic missile defense systems to enable political decision makers the needed time to develop a measured response in the event of an attack. After all, the flight time of a ballistic missile ranges from three to seven minutes, depending on the range.

In order to rehabilitate conventional deterrence, it will become imperative to develop a defensive system capable of destroying offensive weapons while still over the aggressor's territory. A country launching missiles with chemical or other warheads will thereby need to carefully weight the risk of several missiles striking its own territory. Consequently, systems for the interception and destruction of ballistic missiles at the launch and boost phases will be critical to the reestablishment of international stability in several regions of the world.

Even if we succeed in developing suitable counter-measures, we are already facing new concepts of warfare developed as a result of the proliferation of ballistic missile technology. The need for early detection and warning systems, passive and active defenses, as well as long-range offensive systems will bring about many new developments in various fields, including hardware. Those who reach the correct assessments early on and develop appropriate responses will no doubt contribute to regional stability and prevent future conflicts.

His Excellency
Major General (Ret.) David Ivry
Ambassador of Israel to the United States
February 2001

Table of Contents

II. Threat and Response

III. Interoperability, Battle Management, and Strategic Considerations

IV. Guidance and Control in Theater Ballistic Missile Defense

V. Measures of System Effectiveness and Risk Management

Preface

In May 1985, U.S. President Ronald Reagan invited Israel to participate in the Strategic Defense Initiative (SDI) program, popularly known as "Star Wars." This program reflected President Reagan's ambitious decision to develop technologies and weapon systems that could provide defense against strategic ballistic missiles, and the Strategic Defense Initiative Organization (SDIO) was established within the U.S. Department of Defense (DoD) to manage this program.

The invitation to join the program was sent to a small number of countries, all U.S. allies, and all possessing highly advanced levels of defense technologies. The inclusion of Israel amongst those highly developed countries was in itself a compliment and a recognition by the United States of Israel's advanced defense technologies and R&D capabilities. Nevertheless, the decision to join this U.S. initiative was not easy. Scientists in many countries opposed the program for various technological, economic, and strategic reasons. Israel had another consideration—people were concerned that Jewish immigration from the Soviet Union might be compromised by Israel joining a U.S.-led program that was directly challenging the Soviet Union.

Israel also evaluated other aspects of joining the program and assessed the advantages to Israel and the potential contribution Israel could make to the program. The technological community at the Israel Ministry of Defense (IMOD) identified the unique opportunity to become a partner in a very advanced technology program, which would boost and enhance Israel's indigenous technological capabilities, and assessed that Israeli scientists and engineers could make a significant contribution to the United States, despite Israel's relatively small size and population.

It is interesting to note that in those days very few people at the IMOD or the Israel Defense Forces were concerned about the ballistic missile threat as long as the missiles were conventional. IMOD, however, did recognize that joining the program would provide an opportunity to develop technologies that could be applied to ballistic missile defense if and when the need emerged, or if countries hostile to Israel acquired unconventional capabilities. Thus the Israeli government decided to join the SDI program, and in May 1986 a Memorandum of Understanding (MOU) was signed.

Following this decision, a first meeting took place between IMOD and DoD representatives, the U.S. team being headed by Lt. Gen. James Abrahamson, then Director of SDIO. Gen. Abrahamson's message was clear: The technological sky is the limit. Israel is invited to submit research proposals as advanced and as futuristic as it wishes. Proposals accepted by the United States would be funded by SDIO. The only condition was that those research proposals must be relevant to ballistic missile defense.

The IMOD established a new, dedicated, SDI Cooperation Program Office, and that office got to work, soliciting and eventually receiving about 70 research proposals from Israeli universities, research centers, and industries. These proposals were submitted to SDIO; then nothing happened.

It took this SDI Cooperation Office several months to realize that the approach was all wrong. SDIO did not expect Israel to submit proposals in scientific fields that many U.S. researchers were investigating and where Israel did not have a distinct advantage. Rather, it expected Israel to contribute in the one field where Israel had demonstrated its proficiency and excellence: tactical warfare. These were the days following the Lebanese conflict, where Israel had been very successful in attacking and destroying the Syrian surface-to-air missile batteries. The idea was that the Israeli planner, who planned and orchestrated this operation, could very well plan and orchestrate the defense against a multimissile attack, using a large number of defensive assets simultaneously. This is called, in professional language, "battle management."

In parallel, the United States revised its thinking as well. Faced with criticism from Western European allies that, while it was conceivable that the United States could protect its own territory against intercontinental ballistic missiles launched by the Soviet Union, the Western European countries could be attacked by short-range (tactical) ballistic missiles from Eastern Europe, against which the weapons and technologies developed by the United States would not be effective. Thus the United States decided on a new policy: The United States would help its allies defend themselves against their own threats.

This new U.S. policy, plus Israel's realization that its best contribution to the United States would be in theater missile defense (TMD), plus the emerging ballistic missile threat from Iraq and verbal threats made by the Iraqi president, gave birth to the Israeli decision to concentrate on TMD. Thus Israel was the first country to enter this field and eventually attained a leadership role.

Again, the SDI Cooperation Office solicited proposals from Israeli industries, and the proposals were quite numerous. When Gen. Abrahamson visited Israel in 1986, those proposals were presented to him. In his summary comments the general indicated that there was only one way to decide which proposal ought to be supported: Perform an "architecture study" in which the present and emerging threats would be assessed, the candidate technologies and systems would be evaluated as to their potential response to the threat, and the cost of the different solutions would be estimated to arrive at the most cost effective system.

The general's suggestion was accepted by the IMOD, and WALES Ltd. was selected to perform the study. At the end of phase one of this study, WALES recommended a multitier defense system, including UAV-based boost-phase interception (BPI), high altitude, terminal phase, area defense (Arrow) and low-altitude point defense (hypervelocity weapon and high energy laser).

Based on the results of the architecture study and the realization that area defense was more cost-effective than point defense, the United States and Israel decided that the first priority would go to an Arrow demonstration program to prove the feasibility of intercepting an incoming ballistic missile. This decision resulted in a DoD–IMOD Memorandum of Agreement (MOA), signed in 1988, followed by a contract between the U.S. Army Strategic Defense Command and the Israel Aircraft Industries (IAI), which started the Arrow program. Then came the Gulf War and Israel's bitter experience of having its cities attacked by ballistic missiles. As a result of the lessons learned in the Gulf War, Israel decided to take advantage of the Arrow demonstration program and develop the Arrow into a fully operational weapon system. The rest is history.

There are many more aspects to Israel's cooperation with the Ballistic Missile Defense Organization (BMDO, the new name of SDIO), such as development of the Israeli test bed, initial development of the hypervelocity weapon, the BPI concept and risk mitigation studies, and the emerging boost-phase launcher intercept (BPLI) program. However, the Arrow remains the most visible and tangible result to date of this cooperation, the backbone of the Israeli ballistic missile defense system and of the U.S.–Israel interoperability effort.

This joint U.S.–Israel TMD program is now in its fifteenth year and is probably by far the most successful large-scale cooperative U.S.–Israel Defense R&D program to date. Both sides demonstrated a very high level of motivation, commitment, dedication, and professionalism based on a common goal rarely seen in any international program. All meetings, discussions, and negotiations were carried out in a spirit of friendship and sensitivity to each other's positions, always seeking accommodations, mutual benefits, and mutually acceptable solutions. Israel became the most active U.S. ally in TMD, and its recent successes in the Arrow experiments, together with the recent U.S. successes, make this cooperation uniquely effective.

Many good people in Israel contributed to this successful cooperation in the IMOD, the Israel Air Force, and the Israeli defense industries, in particular IAI, Rafael, Tadiran, Soreq, and WALES. But I believe we should all credit and express our most sincere thanks and appreciation to the U.S. DoD, in particular BMDO, the U.S. Congress, and other friends of Israel who made it all possible.

Aron Moss
Israel Ministry of Defense
December 2000

Acknowledgments

Giving birth to this book took much more than nine months. The team effort put together in this volume finally has borne fruit and it is now time to pay tribute to all of those people and organizations that contributed to fulfilling this task.

Maj. Gen. (Ret.) David Ivry, now Israel's ambassador to the United States, served as managing director of the Israeli Ministry of Defense (IMOD) during most of the time the Arrow Weapon System was developed. He is to be thanked for his personal contribution to the Arrow program, and his contribution of the Foreword to this book is very appreciated. Aron Moss is serving with IMOD and, among other tasks, is responsible for carrying out the agreements between the U.S. Ballistic Missile Defense Organization (BMDO) and the IMOD, guiding the BMD programs from their initial phase in 1985 until today. Dr. Moss contributed his experience to the opening section of the book, and his participation is highly appreciated. Gil Naor, Deputy Director of the BMD Cooperation Program Office at the IMOD, is also thanked for his help and encouragement.

In appreciation, and with great admiration, many thanks to the Israeli Aircraft Industries (IAI) MLM Division, and its personnel, for their achievements in the Arrow Weapon System, establishing the framework for the work accomplished by all other participating organizations and persons involved in the BMD effort. Many thanks to Yair Ramati, managing director of MLM, Dani Peretz, Arrow project manager, and Avi Baum for their chapter describing the system and its major milestones. Other industry teams involved in the Arrow project are also cordially thanked. A lot of work that contributed to the contents of this volume was performed in the Israeli test bed (ITB). We would like to take this opportunity to recognize the contribution of the Tadiran ITB team, and in particular Shlomo Azar and Eliezer Kogan.

Many thanks to the IMOD personnel for their continued diligence in setting the requirements for and monitoring the entire Arrow program. Uzi Rubin, who headed the Israeli Missile Defense Organization (IMDO) for more than a decade, contributed a chapter devoted to the history and evolution of BMD efforts and political considerations, and he is cordially thanked for this. Yair Zadik and Asher Wagner are also thanked for their support and encouragement.

The WALES company management, Chava Cohen, Alik Hermetz, and Dror Cohen, realized the importance of a book of this nature and decided to take upon the company all efforts to assist in its creation. They also contributed many of the chapters.

Special recognition goes to WALES Ltd., a privately owned Israeli consulting company established in 1985 by the late Brig. Gen. (Ret.) Michael Cohen of the Israel Air Force. The company has unique knowledge and expertise in the theater missile defense (TMD) arena. Since 1987, WALES has been performing the system architecture study for the Israeli TMD effort on behalf of BMDO and IMOD. Among other large-scale projects in the field is the recently completed definition and risk mitigation study of the Israeli Boost-Phase Interception System (IBIS).

The WALES staff of 50 includes 45 technical personnel; 25% of these individuals have Ph.D.s, and several are retired high-ranking officers of the Israeli Air

Force and Army. Their activities vary in scope from the analysis of nationwide defense structures, through the assessment of system effectiveness on the modern battlefield, to the establishment of detailed requirements for elements of defense system. Over the past five years, current WALES employees presented a total of 21 papers at AIAA multinational TMD conferences.

The entire WALES team incorporated the writing task into their loaded agenda and came up with relevant analysis material based on actual experience. The WALES team did a tremendous task, by no means an easy accomplishment, and is to be given thanks. Author biographies are given in Appendix C.

Other members of the WALES Ltd. team in the past and present, although not actively involved in authoring this book, contributed a lot over the years to the material contained in some of the chapters. We acknowledge Ephraim Bashan, who has been involved in activities relating to the defense process and guidance and control; Maxi Blum, Yuval Karakookly, Lilach Sayag, and Ofrit Schweitzer, who contributed to the material included in Chapters 8, 9, and 14; and Peter Meyer and Menashe Simhi who contributed to the analysis of radar systems and their role in TMD and to issues involved in external cueing. Also, Colin Kessel, of PAMAM Ltd., contributed to the analysis of human factors and their impact on TMD. His work has especially added to the material contained in Chapters 14 and 15.

Many WALES staff were involved in the typing, drawing, and administrative work, and without them the book would not have come to life. All of them have our sincere gratitude.

Moshe Guelman and Joseph Ben-Asher, both of the aeronautical faculty at the Technion, are special consultants to WALES. They contributed and expressed their views on system analysis and guidance and control topics, and are cordially acknowledged. Joseph Shinar, also at the Technion, an old friend who for many years has worked on interception analysis, kindly contributed his recent work to this book and it is greatly appreciated.

Azriel Lorber, a specialist in weapon system development and author of numerous books and articles was engaged by WALES to give the book the correct format. His valued experience assisted the authors in their endeavors, and his work is very much appreciated.

The U.S. BMDO shares responsibility with the IMOD for the Arrow weapon system. They jointly deserve gratitude for the program's abounding success.

AIAA agreed to publish the book and market it via its effective channels, and we are deeply indebted to them. Many personnel from AIAA were involved in the success of bringing this book into being, led by Rodger Williams, Paul Zarchan, and Heather Brennan. We extend to them our thanks for being so helpful, encouraging, and patient. Finally we would like to thank the people who reviewed the book from the technical point of view. They encouraged us to come up with relevant material that we believe has great value to our readers.

Ben-Zion Naveh
December 2000

Acronyms and Abbreviations

ABL	airborne laser
ABM	antiballistic missile
ACES	Arrow continuation experiments
ADP	Arrow deployability program
AEGIS	aerial early-warning ground interception and integration system
AOR	area of responsibility
API	ascent-phase interception
APN	augmented proportional navigation
ARM	antiradiation missile
ASP	air situation picture
ATBM	antitheater (or tactical) ballistic missile
ATC	air traffic control
AWACS	airborne warning and control system
AWS	Arrow weapon system
BET	best estimate trajectory
BMC	battle management center
BMC^3	battle management, command, control, and communication
BMC^4I	battle management command, control, communications, computers, and intelligence
BMD	ballistic missile defense
BMDO	Ballistic Missile Defense Organization (U.S.)
BPI	boost-phase interception
BPLI	boost-phase launcher interception
BSE	baseline system effectiveness
BW	bandwidth
C^3I	command, control, communications, and intelligence
CB	chemical bulk
CBMC	central battle management and control
CEP	circular error probable
CONOPS	concept of operations
CPX	command post exercise
CSM	cluster submunitions
CSOP	combined standing operating procedure
DA	defended asset
DIS	distributed integrated systems
DoD	Department of Defense (U.S.)
DP	defense plan
DPS	defense plan sharing
DSP	defense support program
EAD	extended air defense
ECM	electronic counter measure
EIC	effective interceptor consumption
EMP	electromagnetic pulse
EO	electro-optic

FCC	fire command and control
FCR	fire control radar
FOM	figure(s) of merit
FTAAS	finite-time absolute asymptotic stability
FT-GAAS	finite-time global, absolute asymptotic stability
FWH	fragmented warhead
GBR	ground-based radar
GCC	ground control center
HE	high explosive
HIL	human-in-the-loop
HLA	high-level architecture
HTK	hit to kill
IAI	Israel Aircraft Industries
IBIS	Israeli boost-phase interception system
IBMC	intraconstellation battle management, command, control and communication
IC	interceptor consumption
ICR	interceptor consumption rate
IDF	Israel Defense Forces
IMI	Israel Military Industries
IMDO	Israeli Missile Defense Organization
IMOD	Israel Ministry of Defense
IR	infrared
IRST	infrared search and track system
ITB	Israeli test bed
JSTARS	joint surveillance target attack radar system
KA	kill assessment
KE	kinetic energy
LCC	launch control center
LOS	line of sight
LR	leakage rate or long range
MD	miss distance
MEL	minimum effort guidance
MIRV	multiple independently targeted reentry vehicle
MOE	measure(s) of effectiveness
MOM	measure(s) of merit
MOP	measure(s) of performance
MOU	memorandum of understanding
MR	medium range
MTBF	mean time between failure
MTCR	Missile Technology Control Regime
MTT	mean time to test
MTTR	mean time in repair
NBC	nuclear, biological, chemical
NMD	National Missile Defense (U.S.)
NTW-TBMD	Navy theater-wide tactical ballistic missile defense (U.S.)
ORBAT	order of battle
PAC	Patriot advanced capability
PD	proportional plus derivative

PENAIDS	penetration aids
PLI	prelaunch interception
PN	proportional navigation
PNG	proportional navigation guidance
PPN	pure proportional navigation
PTL	primary target line
R&D	research and development
RCS	radar cross section
RF	radio frequency
RMS	root mean square
ROE	rule(s) of engagement
RSL	reduced sensitivity guidance law
RT	random telegraph
RV	reentry vehicle
SAM	surface-to-air missile
SAT	search, acquisition, and tracking
SDI	Strategic Defense Initiative (U.S.)
SDIO	Strategic Defense Initiative Organization (U.S.)
SIAP	single integrated air picture
SR	short range
SSP_k	single shot probability of kill
SWAT	statistic workload analysis tool
TBM	theater ballistic missile
TBMD	theater (or tactical) ballistic missile defense
THAAD	theater high altitude area defense
TIS	threat information sharing
TMD	theater missile defense
TOF	time of flight
TPN	true proportional navigation
TTG	time to go
UAV	unmanned air vehicle
WMD	weapon(s) of mass destruction
XQ	external cue
ZMD	zero miss distance

I. Some Historic Elements

Chapter 1

Introduction to Theater Ballistic Missile Defense

Ben-Zion Naveh*
WALES Ltd., Ramat-Gan, Israel

I. Introduction

SHORT-RANGE ballistic projectiles have existed since the dawn of human history. The stone, the arrow, the free-flight rocket, the gun shell, and the bomb followed ballistic trajectories to reach their targets. World War II started the era of guided missiles when the people of London and Antwerp were targets to guided ballistic missiles flown out of Germany. For the last 50 years, since that war, guided missile technology has been used extensively in various applications. The rapid development of rocket propulsion systems enabled the missiles to reach every target on Earth and even out in space. The technology developed so well that current missiles are not really limited with regard to warhead types, weights, ranges, or precision.

The Cold War period was characterized by the huge number of ballistic missiles produced by the two superpowers. Those missiles can fly from everywhere (including from submerged submarines), to every target; their warheads are very effective and many were (and still are) aimed against highly populated areas. Today the technology is so well spread throughout the world that many nations can easily equip their arsenals with, at least, a "poor man's" weapon system. The ballistic missile has become a real threat to be considered by all nations. A hostile nation does not need to move forces or share a common border with the target country. A massive surprise attack is feasible in a very short time and can cause severe damage to the target, using conventional and nonconventional warheads.

II. Ballistic Missile Defense

Initially the fast-growing ballistic missile threat was poorly countered. During World War II there were attempts to shoot down the missiles as if they were airplanes, but to no avail. What's more, during World War II there was no warning

Copyright © 2000 by the American Institute of Aeronautics and Astronautics, Inc. All rights reserved.

*Special Consultant and Chief Systems Architect. Senior Member AIAA.

of attack because the technology was not up to the task of discovering an incoming missile. This element was improved somewhat during the Cold War but the main defense strategy remained passive. People were supposed to be warned in time and find a shelter to hide from the attack, as if it were an air raid. As flight and reentry velocity became higher and the explosive force of the warheads became larger, even this method became questionable. In some countries (e.g., the United States, Sweden, and Switzerland) massive shelters against atomic warheads were built following the passive defense concept, assuming people could be sheltered in them in time. In the late 1960s the development of "antiballistic missile" (ABM) missiles was started and stopped. Looking at different aspects of the problem the superpowers understood that such an arms race would be painful to them and signed the ABM treaty to limit the development of these weapons. This fact actually halted the development of technology related to ballistic missile defense (BMD) for more than 20 years.

For reasons not yet entirely understood, President Reagan initiated in 1983 the Strategic Defense Initiative (SDI) program, known as "Star Wars." This program enabled the beginning of development of limited weapon systems to counter some of the ballistic missile threats. (Reference 1 is an excellent source to learn about the ABM treaty, the history of BMD, and the beginning of SDI; see also Chapter 2 of this book.)

In 1991, during the Persian Gulf War, Iraq launched ballistic missiles against neighboring Saudi Arabia and against Israel, where there was no common border, causing loss of lives and property damage. The only existing defense system was the Patriot PAC-2, which was not designed to handle this kind of a threat. All aircraft raids to destroy the ballistic missiles launchers failed, and for many days nothing could be done to stop the ballistic missile attacks. They finally ceased with the end of the war. Fifty years after World War II, the only defense strategy that was helpful was still passive defense.

III. Theater Ballistic Missile Defense

The aftermath of the Gulf War brought to light another factor. As the threat of a massive exchange between the United States and the Soviet Union diminished, it suddenly became obvious that there was a need to defend U.S. expeditionary forces and friendly nations against limited ballistic missile attacks. There were two important differences between the old and new scenarios where one was a global confrontation and the other a relatively limited, local one. The first difference was the absolute size of the attack. Instead of thousands of missiles incoming almost simultaneously, the problem now was of several dozen missiles at most, against which a reasonable level of defense probably would be feasible. The second consideration was that most of the attack, at least for the near future, probably would be conventional (possibly chemical or biological), but would not manifest itself in hundreds of nuclear weapons with a yield of megatons. Thus the term *theater defense* came into wide use, in essence signifying a limited attack against a limited geographic area.

After the Gulf War it also became evident that even for short-range ballistic missiles there was not a good and reliable active answer. As a result the United States and Israel reshaped and accelerated their efforts to develop ballistic missile defense systems.

There are different ways to deal with limited ballistic missile attacks: 1) political deterrence and retaliation, 2) electronic warfare, 3) launching system destruction,

4) boost-phase interception, 5) midcourse interception, 6) reentry interception, and 7) passive defense. To defend a country one may decide to follow all of these paths or only part of them. The tradeoff is between the allowed or acceptable damage on the ground and the cost of the defense. Historically it can be shown that in many encounters on the battlefield an expensive system could be defeated by a cheaper one with the aid of advanced technology; e.g., a tank could be destroyed by an antitank missile or an airplane by an air-to-air missile, and so forth. Here, in the field of missile defense, the cost of defense systems is (for the time being at least) much higher than the cost of the attacking systems. This is a very difficult challenge that requires the defendant to be more sophisticated and, maybe, take more risks.

When the missile is equipped with an unconventional warhead its cost may be higher, but the need to *absolutely* prevent its penetration may make the defense effort considerably more expensive.

In a real attack ballistic missiles may come in salvos and from different directions at the same time. So, the issue becomes more complicated and the defense system needs to engage many threats simultaneously. Another serious problem is the necessity to verify the kill of a ballistic missile after an intercept attempt. If a kill was not assured a second try may be needed. All of these and more issues lead us to look at the defense problem on a national level and design a defense architecture that will be able to handle the various threat scenarios. Because of limited or specific performance characteristics and cost considerations, one type of a BMD system may not suffice, and several types will be needed to devise an architecture that will accomplish the mission. In such a case a whole new issue presents itself: Interoperability among different systems in real (and usually very short) time. If the different systems belong to different nations with different doctrines and considerations, one can imagine how complex the defense against a ballistic missile attack may become.

Each BMD system is planned to engage the threat in a different phase of its trajectory and by this create a series of "defense layers." An acceptable architecture designed to overcome a substantial ballistic missile attack will probably consist of several defense layers. In some cases the defense architectures will need the help of early warning systems. For active BMD systems these early warnings may serve as "external cueing" and help the engagement procedure. For passive defense it is very important to have the alarm given as early as possible, as was demonstrated during the 1991 Persian Gulf War. The incorporation of external cueing and early warning systems into a defense architecture is then subject to interoperability procedures (and problems) and cost-effectiveness performance analysis.

As the cost load on a BMD architecture rises, a kind of measure is needed to better select the optimal architecture. Simple minimum cost analysis is not enough to deal with the problem. Consequently a lot of thought is put into the issue of how to measure the effectiveness of BMD architectures.

The enemy's arsenal and war scenarios are the key factors to define the sizing of the BMD architecture. One can easily sum all of the potential threats and as a result come up with an unaffordable BMD architecture. Special analysis is needed to better assess the threat sizes in different scenarios. Matching threat size to architecture size is based on probabilistic analysis taking into account the allowed "leakage rate."

Analysis by itself, however, is not enough to handle complex situations, and so it is helped by simulations and war game techniques. These techniques were developed for the BMD arena and are flexible to scenario changes. All of these factors are considered to help establish an affordable BMD architecture, but one should know that even at the time of this publication there is not even one system available that has actually proved its value in a real shooting war. The challenge is still with us and we hope that among other issues this book will help a little in the effort to understand the meaning of sound and robust architectures. Reference 2 also provides some views on how to handle the issue.

IV. About the Book

As already mentioned, BMD technologies were late to develop because of international treaties. While the technology base for guided missiles got more and more advanced and known, BMD technologies lagged behind. Since 1950 many books, handbooks, and papers have appeared to help engineer a guided missile; practically none of these resources exist for BMD systems.

This book is intended for engineers and scientists, industry managers, political leaders, military people, and the general public. The book will help to define the unique problems of BMD and will assist in solving them. The chapters have been written by people who gained expertise during the 1980s and 1990s working mainly in the Israeli arena and therefore will focus mainly on defense against tactical ballistic missile threats. The material contained herein is unclassified but still holds considerable relevance.

No attempt has been made to come to grips with political issues, as much material already exists on those topics. The nature of this book is more of an engineering–technological–analytical book; such a book, to our best knowledge, does not exist in the market today. Design solutions to all problems of all systems types are not presented here, but the reader will become familiar with the different issues related to the engineering of such systems.

The book is divided into six parts, each containing several chapters and dealing with specific topics. A summary of each chapter is presented here so the reader will be able to identify areas of interest. Although it is recommended that the chapters be read in the order in which they are presented, one may read chapters separately or in whatever order is desired.

A. Part I: Some Historic Elements

In Chapter 2, "Historical Background," a very brief overview is given from World War II to the SDI. The chapter primarily is devoted to the Israeli story, including interactions with the United States. The local Israeli arena is different from U.S. world-wide concerns. One will become aware of the issues that led a small country to defend itself against ballistic missiles before and after a real wartime experience.

In the mid 1980s a design team in the MLM Division of the Israel Aircraft Industries, led by Dov Raviv, an experienced and innovative engineer, started to develop the Arrow weapon system. The Arrow program is supervised by the U.S. BMDO and the Israeli Ministry of Defense. In Chapter 3, "Arrow System—From Dream to Reality," the reader will become familiar with this weapon system, its development history, and its operational status with the Israeli Air Force.

B. Part II: Threat and Response

The key issue in BMD system definition is threat assessment, and in Chapter 4, "Many Facets of Threat Assessment," a very detailed analysis is presented to show the complexity of this issue. One is not interested only in the types of ballistic missiles the enemy possesses, but also would like to know about their warheads, launching systems, deployment modes, quantities, operational doctrine, and special subsystems. The gathering of relevant information takes a lot of time and the analysis of it is difficult. One has to be very careful, on one hand, not to overestimate the threat (which may cause unnecessary expenditures) and on the other hand not to underestimate it, which may be dangerous. In this chapter the author shows how a reasonable assessment is worked out, taking into account all factors involved.

After determining the threat one has to work out a strategy to defend against it. There are many paths to follow, each with benefits and disadvantages. Even if we broadly understand the nature of the required solution, its implementation will be affected by many constraints: technological know how, cost involved, time to field, leakage (of enemy missiles) allowed, duration of war, etc. In Chapter 5, "Defense Policies and Strategies," some of these issues are considered and discussed. Deterrence, retaliation, defense strategy, and various defense weapon systems are discussed to show the many dimensions of the solution. This chapter in particular should be helpful to decision makers.

In Chapter 6, "Theater Ballistic Missile Defense Architecture Development," the considerations, the process of construction, and the analysis of a defense architecture against a theater ballistic missile threat are presented. This chapter, along with several others in this book, is based on actual studies performed by WALES Ltd. during the last 15 years while working on the Israeli BMD architecture. To flesh out the theory some numerical examples are also presented.

The general process to counter a ballistic missile is common to many defense systems. In Chapter 7, "Antitheater Ballistic Missile Defense Process," a general description of the stages involved in the interception procedure is given. One will become familiar with the interception process, including search, acquisition, identification, target tracking, commitment, and engagement. Also described are important terms and concepts such as kill probability, battle space, second engagement, and footprints. The roles of kill assessment and debriefing systems are brought up.

C. Part III: Interoperability, Battle Management, and Strategic Considerations

The BMD operation is based on a multilayer defense concept and therefore contains more than one defense system. The Arrow and the Patriot together help in defining the actual Israeli defense architecture. Other systems or subsystems are candidates to join the existing architecture. The need to function as a sole integrated system to counter an attack of ballistic missiles requires a lot of coordination levels: technical compatibility of equipment, information sharing, similar work procedures, etc. The many aspects of interoperability among different systems are brought up in Chapter 8, "Interoperability Between Defense Systems," and tradeoffs between performance and cost are discussed. The term "level of interoperability" is formed to explain the different options of interoperability in a given situation.

A very special case of interoperability is the use of external cues to help a defense system improve its performance. In Chapter 9, "External Cueing," different methods of external cueing are described and compared. Calculations demonstrate the contribution of external cueing as well as their optimal use during an engagement.

Air defense battle management systems have existed for a long time. In Chapter 10, "Battle Management," we discover that BMD needs different solutions. The tasks of battle management systems are defined and the different possible setups, depending on different considerations and constraints, are discussed. The human role in conducting a BMD operation is reviewed and simulation techniques and results are discussed.

D. Part IV: Guidance and Control in Theater Ballistic Missile Defense

Chapter 11, "Antiballistic Missile Interception Guidance," is a general review of interceptor missile guidance laws. The review covers classical and modern guidance laws used to intercept ballistic missiles at the reentry and boost phases.

One of the main issues concerning BMD systems is the "end-game"—the final phase of the approach of the interceptor to its target. The effort to obtain a better understanding of navigation and final guidance performance and to translate it into practical terms is still continuing. The end-game part of the trajectory is extremely important for obtaining a kill of the target, by minimizing the distance between the interceptor and the target in the case of an explosive warhead or actually achieving a hit in the case of a hit-to-kill warhead. Chapter 12, "Improved Methodology for Theater Missile Defense End-Games," is devoted to new guidance schemes and to real-time measurements made onboard the interceptor to better predict a target's future trajectory.

In Chapter 13, "Interception of Maneuvering Targets in Theater Missile Defense," the results of a multiyear investigation and analysis of future interception schemes against highly maneuverable reentry vehicles are reported. It is shown that although today it is almost impossible to intercept a maneuvering warhead, a new approach to guidance law design may be used in future theater missile defense systems to overcome this difficulty.

E. Part V: Measures of System Effectiveness and Risk Management

There is not one ultimate architectural solution to the problem of defeating the ballistic missile threat. The nature of the different war scenarios and the need to achieve numerical yardsticks calls for a measurement tool to evaluate effectiveness and compare among different architectures. Chapter 14, "Analytical Methods, Measures of Effectiveness, and Simulations," demonstrates that cost is not the only measure and we should consider issues like leakage rate, interceptor consumption, robustness, and flexibility. The tools to measure effectiveness are explained and used in some examples and simulation techniques are elaborated.

An operational BMD system requires a life cycle logistics analysis. To keep a certain level of readiness one has to evaluate maintenance needs (level and frequency) of the system, the spare parts stocks, maintenance personnel qualifications and training, changing requirements, and so forth. In Chapter 15, "Theater Missile Defense Systems Readiness and Training," the general known logistics, readiness, and training procedures are applied to BMD systems using some special examples and specific considerations. The contribution of this analysis to the total architecture is evaluated.

The development of BMD systems is still a "young" discipline. The programs in work involve large investments of resources and high risks. The risk attached to a given development project has to be assessed, planned for, and continuously managed. In Chapter 16, "Development Program Risk Management: Principles and a Case Study," we learn how to treat risk issues and how to quantify their uncertainties. A detailed example is presented, dealing with a boost-phase interceptor future system.

F. Part VI: A Look to the Future

Offense and defense are highly connected in the age-old see-saw. Improvements in one bring about improvements in the other, and vice-versa. In Chapter 17, "Future Trends in Offense and Defense," we try to foresee future general trends. The technologies of offensive missiles, and the areas in which improvement can be most meaningful from the point of the attacker, are described. Obvious weaknesses in defensive systems, partially derived from the preliminary predictions about future capabilities of the offense, are then described, and some guidelines for improvement are suggested, again with a view to the most cost effective solutions.

Chapter 18, "Concluding Remarks," touches on issues described and discussed in the present volume and rounds out the discussion by briefly reviewing the more important ones. As stated in the chapter, probably the most important issue is that "We believe that by itself the wider dissemination of this knowledge contributes to the deterrence effect, so all this know-how will never have to be utilized in practice."

G. Appendices

Appendix A describes some of the currently more advanced antimissile systems and available technical data.

Although a lot of material was published about the Persian Gulf War, most of it deals with aspects of fighting. Two elements of the war were less discussed. One, for essentially being a failure, concerns the hunt for the SCUD launchers. Appendix B describes some of the reasons for this failure and leads to the second little-discussed issue. Because it was anticipated that some missiles will leak (and all of them did in fact do so) there was a real fear, based on much-publicized threats and statements, that chemical warheads might be used. Appendix B describes the preparations (and some post facto lessons) of the Israeli civil defense organization for this eventuality.

Education and professional experience of the authors who contributed to this volume are detailed in Appendix C.

References

[1]Carter, A. B., and Schwartz, D. N., (Eds.), *Ballistic Missile Defense*, Brookings Instit., Washington DC, 1984.

[2]Stav, A. (Ed.), *Ballistic Missiles, The Threat and the Response*, Brassey's, London, 1999.

Chapter 2

Historical Background

Uzi Rubin*
Israel Ministry of Defense, Tel Aviv, Israel

I. Introduction

THE appearance of the inertially guided, rocket propelled ballistic missiles during the latter phase of World War II instigated an effort, as soon as the war was over, to find the means to defend against them—either by intercepting and shooting them down, or by destroying their launchers. Ballistic missile defense (BMD) programs were launched both in the United States and the Soviet Union during the decades of the Cold War. With the attention of both superpowers riveted to the overwhelmingly destructive power of nuclear tipped intercontinental ballistic missiles (ICBMs), the main thrust of their efforts was aimed to develop adequate defense system against them—efforts that on the whole did not bear any fruit.

While ICBMs were taking center stage during the Cold War, shorter-range ballistic missiles, designed for tactical use in local theaters of future conflicts, were introduced by both superpowers into their arsenals. ICBMs were justly considered as strategic weapons par excellence, but theater ballistic missiles (TBM) were regarded as tactical weapons, a kind of super long-range artillery. This view held forth until the slow but steady proliferation of ballistic missile technology enabled "second rate powers" (so regarded by the superpowers) such as China and India to develop ballistic missiles of their own.

When President Ronald Reagan announced the Strategic Defense Initiative on 23 March 1983, it was already clear to U.S. policy makers that TBMs were more than battlefield weapons, that their threat should be addressed by military technology, and that their spread should be curbed by export controls. Hence, the Strategic Defense Initiative mission included the defense of U.S. allies against ballistic missiles; in other words, it included theater missile defense (TMD).

The history of BMD and TMD is richly documented and deserves a full volume by itself. This chapter endeavors to describe it in broad brushstrokes. Since TMD is closely related to BMD—being in essence an offshoot of it—a short

---

Copyright © 2000 by the American Institute of Aeronautics and Astronautics, Inc. All rights reserved.

*Senior Director for Proliferation and Technologies, Israeli National Security Council. Member AIAA.

history of the latter, and in particular that of the Strategic Defense Initiative, will serve as a backdrop. It will be narrated in a concise form, leading to an equally concise description of the history of TMD at large. This book is written from an Israeli perspective, and hence, the main theme of this chapter will be the history of TMD in Israel, in which the author has had the privilege of being closely involved. We will not recount here the chronology of TMD in Israel. Instead, we will present an overview of the evolution of Israeli doctrines and policies, describe the highlights of the Israeli defense establishment's decision-making processes, and accentuate the debates generated by it. Both the overt, public debate, and the more covert one within the Israeli Ministry of Defense (in particular between the military high command and the political leadership) will be discussed.

TMD as a military art deals with defense against ballistic missiles in all their operational phases: from the destruction of their launchers, through their interception during boost and ascent phases, to their interception and kill during the terminal phase of their flight. The Israeli defense industries have been involved in every one of those aspects at different times, but the main effort has always been focused on the latter, in the form of the Arrow program—the largest single defense program in Israel today, and one of the largest ever undertaken by it. Hence, while the Israeli R&D establishment has recently completed a detailed study of a boost-phase interception (BPI) concept, and while it is currently studying an even more aggressive concept—that of prelaunch interception (PLI)—the section on Israeli history in this chapter will not cover it. Neither will it cover the related Nautilus program, an innovative project for interception of short-range artillery rockets by a futuristic high-energy weapon. Rather, we shall concentrate exclusively on the history of Arrow, as the flagship program embodying the policy, the technological capacity, and the major military response of Israel against the growing threat of theater ballistic missiles posed against her security.

II. Strategic Defense

Ballistic missiles are difficult to shoot down because of their great speed. This became apparent during the closing phase of World War II when two new weapons were used by Nazi Germany against the United Kingdom: "flying bombs" (equivalent to contemporary cruise missiles) and ballistic missiles. While the flying bombs were successfully intercepted by fighter aircraft and shot down in great numbers by fighters and antiaircraft guns, Britain's defenses were helpless against the ballistic missiles. British scientists were quick to develop radar that could detect the incoming ballistic missiles and thus give a rough idea where they were being launched from,[1] but ground attack aircraft failed to pinpoint and destroy the launchers. The ballistic missile attacks terminated only when the allies overran the actual and prospective launching sites.

Both the United States and the Soviet Union were impressed by the German achievement in the area of rocket propulsion and inertially guided missiles, and both hired teams of German experts to achieve successfully what is termed today "technology transfer." The Cold War that quickly followed the end of World War II gave a strong impetus to the advancement of nuclear delivery systems. The

Soviet Union, perceiving its relative weakness in the field of strategic aviation,* made a deliberate decision to rely on long-range rockets for strategic delivery of its nuclear bombs. Thus, while the United States developed super bombers like the B-36, the Soviets were developing what later became the first ICBMs. The growing prowess of the Soviet Union in the field of powerful rocketry (and by implication, technology of ballistic missiles) became evident when it launched the first Earth-orbiting satellite (Sputnik) on 4 October 1957.

The shock of the Sputnik launch, and the string of Soviet "firsts" in the conquest of space that followed, jump-started a spectrum of U.S. rocket and missile programs. Those programs ranged from the prestigious Apollo moon mission that landed a man on Earth's satellite, to numerous ballistic missile programs that yielded a multitude of weapon systems of ever growing capability, from the liquid propellant Atlas and Titan to the solid propellant Minuteman and the naval Polaris missiles. The Soviet Union, in turn, was already graduating from its first primitive ICBMs cum space launchers into an ever more advanced series of long-range ballistic missiles, culminating in the field mobile ICBMs SS-24 and SS-25.

With the realization of both superpowers during the 1980s that defense against ballistic missiles was not technically feasible at the time, both chose deterrence as their key to national survival. The ballistic missile race was on, with (mainly imaginary) "missile gaps" driving each protagonist in turn to more frantic efforts of development and deployment. The response of each side to the appearance of a new missile in the armory of the adversary was to develop better missiles of its own.

This is not to say that the idea of a defensive response, that is, intercepting and shooting down the adversary's missiles, eluded the mind of planners on both sides. Studies on the prospects of ballistic missile defense were initiated almost as soon as the victory in Europe was being celebrated. Initially, however, those efforts were no more than half hearted because of a combination of two factors: First, the requirements for successful antimissile defenses were obviously beyond the technology of the day, and second, it was far from clear during the late 1940s and early 1950s that ballistic missiles could become the powerful precision delivery systems that they were later. In fact, some serious U.S. scientists predicted that ballistic missiles were destined to remain forever short-range, tactical weapons.[2]

Later, when ICBMs graduated into the planet-shattering doomsday weapons that troubled the peace of mind of leaders and peoples alike, considerable effort was made and resources allocated by both superpowers to the technologies and systems needed to intercept them. The most remarkable fruit of this effort in the United States was the Safeguard antiballistic missile system. President Nixon's administration launched in 1969 a full-scale development program of a ballistic missile defense weapon system designed to protect land-based ICBM sites. (For a detailed and fascinating history of the U.S. pre-SDIO ballistic missile defense efforts, see Ref. 3.) This system, impressively advanced for its time, was composed of large radars and two layers of interceptors, the Sprint lower tier and Spartan upper tier missiles. With the relative inaccuracy of the radar systems of the time,

*Soviet World War II aviation was overwhelmingly tactical. Impressed by the achievements of allied strategic bombing, the Soviets managed the feat of copying the design of the U.S. B-29 bomber from aircraft that made emergency landings in Soviet territory. The copied airplanes were mass manufactured under the designation Tu-4.

killing the incoming missiles could only be assured by equipping the interceptors with nuclear warheads—a concept fraught with risks to the defenders no less than to the aggressors. In the Soviet Union, a comparable effort led to the deployment of an antimissile defense around Moscow. Interestingly, the Soviet system was based on modifications of existing ICBMs launched from silos. Because the Soviet interceptors were also relying on a nuclear warhead for target kills, the total effect of the antimissile systems of both sides could hardly be considered as a mitigation of the potential holocaust of a nuclear war between the superpowers; rather, the opposite could be true.

Albeit of doubtful effect, the antiballistic missile (ABM) systems of both sides prompted the development of new generations of ballistic missiles designed to overcome their (probably overrated) defensive powers. The major innovation in this connection was the perfection of the multiple, independently targeted reentry vehicles (MIRVs) designed to saturate the defense systems. New ICBMs now carried several nuclear warheads instead of the single warheads of the previous generations. This, in turn, increased the number of deployed nuclear warheads to such an extent that the leadership of both superpowers became alarmed. The perception that ABM systems were accelerating the arms race rather than slowing it down brought the protagonist to the negotiation table, and in May 1972 a treaty to limit the deployment of ABM systems was concluded. The Safeguard system became operational in 1975, but in spite of being treaty compliant, was subsequently dismantled. Ballistic missile defense reverted in the United States to low priority, back burner, with correspondingly reduced budgets. (The Soviets, however, elected to maintain their Moscow ABM defense system in service. It has been subsequently modernized, and according to Russian sources, its nuclear warheads were replaced with conventional ones. The system, today dubbed A-135, is still operational. For an interesting—but not too revealing—description, see Ref 4.)

Experiments in high-power energy weapons carried out by the Soviet Union during the later part of the 1970s were interpreted by the United States as an effort to develop a more advanced form of ABM defenses. In line with his tough policy against the Soviet Union, alarmed by reports on the Soviet high energy efforts, and strongly influenced by the technological vision of physicist Edward Teller, President Ronald Reagan launched in March 1983 the Strategic Defense Initiative (SDI). The goal of this effort was to make nuclear weapons "impotent and obsolete" by intercepting and killing their major delivery platforms—the Soviet ICBMs and SLBMs (sea launched ballistic missiles).* This initiative, quickly nicknamed by the media "Star Wars" (Alluding to the classic George Lucas fantasy cum science fiction movie released shortly before), surprised the U.S. administration and the military no less than the Soviet government.

The initiative envisaged the deployment of a tight defensive system covering the entire continental United States, permitting a leakage rate of no more than 1 in 1000, although it was not clear how exactly this could be achieved. Although supported initially by public opinion, the SDI encountered fierce opposition from military and academic circles almost from day one. Three major classes of arguments were leveled against SDI: that it was technologically unfeasible, that it was threatening to destabilized the U.S.—Soviet nuclear standoff, and that it diverted resources

*Recent authors speculate that it was the growing threat of the submarine-based Soviet SLBMs, rather than the ICBMs, that precipitated the "Star Wars" initiative. See Ref. 5.

from more urgent national goals (a generic argument used by liberal analysts against development of new weapons of any kind). Regardless of such criticism, the U.S. administration and Congress allocated generous budgets for basic and applied research in a spectrum of candidate technologies, ranging from high-energy lasers of various kinds to supervelocity guns. While all this effort was gaining momentum, the Soviet Union was tottering toward its eventual collapse. With the final dissolution of the Soviet Union at the end of 1991, the *raison d'être* of the SDI disappeared, and it was officially terminated in May 1993 by the Bush administration. Its controlling agency—the Strategic Defense Initiative Organization (SDIO)—was retasked to develop theater missile defenses and was renamed the Ballistic Missile Defense Organization (BMDO).

While the SDI has failed to achieve any of its technological and programmatic goals, its role in the termination of the Cold War and the dissolution of the Soviet Union is regarded as crucial by numerous observers, present author included. Verbal communications from Soviet officials disclosed to this author that the Soviet leadership (attributing to U.S. industry a real capacity to implement SDI as advertised) became pessimistic about the huge outlays of national resources required to upgrade their ballistic missile fleets to penetrate the supposed SDI shield. Furthermore, they doubted their own capability to build a similar strategic defense. The end of the Cold War—and the ensuing demise of the Soviet Union—were the inevitable consequence of the flawed Soviet system, which strained its economic back in a frantic effort to catch up with the increasing military power of the United States. The SDI provided the last straw that broke that back, according to numerous Soviet and Western observers. As bluntly put by Aleksander Solzhenitsyn in 1994: "The Cold War was essentially won by Ronald Reagan when he embarked on the Star Wars program and the Soviet Union understood that it could not take this step. . . ."[6]

Against the backdrop of an ailing Soviet economy, the SDI flaunted America's technological *élan* and her inexhaustible resources in the face of a demoralized Soviet leadership, compelling it to seek accommodation and to pin its hopes on disarmament rather than on further arms races—or so this author believes. However, this view of the role of SDI in the settlement of the Cold War is controversial, and will probably remain the subject of debate in the coming decades.

The concise survey of strategic defense would not be complete without mentioning its recent, albeit strictly limited, resurrection in the form of the U.S. National Missile Defense (NMD). From the fall of the Soviet Union in late 1991 until the end of the decade, U.S. strategists believed that the national territory of the United States would be unreachable by "Third World" long-range ballistic missiles for several decades. A report to the U.S. Congress by a commission headed by Secretary of Defense Donald Rumsfeld warned that the accelerated proliferation of missile technology would pose a "substantial" missile threat to the United States and Europe from radical countries as early as the end of the next decade. Long advocated by the Republican legislators in Congress, this report (as well as a test of a North Korean purported "satellite launcher" that overflew Japan) precipitated the legislation of the NMD initiative. To develop (and perhaps to deploy) a missile defense system aimed to protect the national territory of the United States against ballistic missiles.

There are, however, two crucial differences between NMD and the late SDI: First, NMD's mission is restricted to protection against a limited attack of relatively few, unsophisticated missiles; and second, NMD will rely exclusively on ground-based antimissile missiles, using the technologies of ground-based interceptors from the SDI era. The plethora of futuristic, "Star Wars" like technologies will not be utilized. Still, with all of those distinction and limitations, based on legacy technologies and shackled by the ABM treaty, there is no denying that NMD revives the spirit of President Reagan's original vision, to make strategic ballistic missiles "impotent and obsolete."

III. Theater Missile Defense (TMD)

In the previous section we have seen how the first-generation ballistic missiles of World War II, growing into planet-shattering ICBMs, generated a daring attempt to nullify their threat, by a combination of futuristic weapons, brought together into the concept of the SDI, and how that attempt ceased with the end of the global confrontation between the world's two major superpowers.

While missiles of intercontinental range were being developed and deployed by the United States and the Soviet Union during the 1960s and 1970s, military planners on both sides addressed the use of ballistic missiles for tactical purposes on the battlefield. Side by side with the ICBMs, the military industries of both sides spewed out various models of tactical ballistic missiles (TBMs), the most notorious and, given the Soviet habit of manufacturing everything in prodigious quantities, the most prolific being the SCUD-B, a linear descendant of the German V-2. Simple, robust, and relatively cheap, this 300-km range missile was employed by the Red Army in huge numbers in the role of super long-range artillery, and was also liberally exported to Soviet allies in the Warsaw Pact and the Third World. More potent and slightly longer-range missiles such as the 500-km SS-23 followed, but the SCUD B remained the workhorse of the Red Army's TBM arsenal until the fall of the Soviet Union in 1991.

Tactical ballistic missiles were also added to the arsenal of Western land weapons, albeit in fewer numbers and in a lesser variety. Unlike the Eastern Bloc's tendency to rely mainly on cheap, unsophisticated theater ballistic missile (TBM) designs like the SCUD, the TBMs of the United States and its allies* used advanced technologies borrowed from ICBM designs. Thus, both the Pershing-1 and the Pershing-2 TBMs utilized solid rocket propulsion, modern inertial platforms, and advanced thermal protection. For a time, the Soviet Bloc regarded the Pershing-2 missiles as a strategic threat, countering it by the deployment of the only true "theater" ballistic missile ever developed, the SS-20, a miniaturized version of the MIRVed ICBM, but with a limited range suitable for the European theater. With the conclusion of the INF (intermediate-range nuclear force) Treaty between the United States and the Soviet Union in 1987, all TBMs of both sides were discarded. The service of the Pershing-2, and with it the service of any kind of TBM in the U.S. armory, came to an end.

TBMs of the SCUD generation are relatively simple machines, readily amenable to reverse engineering and modifications by the engineering communities of small, nonaffluent nations. While there are only a handful of countries that can design and produce their own combat aircraft, it is estimated that more than 20 countries, some of them quite backward, are making their own versions of short-range ballistic missiles.

---

*France has developed and deployed a short-range TBM of its own design, the field mobile, nuclear tipped Pluton.

The proliferation of TBMs, initiated by the Soviet Union through its generous export of SCUD missiles to practically all of its client states (including some of the world's poorest nations like Yemen), was later augmented by the proliferation of TBM technology and infrastructure. The threat of the TBMs of the so-called Third World nations became a concern to the U.S. administration in the mid 1980s,* and turned into a global problem during the 1988 "War of the Cities" phase of the Iran–Iraq War. It suddenly dawned on Western military planners that future regional conflicts might see the use of Third World TBMs against their own forces—and with no viable means yet available for defending those forces against that threat.

In the Darwinian-like struggle between weapons and counter weapons that has typified the art of military technology ever since the dawn of organized warfare, it is remarkable that effective antiballistic missiles defenses were not perfected soon after the appearance of the threat. In Section II of this chapter we remarked on the sheer technological difficulty of intercepting ballistic missiles, requiring yet unavailable, extremely advanced, technologies bordering on science fiction. At the same time, the present author believes that the case of defense against TBM was hindered not just by the barrier of technology† but also by complex issues of military conservatism combined with economic issues.

Because ballistic missiles are fired from great distances behind the frontline and approach their targets from above, it has been natural for military planners to regard missile defense as an adjunct to air defense. This view was favored by professional soldiers as well as political leaders because it made economic "sense": missile defense as an addition to the task of air defense promised to be more cost effective than dedicated anti-TBM weapons. Thus, the original specifications for the SAM D, the progenitor of today's Patriot, included both air and TBM defense. The Russian Federation is marketing its two missile defense weapons (to be discussed later) as combined air and missile defense systems. This "extended air defense" concept is the basis of today's Patriot PAC 3 weapon system as well as that of the U.S.–Europe MEADS (medium extended air-defense system) concept.

The extended air defense approach, while intuitively appealing, is technically flawed. In the words of a senior Russian designer, "the substantial differences between aircraft and missiles in their performance characteristics and methods of combat employment, demand the solution of specific and often contradictory problems".[7] Aircraft, whether manned or not, follow radically different flight profiles than ballistic missiles. The latter, once boosted by their short-duration rocket motors, move in high curving, extremely fast, yet easily predictable trajectories. Aircraft, on the other hand, fly at significantly lower altitudes, and follow unpredictable flight paths at relatively slow speeds (relative, that is, to ballistic missiles). For an air defense system, the higher speed of ballistic missiles shrinks the time between detection and engagement, significantly limiting the size of its defended zone. The unpredictability of the flight path of aircraft demand complex solutions, which are not strictly necessary for intercepting highly predictable ballistic missiles, and so on.

*Thus prompting the U.S.-led effort to control missile proliferation through the Missile Technology Control Regime (MTCR), formally established in April 1987.

†In fact, the speed of TBMs, being a fraction of that of ICBMs, permits the use of "conventional" interception techniques such as antimissile missiles. "Science fiction" technologies are not strictly required in this case.

A less obvious, yet even more profound, difference concerns the lethality and kill mechanism. Modern combat aircraft are sizable machines, rich in vulnerable systems that must function continuously throughout the flight. Even one single hit from a fragment of a small warhead might, as often as not, disrupt some vital system and cause a mission scrub, if not an outright loss of the aircraft. In contrast, ballistic missiles are relatively small, and in their descent phase consist mostly of inert structures, their navigation and propulsion systems becoming superfluous after the boost phase. To successfully kill them at this phase, it is necessary to hit their warheads, which usually occupy a small volume at the front end.* Moreover, some types of warheads might be quite hard to destroy, particularly those containing cluster munitions. Hence, the requirements for a successful kill of ballistic missiles are significantly more demanding than those for air vehicles.

American designers quickly came to the conclusion that the two requirements—air and missile defense—were difficult to reconcile. The early requirement for a tactical "extended air defense" system embodied in the late 1960s in the SAM D concept, was reduced in the early 1970s to the pure air defense requirement upon which the original Patriot system was based. It thus fell to the Soviet Union to field the first antitactical ballistic missile—(ATBM) capable weapons systems in history: the SU–300PMU (NATO designations SA-10) and the S-300V (NATO designation SA-12).

In spite of their confusingly similar designations, the only common denominator of these two systems is their dual role as air and tactical ballistic missile defenses—a duality that severely impairs their TMD capabilities as judged according to contemporary standards. The SA-10 have been ordered by the Soviet Air Force, and is based on a single type of interceptor. The SA-12, a much more complicated weapon, was designed for the Soviet Army and utilized two different types of interceptors, a small one for air defense and a heavier round for missile defense. The first model of the SA-10 became operational in 1979, whereas the SA-12 reached operational status in 1986. As air defense weapons, these two systems are formidable; as missile defenses, they are judged to be mediocre by Western analysts. The armament industries of the Russian Federation are currently advertising improved models of the SA-10 and SA-12 for sale in the world arms market—renamed the Favorite and the Antei 2500 respectively.

We have already noted how the initial concept for an "extended air defense" weapon matured into the pure air defense Patriot system. However, by the 1980s, it was becoming clear to European and American planners that theater-type ballistic missiles were a serious threat in future land battles. Furthermore, the huge quantities of Soviet SCUDs in the service of the Warsaw pact forces could jeopardize the belt of Patriot air defenses deployed in Europe. This recognition prompted the return to the extended air defense concept, with the launching of the PAC-2 (Patriot Advanced Capability 2) program in 1982. The PAC-2 just barely made it to the battlefield in the Persian Gulf War, but its use there, initially hailed as a great success, revealed the inherent contradiction in requirements between air and missile defense. Careful scrutiny of engagement results of the Patriots used to

*Missiles with separating warheads are even more challenging; presenting the defense systems with at least two objects only one of which, the reentry vehicle, is the true target.

defend Israel and Saudi Arabia against the Iraqi Al-Hussein missiles* deflated the claims of success made during the war itself. At the same time, the lessons learned during that first attempt in history to destroy ballistic missiles during their descent phase proved invaluable for the sound design of more advanced TMD systems.

While their development started in the early 1980s, TMD really came to the fore in the West after the traumatic experience of the Gulf War. In the United States, the loss of 28 troops to a single Iraqi El Hussein prompted the military and legislative branches to push foreword a spectrum of vigorous TMD programs. In 1991, the U.S. Congress legislated the Missile Defense Act, mandating the administration to develop and deploy TMD systems aimed to defend the U.S. deploying forces as well as to defend U.S. allies and friends. The SDIO was put in charge of this effort in close coordination with the U.S. armed forces.

The flagship and most ambitious program in this effort is the Army's theater high altitude area defense system (THAAD). A dedicated TMD system, designed to engage and kill long-range TBMs with up to 3000-km range, it is a deployable weapon utilizing advanced missile and radar technologies. To tackle the difficult problem of destroying cluster munitions warheads, the THAAD designers chose the novel approach of "hit to kill," i.e., killing the threat's warhead by direct impact of the interceptor, which therefore does not carry a "warhead" of its own. To achieve the phenomenal accuracy required for a body hit of a fast, small TBM warhead, THAAD couples ultra accurate radar, the GBR (ground-based radar), with an optically controlled end-game of the interceptor. The program, launched in 1992, had an ambitious goal to deploy a contingency system by 1996, and to achieve full deployment of several batteries by 2002. However, the innovative technologies embodied in the THAAD proved more difficult to implement than initially envisaged. Whereas the system's various components were developed by 1996, the record of flight tests has had its share of disappointments. By the end of 2000 the THAAD finally achieved two successful interceptions in flight tests and was moving toward its next phase of development. However, deployment of the fully developed version of that system is not expected before the last quarter of the present decade.

Somewhat less technologically ambitious, yet no less important for future TMD, is the Army's PAC-3 program, which uses improved Patriot radar with a brand new, extremely advanced interceptor. Again, the hit-to-kill concept is used, with the end-game of the small, compact interceptor being controlled by an onboard radar sensor. Unlike the dedicated THAAD, PAC-3 is tasked to defeat both ballistic missiles and air vehicles. It is designed to work together with THAAD and to provide a lower tier defense against such missiles that evade the THAAD interceptors. Several recent successes on the test range, and a vigorous flight test program, give hope that PAC-3 will be ready for deployment by the year 2002.

Perhaps the most impressive demonstration of the U.S. decision to regard TMD as a major military challenge has been the engagement of the U.S. Navy in this effort. Ballistic missiles are not normally regarded as a threat to naval vessels, but U.S. Navy ships, deployed to theaters where U.S. forces operate, can offer a

*An extended range version of the SCUD B, locally developed by Iraq during the Iran–Iraq War, made by the cannibalization of Soviet supplied SCUDs.

significant defense to land-based troops and shore installations if provided with suitable ship-borne TMD weapons. Thus, the U.S. Navy has launched two TMD programs of its own, both based on extending the capability of the AEGIS air defense ships. The more immediate one is intended to enhance the capability of the "standard" missile to intercept TBMs at relatively low altitudes. To this end, the AEGIS shipboard radar was enhanced and an improved "standard" interceptor (the Block 4A) was designed. The first flight test of the missile took place in 1997, and a rigorous series of full weapon tests is expected to begin soon, with the goal of achieving operational capability by the early 2000s. The U.S. Navy has recently been authorized to commence the development of a high-altitude TMD system, the "theater wide," which will utilize a new, extended-performance interceptor. However, this program will not yield a fully developed weapon before 2007 or 2008. It is interesting to note that unlike the Army's designers the U.S. Navy elected to use explosive warhead-equipped interceptors for TBM kills, probably because of their need to rely on existing shipboard radar technologies as embodied in the AEGIS naval system.

In this profusion of emerging TMD weapons, none is more ambitious than the U.S. Air Force airborne laser (ABL) concept. Forsaking ground-based radars and interceptors, the ABL hails back to "Star Wars" audacity, aiming to destroy ballistic missiles in their boost phase by the use of an airborne, high-power energy weapon carried aboard a Boeing 747 aircraft. This innovative program, if proved feasible, would revolutionize the art of ballistic missile defense (and the art of military technology at large). It is yet too early, however, to judge whether the tremendous technical obstacles posed by this concept could be surmounted in the foreseeable future.

The deep impression left by the ballistic missiles campaign during the Persian Gulf War, as well as the rapidly evolving ballistic missile proficiency of more Third World countries in east, south, and west Asia, created a demand for TMD by several U.S. allies and nonaligned countries in the world. Japan, threatened by North Korea's No-Dong and Taepo-Dong TBMs, yet hampered by its post World War II antimilitary policy, is carefully evaluating the deployment of national TMD, preferably in a joint venture with the United States and largely based on U.S. systems. Germany is participating in the U.S. Army's PAC-3 program, and in conjunction with other European Union countries, is a leading participant in the MEADS extended air defense program, which is scheduled to enter into a demonstration–validation phase in the near future. France is developing the ASTER system, basically an air defense weapon with a certain antimissile capability. In South Asia, India perceives a threat of TBM both from Pakistan and China, and has reportedly purchased TMD-capable SA-10 batteries from Russia. The United States has recently agreed to sell Patriot batteries to Egypt. Open literature reports attribute TMD requirements to Turkey and several Persian Gulf states.

It is Israel, however, shaken by the trauma of the Iraqi missile attacks in the Persian Gulf War, that leads today the most vigorous TMD effort outside of the United States. The history of TMD in Israel will therefore constitute the substance of the next section of this survey.

IV. Theater Missile Defense in Israel

Proliferation of ballistic missiles into the Middle East started shortly after the ascent of this type of weapon in the rest of the world. In the early 1960s, Egypt launched an indigenous ballistic missile program, leading to the development of two types of liquid propellant missiles: the 300 km El-Zaafar and the 500 km El-Kahir. The program, largely supported by a group of World War II German rocket experts, was terminated after the Six Days War, partly because of heavy Israeli pressure on the West German government. Subsequently, Egypt purchased SCUD B missiles from the Soviet Union, some of which were fired at Israeli positions in the Sinai during the Yom Kippur War. That war saw also a substantial use by Syria of long-range artillery rockets (FROGs) against Israel's air bases. Remarkably, this preview into the significance of ballistic missiles in future conflicts barely gained any attention by Israel's military thinkers.

The introduction of ballistic missiles in massive numbers into Arab armed forces was ratcheted up by the Lebanon campaign in 1982 (Operation Peace for Galilee). The opening phases of that conflict saw a vigorous and innovative Israeli air campaign against the Syrian SAM air defense system, which resulted in its complete neutralization. The Syrian leadership, impressed with what looked like the invincibility of the Israeli Air Force, made a decision to invest in the buildup of a large ballistic missile arsenal, as a strategic response to the perceived permanency of Israel's air superiority. While statements to that effect were made publicly by the Syrian leadership, most Israeli analysts and military planners failed to appreciate the significance of this development.

The next quantum leap in the ascent of ballistic missiles in the region was prompted by the Iran–Iraq War. Launched by Saddam Hussein in 1980 to take advantage of Iran's weakness after its Islamic revolution of 1978, the conflict saw a substantial use of missiles against population centers almost from its beginning. To compensate for Iran's geographical advantage in having launching sites within SCUD-B range of Baghdad, the Iraqis developed an indigenous version of the SCUD missile, dubbed "Al-Hussein," with sufficient range to hit Teheran from Iraqi territory. During "The War of the Cities" in early 1988, Iraq launched nearly two hundred of those missiles at Iranian cities, causing considerable damage and casualties. This highly publicized development—and with Tel Aviv being within the range of the Al-Hussein missiles—stirred some concern in Israeli military circles. However, studies of the effects of such missile attacks on Israel's population centers indicated that unless the attacking missiles carried nonconventional warheads, damage and casualties would be rather limited. Hence, the Israel Defense Forces High Command concluded that the proper response for the missile threat would be a combination of early warning and passive defense. Active defense, although debated, was deemed to be to unwarranted and its expenditures unjustified.

This complacent attitude of Israel's defense establishment remained unshaken by Iraq's attempt of a space launch in December 1989, nor was it revised after Saddam Hussein's threat "to burn half of Israel" in April 1990. With a perception of an overwhelming strategic superiority, most of Israel's political and military leaders apparently believed in their capacity to deter Iraq (as well as any other Arab nation) from attacking Israel's cities, and expressed themselves accordingly once Iraq's invasion of Kuwait precipitated the Persian Gulf crisis. Several top Israeli leaders deliberately and repeatedly made thinly veiled threats of devastating retaliation if Iraq dared to attack Israel's cities. Thus, the salvos of Iraqi Al-Hussein missiles that exploded in Tel Aviv and Haifa at the opening of Operation Desert Storm shocked Israel's government and its military High Command to the core. While Israel had previously made some substantial preparation in the area of passive defense, it did not own any capability to detect incoming missiles, nor did it have any means for thwarting or destroying them. Hasty arrangement with the U.S. government provided a rudimentary link with its global early warning assets, and several batteries of the newly developed Patriot PAC-2, some of them deployed from the United States, attempted to intercept the Iraqi missiles with indifferent results. As the military coalition air strikes against the Iraqi missile launchers failed to halt their fire, Israeli military leaders prepared plans to attack and destroy the Iraqi launchers using Israel's own air and ground forces. Caution, as well as heavy U.S. pressure on Israel to eschew direct military action, finally prevailed. The net result was that Israel suffered attacks, passively and without any effective capability to defend itself, by some 40 Iraqi missiles, which caused light casualties but substantial material and morale damage. This was a searing, traumatic experience for Israel's people and leadership, prompting considerable soul searching as well as a renewed appraisal of the value of active defense within Israel's defense establishment.

Previous to that, at the time when the majority of Israel's defense establishment was still indifferent toward ballistic missile defense, a minority of defense officials and industrial leaders made the first cautious steps to promote it conceptually and technically. When the United States invited Israel to join the SDI, Israel's then minister of defense, Yitzhak Rabin, accepted the offer, and in 1986 a Memorandum of Agreement was signed between the governments to that effect. The first director of the SDIO, Lt. Gen. Abrahamson, visited Israel in February 1986, and upon the invitation of the then chairman of the board of Israel Aircraft Industries (IAI), Lt. Gen. (Ret.) David Ivry, discussed with him the prospective areas of U.S.–Israel cooperation in the SDI. The two agreed that Israel's participation in the field of theater missile defense might be mutually beneficial and reviewed the entire spectrum of candidate technologies: intelligence, passive defense, boost phase and terminal phase interception, and launcher interdiction. Gen. Abrahamson felt that the field of terminal phase intercept held the best promise for practical cooperation, all other aspects of TMD being politically sensitive in the view of the U.S. administration. In addition, the two agreed on the need for a facility to simulate and exercise TMD defenses—a new and untried chapter in military art.

Shortly afterward, Ivry was appointed director general of the Israel Ministry of Defense (IMOD). In his new capacity, he ordered the IMOD to define, together with the SDIO, a joint R&D program along the lines previously discussed by him with Gen. Abrahamson. After a series of meetings, the SDIO formally requested Israel to submit a threefold proposal: first, for an architecture study of an Israeli early warning and missile defense system; second, for an Israeli test bed—a computerized site for studying and exercising architectural and operational concepts involved in such a system; and third, an experimental program for demonstrating endoatmospheric interceptions of surrogate ballistic missiles.

To comply with the third (and most challenging) part of the SDIO's request, the IMOD invited proposals from the two leading missile houses of its defense industries. Rafael's Missile Division proposed the concept of the AB-10, an upscaled version of its Barak ship defense missile, a command to line-of-sight system then in development (and today a mature weapon system in service with several navies, including the Israeli Navy.) The MLM division of IAI proposed the Arrow, an audacious concept for its time, an essentially self-guided antimissile missile with optically controlled, autonomous end-game. Both proposals were based on an explosive warhead kill (rather than hit to kill), and both were presented to the U.S. Army Missile Defense Command and to the SDIO. Upon examination, the

Arrow concept, the bolder of the two, was selected. This, in fact, was the birth of today's Arrow program.

Once the technical outlines and costs of all three tasks were defined, a cost sharing formula was negotiated between the IMOD and the SDIO with the result that the SDIO agreed to bear 80% of the cost, and the IMOD agreed to contribute the other 20%. In 1988 a specific Memorandum of Agreement was signed between the IMOD and the SDIO, covering the three tasks defined by the two governments, and specifying the terms and conditions of the partnership.

The architecture study was allocated by the IMOD, after a source selection procedure, to WALES Ltd., a consulting company led by the late Brig. Gen. (Ret.) Michael Cohen. The Israeli test bed task was allocated to the System Division of Tadiran Ltd., a major supplier of computerized command and control systems to the Israeli military. Because no operational requirement for a missile defense system existed at the time—in fact, the attitude of the Israeli High Command was outright hostile to such a requirement—the development program of the Arrow missile was contracted directly by the SDIO to the IAI. That contract was signed in 1988, and under the energetic leadership of the then manager of the MLM division of IAI, Dov Raviv, the development of the missile was pushed toward a first flight test two years after receiving the contract. This test (a flyout of the prototype Arrow, no target interception being attempted yet at this stage) took place in August 1990. The test failed because of an erroneous destruction command transmitted by the test range safety system. Undeterred, IAI performed two more tests, both ending in failures that exposed significant design weaknesses in the Arrow missile. With the active participation of U.S. "red teams," the design failures were corrected, and after a further series of tests, the Arrow missile succeeded, in the summer of 1994, to intercept and destroy a surrogate ballistic missile target.

While the Arrow missile was approaching its first test in 1990, a change of watch in Israel's government brought Moshe Arens back to the post of Minister of Defense, replacing Yitzhak Rabin. Reviewing Israel's future needs in air and missile defenses in the summer of 1990, Arens directed the IMOD to initiate the development of a missile defense system based on the U.S.-sponsored Arrow experiment, to establish a dedicated program office to this end, and to include the Arrow weapon system in the IDF's long-term budget plan. Accordingly, a program office was established by the IMOD in early 1991 and the first cut cost projections for a full-scale antimissile defense system development and acquisition were presented during that year. However, because of severe cuts in the defense budget and the staunch opposition of the IDF's High Command, no firm decision was made. Defense Minister Arens approached the SDIO with a proposal to share the development of a dedicated fire control radar for the Arrow, but this was rejected by its second director, Ambassador Hank Cooper, on the grounds of the unsuitability of the proposed technology to U.S. needs. Instead, Cooper proposed that Israel should participate in the development of a U.S. TMD fire control radar. Arens felt that this would rob Israel's own electronic industries of the opportunity to leapfrog into the future. Accordingly, and in the face of a protest by the IDF's general staff, Arens approved the full-scale development of a fire control radar for Arrow (later dubbed Green Pine) to be funded in full by Israel and without any U.S. support.

Defense Minister Arens' directive in the summer of 1990 to engage in the development of an Israeli antimissile weapon system, although not officially disclosed to the press, provoked a heated public debate about its merits. Like their counterparts in numerous countries in the West, officers of the IDF often use media commentators to voice their covert criticism of political leadership directives. In the case of the Arrow, the high command found its most eloquent spokesman in Reuven Pedahzur, a former Israel Air Force combat pilot who, after retiring from the military, became a prolific and respected commentator on security affairs.* Under the academic sponsorship of the prestigious Yaffe Center for Strategic Studies, Pedahzur published in 1993 a lengthy and detailed paper that expressed in essence the IDF's High Command rebuttal of Arens' directive.[8] In his paper, Pedahzur warned that:

> The decision to put Arrow at the top of the list of defense priorities has a significant strategic impact, and direct implications to the IDF force structure, to Israel's national economy and to the entire defense doctrine of Israel. Those implication will become apparent during the next decade and perhaps even beyond it. The development of an Israeli ATBM system demands the updating and modification of other components of Israel's entire defense policy.

He then went on to question the ability of Israel's electronics industry to develop the sophisticated radar needed for a missile defense system, and predicted that the definitive form of the Arrow weapon system would not be fielded before the year 2010. That such statements are revealed today as a gross misjudgment is immaterial for the purpose of this narration. Their significance lies in their articulation of the IDF's concern over Defense Minister Arens' directive. As elucidated in Pedahzur's paper, the High Command evaluated the threat from conventional ballistic missiles as negligible, and believed that Israel's already existing strategic capabilities should be brandished as a cost effective deterrence against future nonconventional threats. Missile defense, in the prevailing view, was a waste of scarce budgets and a danger to the IDF's future acquisition of modern arms.

However, there was a deeper cause for the IDF's alarm. To appreciate it, attention must be paid to the key phrase in Pedahzur's statement: "The decision . . . has . . . direct implications to . . . *the entire defense policy*" [emphasis added]. With its small population, miniscule area, and indefensible borders, Israel's classic doctrine called for an aggressive stance and stressed the need to fight her wars in the enemy's territory. Ever since the establishment of the Jewish state in 1948 and the costly victory in the hard fought conflict that followed it, Israel's top soldiers have considered this policy axiomatic. The force structure of the IDF reflected this policy, being rich in strike weapons and relatively poor in defense systems. As recently asserted by Lt. Gen. Israel Tal,[9] the Israeli military establishment prefers "the power to strike (i.e. offensive capability)" to "the power to withstand (i.e. defensive capability)." †

---

*While not alone in his criticism of Arrow and active defense in Israel—he was later joined by A. Shtiglitz, M. Van Kreveld, and A. Stav, among others—Pedahzur has been, and still is, its most eloquent and persistent critic. We shall therefore refer to his criticism as typical and representative throughout this narration.

†To be sure, at the time of Aren's directive, Israel's Air Defense Command was operating light and medium antiaircraft artillery and Hawk guided missiles air defense batteries. It was also preparing to accept the recently acquired Patriot system. However, the allocations for air defenses were always a miniscule fraction of the Air Force budget. In fact, the decision to buy Patriot was as fiercely resisted within the Israel Air Force as the later decision by Arens to authorize the development of Arrow.

Now Arrow represented the first major-scale R&D program in Israel dedicated to a purely defensive weapon system.* In the words of Gerald Steinberg, "After four decades in which Israeli doctrine focused on offensive strategy and deemphasized defensive weapons.... This approach [the deployment of missile defense]... would represent a fundamental change."[10] Notwithstanding the harrowing experience of the Gulf War, the rationale of the Arrow program contradicted one of the basic tenets of Israel's armed forces. The objections of the IDF High Command thus stemmed from deeper motivations than the usual "battle of the budget" *a la* the freshly cancelled Lavi fighter aircraft program.† While this conservative attitude could be understandable, it had an adverse impact on the progress of the Arrow program, as will be described further on.

When Yitzhak Rabin came back to the Ministry of Defense in the summer of 1992, his immediate agenda included the fate of the Arrow program. In the previous year, MLM's energetic general manager, Dov Raviv, negotiated with the SDIO a second Arrow contract, dubbed ACES (Arrow Continuation Experiments.) The main thrust of this program was the development of a new version of the Arrow (later called Arrow II), based the same principles of the previous version but correcting its inherent design weaknesses (mainly in the areas of heat shielding and thrust profile) and utilizing more advanced technologies. With the agreement of the IMOD to contribute 28% of the $320 million cost of the program, a second contract was signed between the SDIO and MLM, and a four year program was launched. It was, then, Rabin's dilemma whether to uphold his predecessor's directive to develop a full weapon system around the Arrow missile, or to let Arrow linger as an exercise in advanced R&D.

The debate, which took place in the fall of 1992, was fierce, with the High Command voicing its resolute objection to moving forward with a full weapons system. They argued that the events of the Gulf War were a kind of aberration unlikely to be repeated in any "normal" future war between Israel and its Arab foes. As a compromise, the High Command proposed to purchase the THAAD missile defense system (the development of which was being initiated at the time) once that system became available for acquisition. Both the deputy minister of defense, the late Mordechai (Mota) Gur, and the incumbent director general of the IMOD, David Ivry, supported a limited Arrow weapon system program. Rabin, who during his previous term in office had already expressed his alarm over the growing threat of ballistic missiles in hostile Arab countries and saw it as a potential strategic threat, accepted the view of Mota Gur and David Ivry. He therefore overruled the objections of the High Command and authorized a five-year program, with the limited objective of developing and integrating a complete weapon system, but without its acquisition or deployment. Following this decision, the Green Pine program was stabilized, and the development of a dedicated fire control center, later dubbed Citron Tree was initiated. In addition, several essential supportive programs

*This is not entirely accurate. The Barak antimissile ship defense system was already being developed at the time. However, the Barak was perceived as a modest program, destined to remain so by the Israel Navy's minor share of the IDF budget.

†This attitude lingers among some of Israel's top officers (see Ref. 11). Discussing the merits of a new concept for launcher destruction (BPLI), an unnamed senior official enthused that "a BPLI capability.... [will] shift the battle from our homeland to enemy territory, where it belongs."

were initiated, including the development of the operational configuration of the Arrow II and its launcher, and the establishment of an integration laboratory and a high fidelity engineering simulation site.

The first two flyout tests of the Arrow II took place in 1995 and early 1996 and were on the whole quite satisfactory. Buoyed by that achievement, IAI conducted the first interception test in the summer of 1996 with a gratifying success. In the next interception test, in spring 1997, the Arrow hit the target missile and destroyed it, albeit in a "hit-to-kill" mode, due to a malfunction in the fusing sequence of the warhead. That test saw also the first use of the recently delivered (in record time) Green Pine radar, which observed the flight and the interception in a "shadow mode" (i.e., without intervening in it). The next test, in summer 1997, failed completely because of a malfunction of a subsystem in the Arrow interceptor, which sent it into an uncontrolled spin and required its destruction by the safety officer.

It is useful, for the purpose of this narration, to note that the public debate about the Arrow program did not cease after Rabin's decision of 1992, neither did the IDF desist from its (muted) objections. The failure of the fifth Arrow test was greeted by the leading Israeli daily *Ha'aretz* in banner headlines, and Pedahzur as well as other commentators suggested that the occasion justified a reevaluation of the need for the program. Shortly after the test, Pedahzur stated in a radio interview that:

> The Israel Air Force does not believe in [the Arrow] program. The budgets needed for the program are so immense that they will bite into the acquisition programs of the IDF and the Air Force. In addition, the Israel Air Force does not believe in the effectiveness of the Arrow . . . that would justify such huge outlays . . . the Budgets and Allocations Committee of the U.S. Senate estimated the cost [of Arrow] at up to 10 billion $U.S.*

Obviously, the thrust of Pedahzur's argument revolved around his projected $10 billion cost of Arrow. Such a staggering expenditure (in Israeli terms) could undermine the entire long-term planning of Israel's force structure, necessitating a reduction in the level of preparedness of the IDF as a whole. Although Pedahzur did not disclose his source material, nor did any report about the Arrow projected cost by "the Budget and Allocations Committee of the U.S. Senate" ever surface, his allegation gained currency in Israel and in the United States. To address this issue, Ivry authorized a press conference on Arrow in May 1996, where the IMOD's own cost projection of $1.6 billion (for two Arrow batteries) was disclosed. Pedahzur did not accept this estimate, arguing that Arrow could not be much cheaper than the comparable U.S. THAAD program, the cost of which was estimated at the time at $12 billion.† Accusing the IMOD of hiding the truth, he

*Dahlia Yairi interviewing Reuven Pedahzur, IBA radio channel 2, 21 Aug. 1997.

†The comparison reflected a lack of appreciation of the profound difference between the two programs. The Arrow weapon system is on the whole less technologically stressing than the THAAD system. For example, the Green Pine radar, operating in the longer L band, requires about one tenth of the transmit–receive modules of the THAAD's X band GBR, making it significantly cheaper. The scope of the Arrow program, limited at the time to two batteries, was incomparably more modest. Pedahzur also disregards the fact that R&D in Israel is usually less costly than in the United States, as demonstrated by Israel's highly competitive position in the area of high technology.

angrily wrote:

> They [IMOD officials and IDF ranking officers] know that the sum needed to complete the system is several times higher than what has been officially disclosed by the IMOD; they know that the disclosed timetable is unrealistic, yet they remain silent, thereby participating in the deception of the public.[12]

Arrow's anticipated cost also worried its U.S. supporters. In 1994, the U.S. Department of Defense (DoD) conducted an independent cost projection on Arrow, conducted according to its own procedures evaluating R&D, manufacturing, and deployment costs. The result was never disclosed to the IMOD, but DoD sources assured the Israelis that the result was a mere fraction of Pedahzur's alarming figure. One year later, Undersecretary of Defense Paul G. Kaminski, wrote that:

> "... Some predict that the Arrow system will ultimately cost up to $10 billion ... a classified estimate of the costs for the Arrow Weapon System was prepared by the Department of Defense and forwarded to Congress in the April 1994 Arrow System Report to Congress. The estimate, which followed the Department's cost estimate standards, was significantly below $10 billion."[13]

In general, criticism of Arrow in Israel echoed the main themes of the 1980s objections against the SDI in the United States: That TMD was technically unfeasible (or, in another permutation, that it was easy to defeat), that introduction of active defense in Israel would destabilize the Israeli–Arab confrontation, and that it was economically unaffordable. To those three "classic" arguments, a fourth and uniquely Israeli argument was added: That Arrow contravened the long-standing Israeli defense doctrine of preferring offensive to defensive weapons. One noted Israeli analyst, Arieh Stav, pronouncing Arrow "a strategic and conceptual error," argued the point eloquently in a recent book.[14] In contrast, Israel's general public expressed its enthusiasm for the Arrow program—as could be testified by this author from personal experience—and Israel's legislative branch, the Knesset, gave it its full support. Obviously, and not unlike what transpired in the United States during the "Star Wars" era, Israel's "man in the street" preferred his own gut feeling and common sense to the erudite arguments of commentators and analysts. Simply put, the general public clamored for defense against a recurrence of the Persian Gulf War experience, and was ready to pay for it.

To return to the chronological sequence of this narration, it is now necessary to review the chain of events that melded the ACES contract with the IMOD's parallel and complementary program. With the ACES contract on track, the managements of IAI and IMOD initiated discussions with their U.S. colleagues about a possible continuation joint venture. Various limited-scope programs, involving the integration of the Green Pine radar, the Citron Tree fire control center with the Arrow II missile were suggested, attracting rather lukewarm response from the U.S. administration. It was the impression of the Israeli side that the U.S. administration was skeptical of Israel's commitment to develop an Arrow-based TMD system. This feeling was compounded by a highly critical U.S. Government Accounting Office (GAO) report, published in 1993, which faulted the procedures for safeguarding U.S. technologies employed in Arrow. Antagonistic observers could construe such criticism as an indication that Israel's true agenda was the quest for classified U.S. missile technologies, the Arrow program being exploited as a cover story to obtain them.*

In the fall of 1994, David Ivry decided to bring the matters to a head. In a meeting with then Deputy Secretary of Defense John Deutch, held in November, Ivry disclosed the full scope of Israel's effort to develop a fully capable, Arrow-based TMD system. The Green Pine and Citron Tree programs were described, as well as the recently initiated R&D effort to convert the Arrow into an operational missile and to develop an operational rather than a test launcher. The independent funding by Israel of those efforts was stressed, and Ivry pointed out that as he was speaking Israel was already spending more money on the operational Arrow weapon system than the United States investing in the ACES contract. Moreover, Ivry made his U.S. colleagues realize that Israel would go on with the complementary programs, with or without U.S. financial support.

Ivry's presentation and arguments made a deep impression on the U.S. side. This, in fact, was the very first time that the true scope of Israel's own effort to develop a viable TMD system (rather than experimenting with a test missile) was exposed to the highest levels in the Pentagon. The timing of the meeting was propitious; U.S.–Israel relations were at one of their warmest peaks ever, thanks to Yitzhak Rabin's initiative in forcing the pace of the peace process, and Israel was clearly in need to allay her fears over the risks she was taking to achieve peace.

Thus, when David Ivry proposed that the United States join Israel in turning the Arrow into a weapon system, his proposal was favorably received, and the deputy secretary of defense pledged the sum of 200 million U.S. dollars to that purpose. With this agreement in his pocket, and with a growing alarm at the massive buildup of the Syrian ballistic missiles force, Ivry instructed the Arrow program office in the IMOD to draw up a comprehensive 10-year plan for the development, manufacturing, and deployment of two full-size Arrow weapon system batteries. The bold feature of that program was the prompt initiation of series production of the Arrow missile well before the completion of its development tests—in fact, even before the first interception test was to take place. It is little wonder that this instruction drew fire from the Israel Air Force, which voiced its forceful objections to the extreme and unorthodox "telescoping" of the proposed program. However, David Ivry's logic prevailed, and a full consensus with the IDF High Command was now reached. In April 1995, supported by this consensus, Ivry obtained Yitzhak Rabin's approval for his 10-year program plan. The United States was to contribute 36% of the expenditures between 1996 and 2001, after which Israel would continue to fund the program on its own until 2005.

The consensus and the endorsement of the program by the IDF's High Command put an end to all internal disputes within the Israeli defense establishment. Once let loose by their superiors, the officers of the Israel Air Force's Logistic and

*A certain mistrust between the United States and Israel was still lingering at that time, following U.S. allegations that Israel had transferred Patriot technologies to China during or after the Gulf War. Although a full-fledged U.S. inquiry into the matter, including challenge inspections in Israel Air Force installations, failed to turn up any evidence for such misconduct, Secretary of Defense Dick Cheney maintained that the United States possessed "hard evidence" to support the allegations. The mystery of this affair remains a puzzle to date.

Air Defense Commands joined enthusiastically with IAI and the IMOD Arrow program office to form what was perhaps the most effective development team in the history of Israel's military programs. With the willing support of the U.S. Arrow Program Office in Huntsville, Alabama and the BMDO, the Arrow contract was harmonized with the IMOD program and configured into a single unified effort, dubbed the Arrow Deployability Program (ADP).

A new Memorandum of Agreement formalizing the program's scope, cost, and management structure was signed on March 1996. Upon U.S. request, the ADP program included a special integrative task to make the Arrow interoperable with peer U.S. TMD systems, once such systems were deployed to the Middle East. The team effort was channeled into three parallel directions. first, to reconfigure the Arrow missile itself from a pure test configuration (as developed for the ACES program) into an operational missile and to develop an operational launcher, second, to integrate the various components into a cohesive weapon system (a formidable task considering that each component started its development cycle in separation), and third, to develop the technical link that would allow the Arrow weapon system to be interoperable with U.S. TMD assets such as Patriot, THAAD, and future naval systems.

Progress became subsequently smooth and steady, although marred to some extent by a fire in the MLM plant of IAI, which destroyed several key laboratories, thus delaying development and manufacturing effort. Nevertheless, by the end of 1997, the Air Defense Command of the Israel Air Force established the initial Arrow operational unit and started the training of the troops. In early 1998, the Green Pine radar achieved initial operational capability for early warning, and Israel became the third nation after the United States and Russia to deploy its own indigenous early warning assets against ballistic missiles.

The new team that took over the top positions in the IMOD following Israel's general elections of 1996, Minister of Defense Yitzhak Mordechai and his new director general, Ilan Biran, continued the supportive policy of their predecessors regarding the Arrow program. Biran convinced the United States to increase its contribution to the ADP program by $48 million to address interoperability testing requirements. Under his direction, the IMOD Arrow program office studied the problems arising from the Iranian long-range threats and, together with the BMDO, recommended an increase in the Arrow deployment from two to three batteries and endorsed a further contribution of 169 million U.S. dollars for the acquisition of the third battery. In May 1998, Mordechai conducted a top-level review of Arrow program, in which he approved its technical objectives but directed its extension to the year 2010 and its increase to a three batteries architecture. In September 1998, an Arrow flyout test using the fully integrated suit of the weapon system components achieved a resounding success. Two months later, in November 1998, the first operational Arrow missile left the newly established production line and was handed over to the IMOD.

In October 1999, a live interception test involving the entire Arrow weapon system achieved a resounding success, with the fire control radar, battle management center, and Arrow interceptor missile itself performing harmoniously and flawlessly, convincingly demolishing a surrogate TBM target over the Mediterranean sea. Subsequently, in March 2000, the Israel Air Force formally rolled out the core of its first Arrow battery, thereby signifying the transition of the program from the R&D phase to the deployment phase. Thus, Israel is in the process of becoming the first nation to deploy a new generation, nation-wide missile defense system, albeit—for the time being—limited to contingency operational capability. With production lines at IAI and other Israeli defense industries humming, a fully operational status of the Israeli national missile defense system will probably be achieved soon.

V. Summary

We have described in some detail how the inception of the Arrow was far from unopposed and have charted its rocky development history. Still, after all is said and done, Arrow might well be the first of the new crop of antimissile weapons to see operational status. That this happens in Israel—one of the smallest and least affluent countries in the industrialized world—should not be surprising. Of all of the industrialized nations, Israel is facing the most extensive threat of ballistic missiles; moreover, it alone of all industrialized nations has recently experienced the trauma and humiliation of an indiscriminate, unstoppable ballistic missile attack on its major population centers. More ominously, the threat is now becoming even more pronounced and deadly with the transfer of North Korean and Russian ballistic missile technologies to Iran, heralding the appearance of more capable, longer-range threats. It is only natural that, in spite of the bitter disputes, the combined wisdom of the leaders of the Israeli defense establishment brought forth the development of an audacious, yet technologically and financially feasible measure of defense.

The opposition to Arrow is not yet over. It can be expected that the almost inevitable failure in some future flight test would rekindle public debate as well as internal criticism within the defense establishment. Yet, whatever future criticism is leveled at Arrow, it will not be synonymous any more with the rejection of the need for missile defense; rather, the debate will revolve around the optimal way of achieving it. The manifest appetite of the region's radical regimes for ballistic missiles forced a shift in the priorities of Israel's high command. In the recent words of its present chief of staff, Maj. Gen. Shaul Mofaz:

> One of the threats to Israel comes from ground to ground missiles. In our judgment, it is quite probable that such missiles will be used against us in any future conflict. We believe that Israel will thus face a major difficulty in accomplishing the timetable of mobilizing the reserve forces. If this threat is realized, Israel's rear areas, military installations and air force bases will be exposed to attacks by such missiles, conventionally armed or otherwise . . . ."[15]

Thus, Arrow's basic mission has now become embedded in Israel's contemporary defense policy. In spite of the dire predictions of naysayers like Pedahzur, Arrow proved to be a financially affordable program. Consequently, it did not obligate the sacrificing of any long-standing Israeli military doctrines. Its pursuit, however, necessitated some relaxation of rigid mindsets in Israel's High Command and a shift in the perspective of its ranking officers. The role of the United States in this story had been crucial and decisive. Yet, at the end of the day, it was to the credit of the people of Israel that a small group of its leaders was perceptive enough to contest the conventional wisdom of their peers. The technological vision of Dov Raviv, the far sighted statesmanship of the late Yitzhak Rabin, and the wise and astute leadership of David Ivry thus came to the fore at the appropriate junctions in time, to provide the nation with a defensive response to what is perhaps destined to be its major strategic threat in the coming decades.

References

[1]Collier, B., *The Battle of the V Weapons*, Morrow, New York, 1965.

[2]Bush, V., *Modern Arms and Free Men*, Simon and Schuster, New York, 1949; courtesy Lorber, A., *Science, Technology and the Battlefield*, Kronenberg Professional Books, Tel Aviv, Israel, 1997.

[3]Moteff, J.A., *Review of US Research and Development Programs in Ballistic Missile Defense*, CRS Report for Congress, March 1, 1989.

[4]*Russia's Arms Catalogue*, Vol. VI, Military Parade Edition, Moscow, 1997.

[5]Sontag, S., and Drew, C., *Blind Man's Bluff*, Harper, New York, 1998, pp. 339–341.

[6]David Remick, D., "Profile: the Exile Returns," *New Yorker*, Feb. 14, 1994.

[7]Svetlov, V., General Designer of Fakel Engineering Design Bureau, "Russian Desert Fox Hunters," *Military Parade*, March–April 1999.

[8]Pedahzur, R., "Arrow and the Active Defense System Against Ballistic Missiles—Challenges and Problems," Paper 42, Yaffe Center for Strategic Studies, Tel Aviv Univ., Tel Aviv, Israel, Oct. 1993.

[9]Tal, I., *National Defense: The Few Against the Many*, Dvir Publ., Tel Aviv, Israel, 1996.

[10]Steinberg, G.M., "Deterrence, Defense or Arms Control? Israel Perceptions and Responses for the 1990's," California Seminar on International Security and Foreign Policy, Paper 117, Santa Monica, CA, July 1990.

[11]Opal, B., "Israel Proposes Mission to Target Missile Launchers," *Defense Weekly,* 29 March 1999.

[12]Pedahzur, R., "Who Shall Proclaim that the King is Naked?" *Ha'aretz,* 12 Dec. 1998.

[13]Letter to Congressman Bob Livingston, Chairman of the Committee on Appropriations, U.S. Congress, 25 July 1995.

[14]Stav, V. (Ed.), "*Ballistic Missiles, the Threat and the Response, the Principles of Defense Against Ballistic Missiles,*" Ariel Center for Policy Studies, Yediot Acharonot and Chemed Publ., Tel Aviv, Israel, 1998. (For Stav's view of Arrow, see Editor's Introduction.)

[15]Mofaz, S., "The Israel Defense Forces in the 2000's," *Ma'arachot*, May 1999 (present author's translation).

Chapter 3

Arrow System—From Dream to Reality

Yair Ramati,* Dan Peretz,† and Abraham Baum‡
Israel Aircraft Industries, Be'er Ya'akov, Israel

I. Introduction

AT THE beginning of 1986, U.S. Gen. Abrahamson, head of the Strategic Defense Initiative Organization (SDIO)/Ballistic Missile Defense Organization (BMDO), presented a major challenge to Israeli industry and the Israel Ministry of Defense (IMOD): open and genuine participation in the fight against ballistic missiles. Israel Aircraft Industries (IAI) MLM Division, led by Dov Raviv, then general manager of the plant, initiated an accelerated examination of a system of solutions that would satisfy Israeli requirements and provide an answer to typical threats in the Middle East.

A thorough analysis performed by IAI/MLM on the problem of intercepting theater ballistic missiles (TBMs) showed that a window of opportunity had opened with regard to technological availability, operational requirements, and business prospects.

II. How was the Program Implemented?

The feasibility of intercepting a TBM with a hypersonic missile was not established at that time. Therefore demonstration/validation (Dem/Val) projects were initiated, both in the United States and in Israel. They were designed to express the essence of the engineering ability to launch hypersonic interceptors to various heights (from a few kilometers to space) and intercept simulated targets. The second step would be the development of the ability to produce operational configurations.

In the two years following Gen. Abrahamson's visit, up to the signing of the Dem/Val contract between the U.S. Government and IAI/MLM, two conspicuous events took place in the Middle East. The first was the launching of Libyan SCUD missiles (in April 1986) toward the Italian island of Lampedusa in

Copyright © 2000 by the American Institute of Aeronautics and Astronautics, Inc. All rights reserved.

*General Manager. Member AIAA.
†Director, Arrow Program. Member AIAA.
‡Manager, Research Projects.

retaliation for an attack by U.S. forces against Libya. This act showed how fragile deterrence was as a central premise in the war against TBMs. The second event was the "War of the Cities," between Iran and Iraq, January–April 1988. At that time it became apparent that attacks by conventional TBMs against population centers could affect the outcome of even quite bloody wars. Something else observed in that war was the sight of millions of city dwellers fleeing urban centers. It became clear that TBM attacks constituted a process that exerted pressure on the formulators of national security policy, even in countries like Iraq and Iran.

These events strengthened internal support for the need to counter TBMs in general and support for the Arrow interceptor in particular. Senior political circles in the National Unity Government (the prime minister, minister of defense, MOD director general, etc.), key figures in the Knesset, in industry, and in a limited circle of political commentators declared their support for the idea. On the other hand, at that time there was no widespread support for or recognition of such a need in certain segments of the military and the defense establishment.

III. Formulation of the System Solution

The design of the Arrow system was based on a number of key considerations (which were verified only later) and enabled it to be introduced into operational service ahead of several of its competitors. It featured simple and robust concepts that were intended to make it effective against a wide range of threats.

1) *Area defense:* Maximum defense of population centers was desired with a limited number of batteries as an alternative to "point defense" (a city, for example), which requires deployment of a large number of systems.

2) *Dual-purpose radar:* In contrast to the "classic" solution, which uses separate detection and fire control radars, was chosen for detection, warning, and fire control. Furthermore, in the 1980s, as a lesson learned from the environmental opposition to the Voice of America project, it was clear that there was no possibility of locating a great number of electromagnetic transmitters in Israel. The radar and missile design was, therefore, subordinated to environmental and price considerations.

3) *Interoperability:* Keeping the option to include the use of additional assets, such as U.S. satellites, additional types of radar, etc., was an important feature of the system.

4) *A single interceptor:* In conventional design it is easier to develop an interceptor to work at a low altitude or an interceptor for area defense at high altitude. It is far more difficult, from the technological and system aspects, to develop a dual-purpose interceptor, as was done for the Arrow system.

IV. Gaps in Knowledge

Already at the early stages of the project, the development team, which was formed in 1986–1987, had to identify and confront the main gaps in knowledge, as estimated by the Israeli design team and the U.S. entities involved. Agreement was not reached on every subject, but ultimately and with the help of two "red teams" for Arrow I and Arrow II, on which most senior U.S. scientists served, the following principal gaps were identified.

1) The ability to develop a hypersonic interceptor (including such processes and subsystems as heat transfer, booster, sustainer, etc.). These gaps were "closed," so to speak, while still in the demonstration and validation stage.

2) Advanced homing heads.

3) The capability to test the complete system under Israeli geographic limitations.

4) The lethality against a range of enemy missile warheads by the use of revolutionary destruction mechanisms.

V. Methodology

The method employed in the solution gave complete priority to existing subsystems rather than development of "optimal" technologies. For example, the L-band frequency fire control radar implements know-how from another program, and the Arrow I demonstration interceptor was based on the Shavit satellite launcher subsystems (first launched in September 1988). On the other hand, the mobility of the battery and the size of the systems were from the beginning identified as secondary considerations. Therefore, when considered in relation to the system as a whole or the technological points of view, the designers were released from these aspects. Maximum use of commercial equipment (C.O.T.S.) was implemented. It included computer hardware, standard communication protocols, etc. This stage had far-reaching implications from the standpoint of simplifying integration, reducing costs, and the possibility to distribute work among several subcontractors.

Another important point was the earmarking of dedicated work teams at the main contractor and other leading industries (Rafael, Israel Military Industries, Tadiran, ELTA, etc.). The Ministry of Defense and the Israel Air Force maintained harmonious working relations and guided the project through crises, test failures, and development difficulties, and showed an absolute commitment to rigorous inspections and tests: "Test as you fly."

VI. Interception Process

To better understand the various subsystems that will be described, a few words on the interception process are in order. The interception concept used by a weapon system is based on a succession of preplanned events, beginning with detection and ending with warhead fragments hitting the target. The design of the present system was carried out so that not only a single interceptor could be fired against a threat. The comprehensive concept though is still based on the single interceptor. Figure 1 shows the basic system concept.

The interception process includes 1) radar detection of the target, 2) radar classification (TBM or other target), 3) transfer of data to fire command and control (FCC), 4) decision to intercept, 5) preparation of a defense plan, 6) decision and order to intercept, 7) radar acquisition of the interceptor, 8) radar tracking of the target, 9) updating interceptor with real-time data, and 10) interception.

VII. Transition From Arrow I to Arrow II

A. Arrow I

Arrow I, intended to demonstrate ballistic missile interception during penetration into the atmosphere, was chosen for the relatively simple and effective conical single-stage configuration. The objective, which was defined for the developers, focused on a minimum development time and maximum use of off-the-shelf equipment. Based on these requirements, use was made of a powerful motor to give

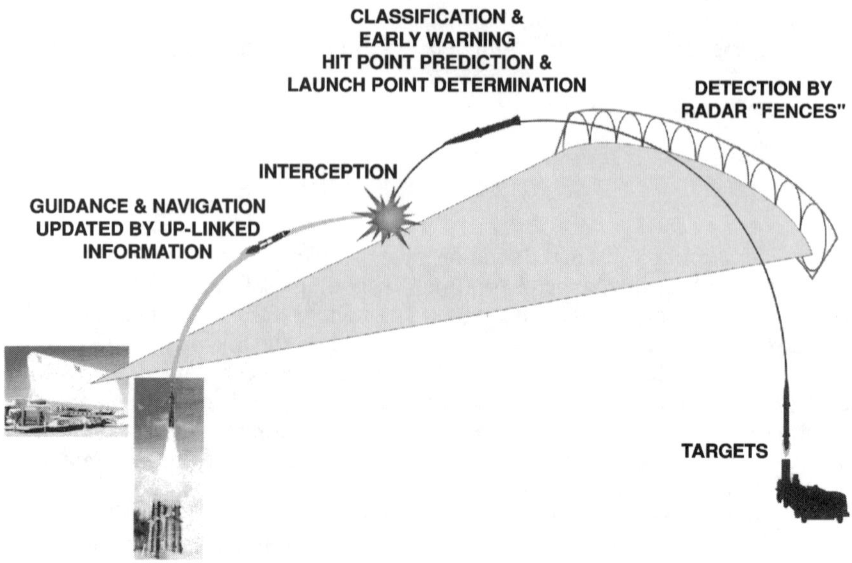

Fig. 1 System concept.

maximum velocity and enable maximum maneuvering at the interception stage. The points of interception were determined during the first stage, while still in the atmosphere, so that a powerful single-stage configuration was obtained with aerodynamic steering.

B. Arrow II

When the project was continued with the operational configuration (Arrow II/ACES) the necessity to increase the "footprint" (the area defended against attack) defined a need for long-range interception in and out of the atmosphere. In addition, certain improvements were demanded, and also the ability to launch from a canister while achieving a fast response time, starting at the request to launch a missile, was desired. [Figure 2 shows the Dem/Val and Arrow continuation experiments (ACES) missile configurations.]

VIII. Arrow Weapon Systems and Subsystems

Following development and tests, which lasted about a decade, the complete system solution was formulated. It currently includes Arrow II launchers, a transportable shelter for launcher control, a fire control unit, and detection and warning radars. See Figs. 3–5 for depictions of the battery configuration, Arrow liftoff, and the interception procedure.

A. Arrow II Interceptors

Because of the need to intercept targets at long ranges and high altitude (with no atmospheric effects), and in light of the radar accuracies, the booster-sustainer, two-stage configuration was chosen.

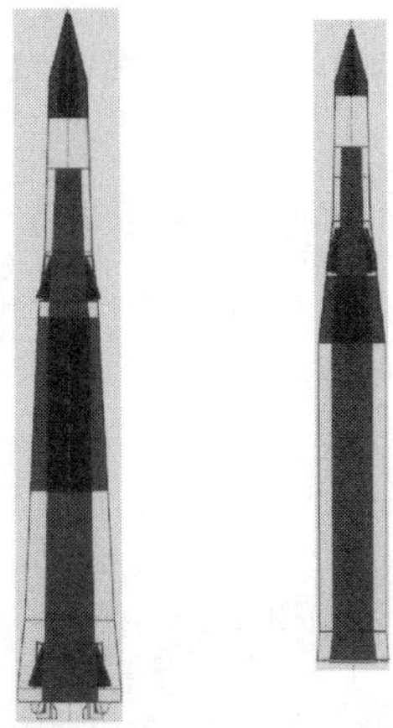

Fig. 2 Arrow configurations.

The booster quickly brings the interceptor to hypersonic velocity, the steering system (thrust vector control, or TVC), stabilizes the path of the missile, and the canard wing configuration enables navigation during the powered stage of the flight and after it. Toward impact, when the interceptor is autonomous, the booster separates. The second stage is ignited and the interceptor's sensors now acquire the target according to data transmitted from the fire control radar. The high impact velocities (three times higher than that of kinetic penetrators fired from tank guns) and the power of the interceptor's warhead ensure the destruction of the target and any type of warhead carried by it.

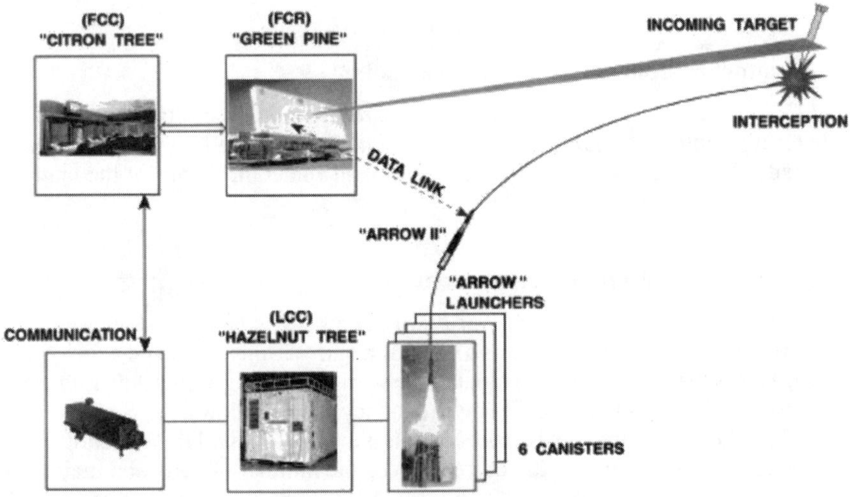

Fig. 3 Battery configuration.

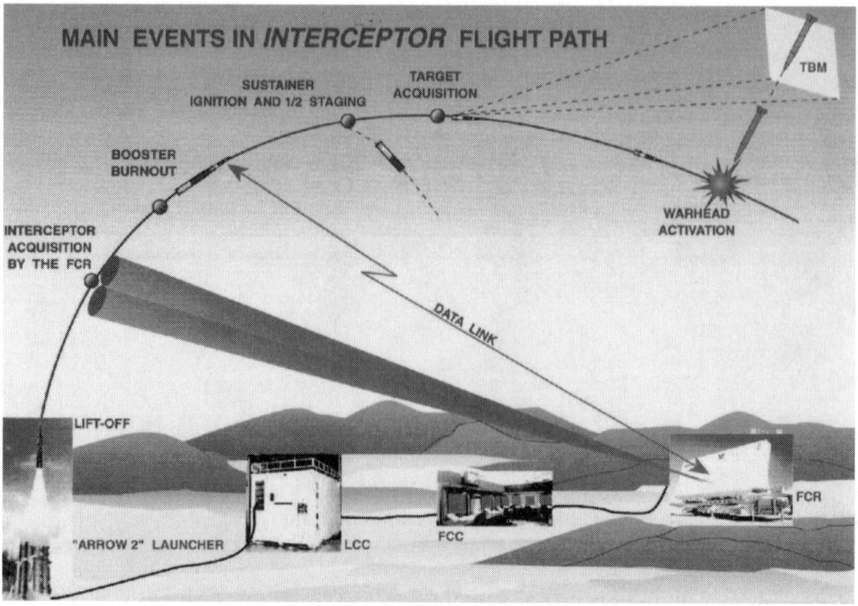

Fig. 4 Interception procedure.

B. Arrow II Launcher

The towed launching vehicle is characterized by its simplicity and operating flexibility. Every vehicle carries six missiles in canisters. In an operational situation, the launching vehicle is supported on legs with the canisters in the erect position. (See Fig. 6.) Its principal characteristics are as follows: 1) all electrical, 2) simple in construction, 3) standard interfaces, and 4) independent of positioning azimuth.

C. Launcher Control Transportable Shelter

LCC—Launch Control Center (Hazelnut Tree): Standard military transportable shelter for control of a group of Arrow launchers is provided, with up to eight on each site. The shelter also contains the command and control unit for the launcher unit.

D. Detection and Fire Control Radar

FCR—Fire Control Radar (Green Pine): The FCR is an L-band–phased array radar that is used simultaneously as a detection and warning radar and a fire control radar. This is the first fire control radar in the world operating at such low frequency. The implications of choosing the low frequency are as follows:

1) The number of transmission/reception units (*Tx/Rx* module) depends on the frequency. A low frequency therefore reduces the number of parts and mainly the price.

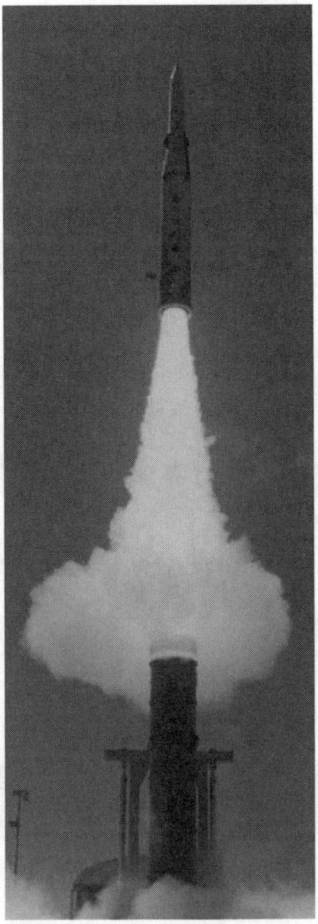

Fig. 5 Arrow liftoff.

2) The unit is an improved subsystem that was used in another program.

3) The low frequency enables scanning of large areas of space and implementation of the early warning option. On the other hand, the design of the Arrow missile enables it to cope with the reduced accuracy that results from the choice of this frequency.

The Green Pine radar, which was developed and produced by IAI/ELTA, enables cooperation with additional radar systems for the detection of TBMs and may be assisted by external indication such as cueing. The first and second radar systems already have been positioned on sites in Israel. (See Fig. 7.)

E. Fire Control Radar Transportable Shelter: Golden Citron

FCC—Fire Control Center (Citron Tree): The mobile fire control system is installed in the transportable shelter and uses standard civilian computer equipment.

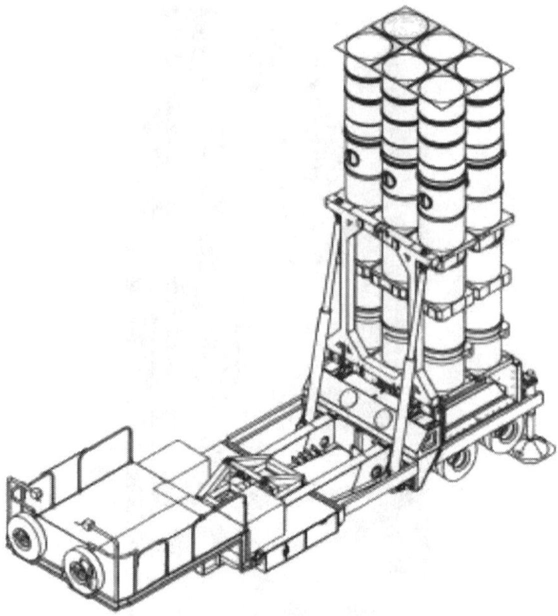

Fig. 6 Arrow launcher.

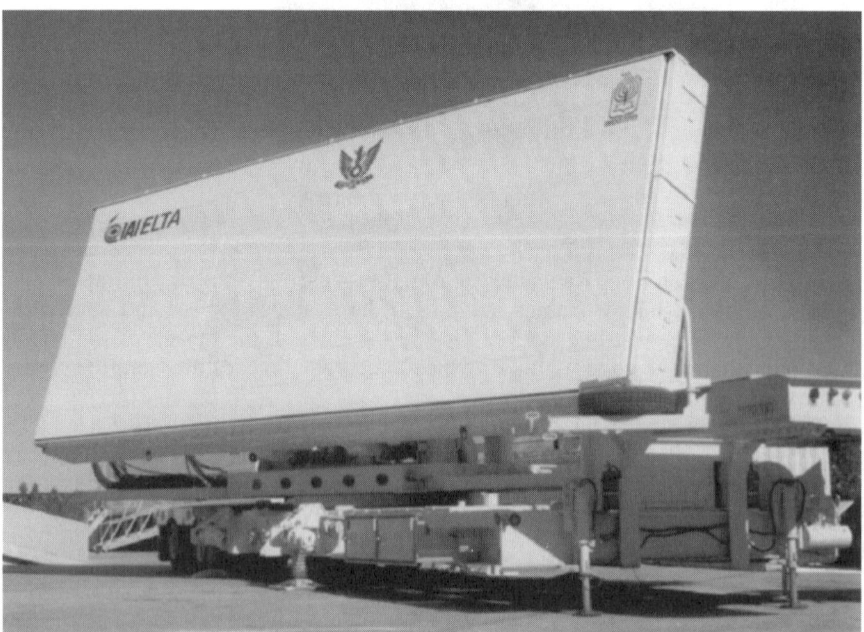

Fig. 7 Green Pine radar.

System characteristics are 1) automatic processes, 2) operating flexibility, 3) communication with other sites in the country, and 4) in-depth debriefing and play back.

The first transportable shelters, manufactured by Tadiran, are already deployed at their designated sites in Israel.

IX. Future Developments

The current plan is to complete development and production of three Arrow weapon system batteries. This will enable the stabilization of most of the active defense layers in Israel, based on the initial definitions, which were formulated by the Israeli Air Force. On the other hand, the expected development of threats and the desire to carry out additional flight tests will enable Israel and the United States to crystallize a continuation program known as ASIP (Arrow System Improvement Program).

The future directions of these activities will broaden the activity envelope with quantity, quality, and accuracy in relation to future long-range threats. Against these threats, the counterforce alternatives are less effective and are also problematic in the political arena because of the need to commit to early entry into enemy territory.

X. Conclusion

It seems that not one of the Arrow weapon system critics has admitted that this is an impressive technological and program success that places Israeli industry (led by the IMOD and IAI/MLM) side by side with the most prominent European manufacturers. Several factors contributed to the success of the program, of which the principal ones are as follows.

1) High technical know-how based on an excellent engineering infrastructure in Israel.

2) A work ethic in the development teams during long years, coordinated by the Israeli Air Force (user), the Ministry of Defense (customer), industry (supplier), and the United States (partners).

3) The courage of the initiators who made the correct choice of subsystems, working points, and development processes (any mistake in this aspect would have caused the project to fail).

4) High industrial control at the level of complex integration.

The strenuous work that was performed at a high rate and that started with maximum emphasis on development and tests is today gradually moving in the direction of system integration, production, and testing. This new phase reflects the progress of the project and the closing of the gaps that characterized it in the beginning. It is also appropriate to acknowledge the importance of the work with the U.S. establishment. Development of the Arrow system was the first opportunity that Israeli experts had to work hand in hand with the best brains in the United States. U.S. industry, consultants, and government infrastructures participated in this process with particular emphasis on development of advanced ground-testing equipment.

The completion of the Arrow weapon system is expected to provide the State of Israel with a suitable answer to the threat of TBMs, and in addition it will give fundamental support to others engaged in pinpointing enemy missile trajectories and predicting the point of impact.

The latent interoperability capability with U.S. and other systems will also serve as an important defense layer, technical as well as political, and will enable a broadening of the response to the threat of TBMs in the Middle East.

Acknowledgment

The authors of this chapter want to take this opportunity to thank the marvelous team working on the project, in industry and in the defense establishment (in Israel and around the world), who enabled IAI/MLM to gradually transfer the Arrow weapon system to the Israeli Air Force, and above all, to Dov Raviv who initiated and led the project during its first years.

II. Threat and Response

Chapter 4

Many Facets of Threat Assessment

Reuven Eyal*
WALES Ltd., Ramat-Gan, Israel

I. Introduction

THE possible employment of TBMs (theater ballistic missiles) in a conflict stimulates worry since no battle-proven defense systems have been developed and fielded to successfully counter them. In spite of their first operational appearance in World War II, no systematic effort has been conducted over the years to develop suitable countermeasures and appropriate defense doctrines. In Operation Desert Storm neither suitable weapons nor concept of operations (CONOPS) were available to destroy TBM launchers or the TBMs themselves during boost-phase or reentry. Mobilization of the Patriot surface-to-air missiles (SAMs) for this task can be considered, at best, a hasty expedient for lack of a better solution.

By their very nature, TBMs are purely offensive weapons, whereas the theater ballistic missile defense (TBMD) systems that are in various stages of development do not pose any threat except to those missiles. The TBMD is, therefore, defensive in its nature both in the strategic and the tactical sense. TBMD is an answer to a very specific problem and is limited to the single task of intercepting TBMs only. As such, TBMD turns out to be problematic from a cost-effectiveness point of view, unless its operational achievements are satisfactory and exceed a fairly high performance threshold, yet to be defined, and are measured by the potential damage spared on the ground as a result of TBMs destroyed in the air.

It is true that several defense systems in the development phase attempt to deal with both air defense and TBM defense in what is sometimes called EAD (extended air defense). However, even in these systems there are significant differences in the characteristics of distinct interceptors designed for the different tasks. Furthermore, compromises (for example, in the selection of the ideal deployment site of the firing unit) are likely in order to satisfy two sets of operational specifications, thus preventing the attainment of ideal performance in either one.

The defense system's design must be optimized to justify the cost and engineering effort intrinsic in the development of so specialized a system. The reference

Copyright © 2000 by the American Institute of Aeronautics and Astronautics, Inc. All rights reserved.

*Senior Threat and Operations Analyst. Member AIAA.

threat must therefore be as close a representation as possible of the actual threat with which the defense system will have to contend. Bearing in mind that the development and fielding of such defense systems take many years, the threat assessment and description require an accurate long-range forecast, which is a formidable task. This task is further complicated by the fact that technological issues that must be considered are very often influenced by the political environment. For threat assessment to contribute significantly, forecasts must be updated and corrected in line with changes observed over time (in the evolving threat) and their implications must be manifested in adaptations of the defense systems' design. Of course, long-range forecasts should a priori have reasonable, but not exaggerated, safety margins, also subjected to periodic amendments.

Defense against worst-case forecasts and scenarios, if presented as precautionary measures and safety nets, can mitigate the operational risks but may carry a high price tag that could turn out to be prohibitive, possibly leading to an unjustified abandonment of the whole TBMD project.

Because the threat, real or perceived, is the basic driver, and the *raison dêtre* of all TBMD projects, its portrayal has a decisive impact on all decisions that govern TBMD doctrines and technological developments, as well as their massive budgeting. Any mistake or misjudgment in threat assessment can mislead decision makers and system developers and result in waste of efforts to a degree that might jeopardize the entire defense system or severely curtail its effectiveness. Yet, the existing experience with systematic TBM threat analysis and its presentation in terms convenient for the formulation of concrete defense concepts and systems' design, seems to be very limited. It is, definitely, much more restricted than analyses regarding ICBMs or traditional air-breathing threats, the former having been studied thoroughly for nearly half a century, and the latter since World War I.

It is high time to attempt to offer a systematic approach to the challenge, or at least to point out some of the basic topics entailed in such an effort and the order in which they might be tackled, even if there is no guarantee that such an approach will lead to quick, final, and perfect answers. Different approaches can be adopted and could provide further development and streamlining of analysis tools. So far, however, few have dealt in depth with the issue and very little has been published openly on this subject.

This chapter is intended not only to suggest an approach but also to trigger reactions, objections, reservations, criticism, and so forth, and initiate a fruitful debate regarding TBM threat assessment methodology.

II. Threat Assessment as a Cornerstone to TBMD Development

Threat assessment entails a wide variety of topics, starting with basic conceptual aspects, all the way down to technical and operational details that influence the outcome of individual interceptions and engagements, or statistical results of engagements in large scale scenarios. It addresses TBM force buildup long before the force is operationally ready for combat, as well as combat intelligence in the final minutes prior to the TBM launch and its engagement.

Figure 1 summarizes the possible contribution of threat assessment at various stages of an assumed enemy's activities along the time axis, from TBM force buildup until close to TBM launch in wartime. Each of the topics in the diagram represents an entire area of analysis that requires special effort, time, and

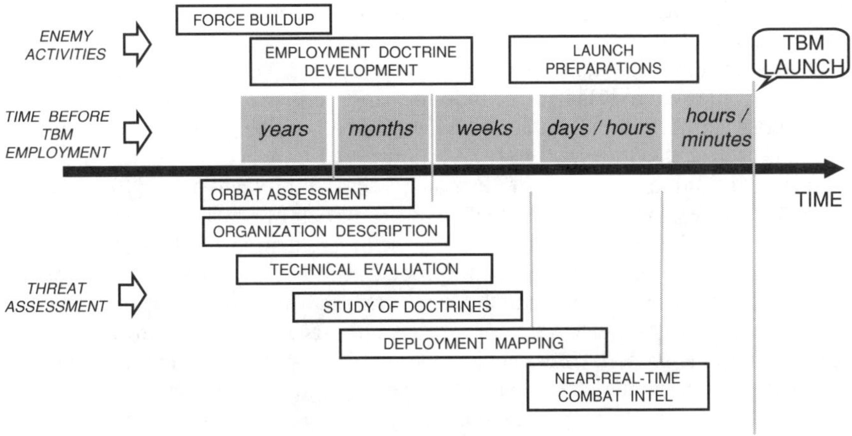

Fig. 1 Typical activities along the time axis.

expertise. Each subject can be subdivided into many elements that prescribe collection requirements or means, and that influence the quality and resolution of the intelligence analysis process. All of them together form a continuum in which each element contributes its share to the complete, accumulated threat picture.

This basic model seems to be valid for all theaters and all TBM types. Differences between theaters and TBM types appear when the model is further elaborated to a higher level of resolution.

A. Examining the Threat

Examples of how each of the topics listed in Fig. 1 can be further broken down to more elementary activities follow. Force buildup on the enemy's side includes procurement or production of TBMs, construction and development of infrastructure, establishment of operational and logistic units, training facilities, etc. Employment doctrine development contains the conceptual aspects as well as trials, training, and assimilation of procedures. On the threat assessment side, order of battle (ORBAT) assessment addresses types, quantities of TBMs, and launchers, as well as the logistic setup that is supposed to maintain the equipment in serviceable shape and support the launch units in wartime. Technical evaluation includes performance, signatures, vulnerability of components, trajectory profiles, warhead types, penetration aids, etc.

In many cases the level of required assessment details can easily be blown up to unmanageable proportions, but in practice only the really essential aspects must be addressed. Perfection can be the goal but much less may suffice for the purpose of defense systems design.

The near-real-time activities that appear on the right-hand side of the timeline, in Fig. 1, border on early warning. Under most conditions the acquisition and timely processing of intelligence at this stage becomes more difficult and its contribution is limited. A more detailed discussion of this phase exceeds the scope of this chapter, and it touches on sensitive aspects of threat assessment and near-real-time or real-time monitoring of an enemy's activities. It more appropriately belongs in the category of external cues, which are covered in a separate chapter later in this book.

Obviously, the presented model does not have a clear beginning and end. During hostilities, after each TBM salvo, mobile firing units are likely to vacate launch sites, hide, and redeploy for the next salvo. Locating these units thus becomes a continuous process. Information from an observed impact of a missile salvo, and remnants of fired missiles, might generate an opportunity and a need to reevaluate enemy doctrines, practices, and technical properties of his TBMs. Massive employment of TBMs in wartime might offer the first real opportunity to study enemy operational and logistic doctrines and procedures in real-life environment and to validate or reassess previous conclusions. Thus the process in Fig. 1 becomes a cyclical one that is repeated as more information is gathered as a result of more missiles being launched. Conclusions from previous engagements serve as inputs to new threat assessments and forecasts regarding future TBM strikes. In wartime, the analysis must be accelerated to enable conclusions to be implemented in time to counter the next TBM salvo.

B. Limitations and Uncertainties

One of the undeclared responsibilities of the intelligence community and the threat analysts is the education of the intelligence consumers as to the limitations and uncertainties that characterize threat analysis and the caution which is appropriate when the outputs are used. Threat assessments and forecasts, in their broader perspective, are not prophesy and are not necessarily based on mathematical laws and scientific principles. They are normally an estimate supported by somewhat limited knowledge, by many assumptions and much logical reasoning. The process is never fully completed, and at any point in time the assessment is only a basis for future amendments that serve as a recommended temporary design point for system developers and defense strategists. How to read threat assessments is no less important than how to generate them, and not all intelligence consumers are masters of this art.

Uncertainties and possible misjudgments are a feature of all aspects of intelligence work, but there are certain inherent differences between the technical and the nontechnical aspects. In the technical field the laws of physics set limits to possible tradeoffs between payload, range, weight, guidance principles, accuracy, etc. This process ensures that technical estimates will converge to within certain reasonable limits accepted and adhered to by all knowledgeable engineers. The sharing of technical intelligence on specific TBM types, among countries faced with a common TBM threat, will normally shorten the time required for technical familiarization with the threat. Significant engineering modifications of TBMs take years to implement so that technical intelligence remains valid for a relatively long period of time. It is the task of intelligence organizations to keep track of later major modifications to ensure that assessments regarding the technical aspects remain up to date. On the other hand, assessment of deployment doctrines and TBM employment profiles, for example, is fraught with a higher degree of uncertainty and more prone to error. A number of reasons why this is so are presented here.

1) Although enemy countries in different theaters operate the same TBM types, each theater might differ in terrain, in doctrine and employment modes, in deployment strategies, in support measures, proficiency of personnel, and so forth.

Basically, each threatened country is on its own in assessment of these aspects of the threat and the value of exchange of information on some of the theater-specific topics can be limited. Also, the perception of the threat and its effect will vary from country to country.

2) An enemy's doctrines and TBM employment modes are less rigid than technological factors and can change relatively quickly, and this can have a very strong impact on the effectiveness of the defense, at least until such changes and their operational logic are well understood. In general, military doctrines and modes of operation do change with time and such changes are characterized, at least in theory, by *relatively* short time-constants. It is practically impossible to predict the full spectrum of imaginable employment modes and prepare appropriate answers and protective measures against all of them.

3) All implications of TBM launches in large numbers might become apparent only in war as trials and exercises in peacetime never involve more than one or two TBMs. Several concurrent launches against the same target, or closely located targets, introduce certain complicating elements that have also a qualitative impact exceeding the total effects of individual launches, for example, a salvo of multiple simultaneous launches obliges the defense system to associate between targets seen by several sensors and fusion of the data into a single coherent sky view. The combination of parameters in feasible launch scenarios can lead to surprises in some unforeseen dimension.

4) Two of the basic parameters in any multiple launch scenario in the Middle East are the number and identity of all conceivable enemy countries that might participate in the war, or in a specific scenario, in the case of a coalition of enemies. These determine, among other things, the directions from which missiles can come and which must be covered by the defense systems.

A superpower with global responsibilities is faced with another kind of uncertainty, namely, definition of the reference theater. It is desirable but practically impossible to prepare today for TBM launch scenarios in a war that will be fought in some still unknown corner of the world, 10 or 15 years from now. How can the threat be assessed at all in this case, beyond the study of the TBM types and some basic familiarization with the ORBAT in various unfriendly countries? The real assessment must be postponed to a later point in time when a realistic chance of a confrontation emerges.

Uncertainty and obvious difficulties in TBM threat assessment are not an excuse for not attempting to do the job. Defense system developers need a design point for their R&D and system engineering work, and they cannot be required to complete the threat assessment by themselves. Intelligence analysts must face the challenge and do their best.

III. Possible Classification of Theater Ballistic Missiles

Classification of TBMs is more a matter of convenience than of necessity. The main reason behind classification is the variety of intelligence consumers who need information about these types of weapon, each with a specific field of interest and unique responsibilities.

The organization responsible for the threat assessment, and also responsible for the presentation of its findings to different audiences, will find it very helpful to group the information in a manner that coincides with the needs of these audiences. Not only does this save time but it also serves as a guide during collection, exploitation, editing, and dissemination of the data. It certainly helps in computerized interaction between intelligence producers and intelligence consumers. Not all consumers need the same set of data. For example, there is a big difference between the needs of units involved in passive defense (civil defense), units responsible for active defense, and combat units tasked to strike and destroy the launchers and the infrastructure of the TBM force.

A. Criteria

Classification is possible according to various criteria, some of which are listed here:

1) Objective (tactical or strategic).
2) Adapted (yes/no) for conventional/unconventional warheads.
3) Range (normally refers to maximum range, although minimum range has its implications as well).
4) Mobility of the launchers (static, transportable, or mobile).
5) Proliferation (countries that operate the various TBM types).
6) Technological complexity.
7) Accuracy (circular error probable).
8) Quantity (number of TBMs, launchers, and warhead types in ORBAT).
9) Number of motor stages (single or two stages).
10) Type of propellant (liquid or solid).

Other criteria could be suggested, but the question is whether they all, including the listed ones, have any operational or practical significance. Some have, as shown later, and some do not, and they are mentioned only for methodological purposes. A few examples of classifications that have a practical meaning are worth mentioning.

1. *Maximum Range*

The maximum range of a TBM immediately indicates the limits of the area within which the TBMs must deploy to place them within effective range from our own potential targets or borders, and it also reveals the maximum anticipated velocity along the trajectory, especially during the critical reentry phase. Range to the expected deployment sites is an essential input for counter-force operational planning, or for estimation of expected detection range of an incoming TBM and calculation of the expected warning time available for civil defense purposes.

2. *Types of Warheads*

Identification of warhead type as conventional, unconventional, cluster warheads, or some other sophisticated type, is an essential input for defense assets allocation, engagement prioritization, and formulation of appropriate defense strategies, especially in cases in which unconventional warheads might be employed. Obviously, considering the dangers posed by the different warhead types, especially unconventional ones, the availability of such information and its orderly presentation to decision makers, will, no doubt, affect not only defense measure development and an appropriate prioritization of budget allocation, but also diplomatic activity and further intelligence collection efforts. Of special interest are the parameters that can contribute to detection and identification of unconventional warheads in flight, or can alert the battle managers as to the probability that such warheads are being used or that their employment is imminent. Some of these topics give rise to technical intelligence requirements, or essential elements of information, that must be addressed even if success is not guaranteed.

Cluster warheads pose a special challenge since their intercept is practically impossible after the bomblets have been dispersed. This implies that special defense systems must be developed and tailored for their destruction before the submunitions are dispersed.

3. *Circular Error Probable*

Circular error probable (CEP) is a common term that denotes TBM accuracy. (It denotes the radius of a circle into which 50% of the fired ordnance will fall, and it serves as a standard criterion for weapon system accuracy and ordnance dispersion.) CEP is very helpful in determining possible uses of such missiles; e.g., whether against small or large targets, whether against military installations or large urban areas, and for population terrorization. There is always the possibility that unconventional warheads with huge destructive effect will be developed or procured to compensate for reentry vehicle (RV) inaccuracy. Validation or refutation of this possibility is another responsibility of those tasked with threat assessment.

4. *Design Elements*

Motor characteristics, number of stages, separable or nonseparable RVs, etc., are very important pieces of information and helpful inputs for engineering teams responsible for sensor specification and design and for development of discrimination algorithms. Intimate knowledge or reliable estimates of such characteristics together with information on physical dimensions and other properties are essential for identification of the warhead in the presence of other closely spaced objects. Motor behavior is a critical input for boost-phase interception (BPI) or ascent-phase interception (API), and it will determine, for example, the specification of the interceptor that is designed to carry out such missions.

B. Example Case

Obviously, the preferred classification of TBMs depends on the uses such information is supposed to serve, and different analysts in different organizations might favor different criteria. More than one classification method may be used in parallel, and in many cases simultaneous classifications, according to two different sets of parameters, lead to additional insight and enlightening conclusions.

Take for example a simple case, depicted in Fig. 2, of a two-dimensional correlation matrix. In it, one dimension represents (conventional) warhead weight, which has some correlation with the yield, and the other dimension indicates CEP or predicted impact point accuracy (a large CEP being on the order of several kilometers). CEP and warhead size are outputs of technical intelligence. In the matrix, three types of TBM, designated A, B, and C, are presented. An immediate conclusion is that TBM type B, because of its poor accuracy, is not effective against small targets such as typical military installations, but it poses a threat against large targets—urban areas for example. Its warhead size could enable some future upgrade and sophistication to compensate for the inaccuracy even if this would entail

CEP / W/H WEIGHT	SMALL	MEDIUM	LARGE
LIGHT	TBM TYPE A		
MEDIUM			TBM TYPE C
HEAVY			TBM TYPE B

Fig. 2 Two-dimensional TBM characteristics correlation matrix.

a weight penalty. On the other hand, TBM type A, with a small CEP (say 150 m or even less) seems to answer requirements posed by typical, relatively small, but not hardened military targets.

To confirm the validity of such preliminary conclusions, more specific information will be needed, based on intelligence collection regarding stocks, doctrines, exercises, etc. However, once the first assumptions are clearly phrased, they can serve as guidelines that focus all further data gathering and analysis efforts on specific topics that seem important. Much care must be exercised not to reach hasty and unfounded conclusions that can bias future, more intensive, analysis.

To take the presented methodology one step further, this correlation matrix can be expanded into a multidimensional matrix in which several properties of specific missile types are mapped and their suitability for specific tasks is evaluated. More than three dimensions (because of graphic constraints), necessitate a purely conceptual process that follows the same logic in principle, but three dimensions enable some further graphic elaboration, as shown in Fig. 3. In this example another parameter "range" is added to the information contained in Fig. 2. Range is specified as either short, medium, or long, and is depicted as a layer in the three-dimensional diagram.

For further discussion let us assume that short range, in the present example, represents tens of kilometers, medium range stands for hundreds of kilometers, and long range covers TBMs with a range more than 1000 km.

The new additional preliminary conclusions that can be drawn from this three-dimensional presentation are as follows.

1. *TBM Type A*

TBM type A seems to suit mainly tactical needs on the battlefield because of its short range and high accuracy. This does not rule out its employment against strategic targets if they are within range. Range to such potential targets must be checked, and the targets listed for planning their appropriate defense. The short-range, and therefore relatively slow reentry velocity, does not put severe stress on the defense requirements, but the relatively short flying time (not indicated in Fig. 3) might do so. This time needs further investigation and should be considered an essential element of information (EEI).

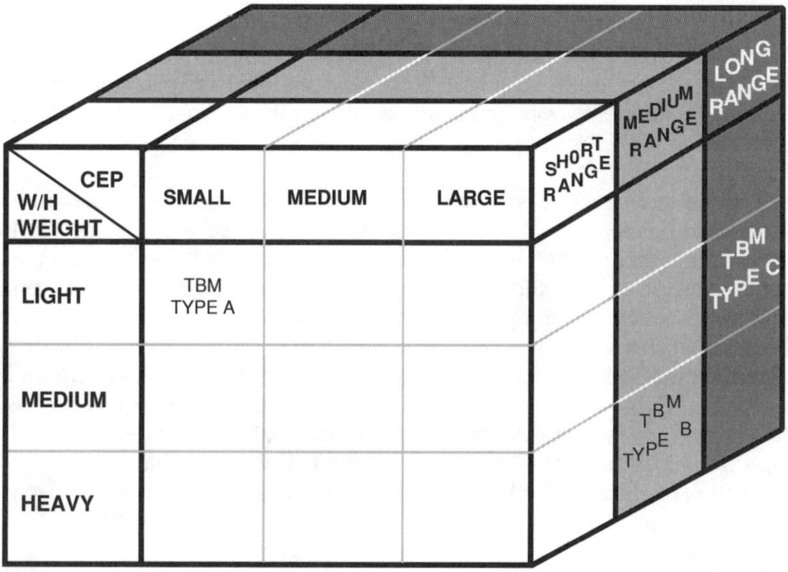

Fig. 3 Three-dimensional presentation of TBM characteristics.

2. *TBM Type B*

TBM type B has the same properties as type C except in range, but its bigger payload leaves room for technological sophistication in the future. This finding justifies an analysis of the minimum range for type B TBMs from possible, enemy launch sites to potential targets. The issue is important if the maximum range of the missile is less than the distance between the potential launch sites and important targets, thus necessitating a modification in the missile in order for it to pose a threat. One should be aware that there is a tradeoff between warhead weight and TBM range. Weight saved by warhead weight (and yield) reduction can be used for additional propellant, and thus for attainment of longer range.

3. *TBM Type C*

TBM type C, due to its long range seems, at first glance, to serve strategic needs, but has limitations imposed by accuracy and warhead yield. It can be assumed to be a candidate for future upgrade and modifications, one possibility being to fit an unconventional, chemical or biological warhead, for which accuracy is not critical, and a "medium size" payload delivery capability is sufficient. Such a speculation would lead to various questions regarding development of weapons of mass destruction in the enemy's countries, which is another (complementary) threat assessment issue.

A special case where the correlation between range, accuracy, and yield is enlightening refers to two belligerents with no common border, separated by a third country, and *slightly* out of TBM range.

C. Summary

As already stated, classification of TBMs according to various criteria, and comparison of the results, can lead to some additional insights and previously hidden perspective. However, great care should be taken not to automatically adopt the preliminary conclusions reached in this way: use them only as road maps for further investigation.

Organizational structure and subordination of units operating a certain TBM type can also be used as a classification criterion. The decision-making level and chain of command might serve as an indicator of the strategic importance and possible strategic tasks of the TBM types. For example, units that operate unconventional warheads may enjoy a privileged position in the organizational structure and command chain.

Classification of TBMs according to the various criteria is always helpful, even if it serves only for documentation and reference, but whether it can be used as a tool for defense system development or operational considerations depends on the specific needs and questions to be answered. The analyst has to decide when classification has an added value and what is the most logical classification to work with for some specific purpose.

IV. Possible Model for TBM Threat Assessment

As already mentioned, threat assessment serves as an essential and central input for the various teams responsible for development of defensive measures. The assessment is not an end in itself, but rather an output produced for and provided to other teams. These teams include politicians, scientists, military personnel, civil defense experts, and others.

The TBM threat is a dynamic entity that develops and changes with time, and it is reactive in the sense that it in turn responds to defense measures acquired or developed against it. This is true both in peacetime and in war, but in war the dynamics of the process are much faster for three main reasons:

1) Much additional and more reliable information becomes available as an enemy's practices and doctrines are revealed and pieces of hardware (TBM remnants) become available for examination. The understanding or the perception of the threat changes even if no changes in TBM employment, or in the weapon itself, occur in practice.

2) The enemy might react to a defensive measure if lessons can be learned and conclusions drawn, and if time is available to implement changes in the modus operandi.

3) As a result of battle damage and other attrition factors, a reduction in launch intensity, and a corresponding change in the employment mode, might become necessary. On the other hand, rapid resupply of launchers/missiles or reinforcement of the ORBAT by expeditionary TBM units from a third country would enable an increased launch rate.

The threat assessment, therefore, must address such possible developments and present to the various teams that rely on the assessments possible courses of action and possible or likely developments. This is necessary to imbue the defense systems and procedures with adequate flexibility and robustness to deal with unexpected deviations from a defined baseline threat.

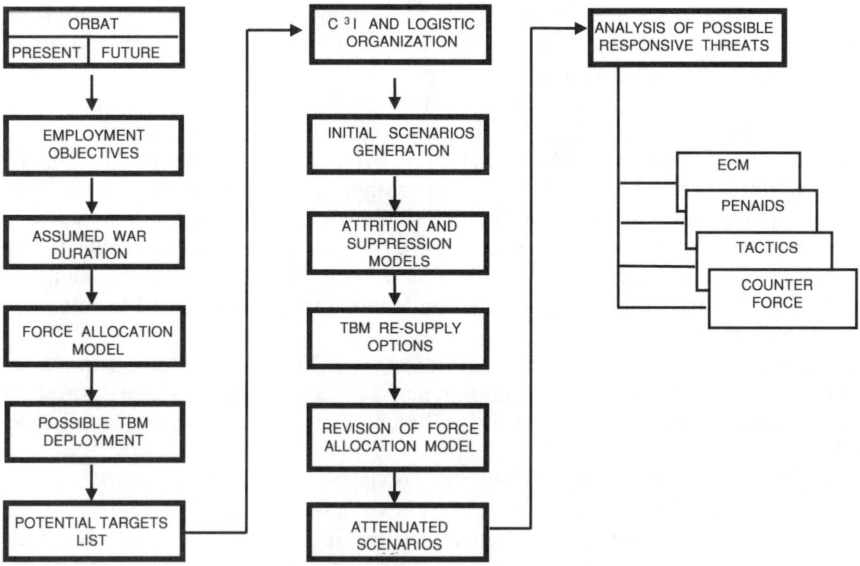

Fig. 4 Possible threat assessment sequence model.

A possible basic threat assessment model is presented in Fig. 4. Two remarks, regarding this figure, are appropriate at this point:

1) The arrows joining the various steps do not necessarily indicate dependency, but rather a suggested sequence in which the steps should be handled.

2) The model presented is for use in the design of TBMD systems and is limited in its scope for this purpose. If, for example, it were to be used for TBM launcher strike planning, it would need some additional modules not included in the Fig. 4.

The complete process is supposed to culminate in the generation of reference scenarios representing series of TBM attacks or possible courses of action in which conventional and/or unconventional warheads are employed. These scenarios must support defense command and control functions, various levels and types of simulations, defense setup sizing decisions, defense doctrines evaluation, sensitivity studies, etc. To cover the most likely as well as the most dangerous, even if less likely but still possible, developments, several scenarios must be produced and presented. Care must be taken to distinguish, both in the analysis and in the presentation of the results and the recommendations, among the various cases: those that represent the most likely scenario, the worst but less likely case, and the one that can be repeated many times as opposed to the one that is very specific and probably a single event scenario. The last one, for example, fits an opening scenario at the outbreak of a war when everything is still under full control, and all activities of all TBM units can be coordinated and fully synchronized.

The first step in the model is to define the ORBAT, an intelligence building block that is very often available within reasonably accurate limits, and in most cases is the most stable anchor from which the assessment can be initiated.

The next step in the model addresses TBM employment objectives that might be known from solid sources or must be assumed based on strategic analysis and overall military force structure study.

An assumption regarding the duration of the war is necessary for calculating daily TBM consumption. Daily TBM consumption, or daily apportionment, is a difficult question to answer, but it cannot be bypassed. It is a vital factor in determining reference scenarios. The daily consumption, as well as the overall TBM consumption profile throughout the war, obviously depends on the assumed war duration and is a function of war objectives, political constraints, available TBMs in stock, envisaged/available resupply sources, etc. Because of the uncertainties, more than one assumption may be made and a wider spectrum of possible outcomes may be used for further analysis.

The force allocation model refers to allocation of TBMs to targets both quantitatively and by TBM type. If solid intelligence is not available, reasonable estimates can be made on the basis of the TBMs' characteristics (such as warhead yield and CEP).

Clearly, the locations from which the TBMs are fired are a necessary input in the generation of a scenario. Generally, it is sufficient to provide a representative deployment location for an entire unit and to specify a doctrinal range of distances between launchers when firing, if this information is essential. More detailed and more specific descriptions might be required for design of defense systems tailored for launch detection and APIs, for example.

The potential targets list is an additional input that must be prepared. Two approaches are possible for preparation of such a list. The first one defines target priorities from the adversary's point of view, as *assessed* by the intelligence community. The second approach prioritizes targets according to the value attributed to them in our own view. The two do not necessarily coincide. To provide a safety margin, doubtful targets may be included in the list of targets that must be defended even if the logic of the need is not fully understood.

Command, control, communications, and intelligence, as well as logistic organization, affect force employment efficiency and maximum possible firing rates. Knowledge of these factors is helpful, alongside other parameters, for estimating the conceivable upper limit of TBM launch rate by the various units.

Using the information listed, together with the technical information necessary to generate TBM trajectories, scenarios of launch salvos can now be generated. However, for these scenarios to faithfully simulate real-life TBM strikes, they must be adjusted to take into account effects that can be expected to occur in wartime.

The enemy's ORBAT, mentioned as the first step in the model, refers to the ORBAT at the outbreak of hostilities only. This ORBAT, however, can be affected by attrition and its operating capability can be reduced, for example, by allocating forces to suppress the launchers' freedom of movement. On the other hand, resupply can increase the ORBAT and launch capacity. Therefore, attrition and resupply factors should be introduced into the model and their possible impact on the outcome should be evaluated. Alternatively, these factors can be addressed in the context of sensitivity analyses in which excursions from nominal models, and implications of such excursions, are studied and possible corrective measures considered.

The responsive threats, an all-inclusive name to enemy actions intended to reduce the effectiveness of the defense systems, might contain not only development and employment of additional sophisticated hardware, or changes in specific TBM employment modes and operational tactics, but also employment of counter-force means and methods against TBMD elements. Because of its potential effect on a critical part of the overall defense effort, its danger should not be underestimated. Ordinary bombs, precision guided munitions (PGMs), antiradiation missiles (ARM), or artillery are representative examples. Furthermore, this threat could be manifested before employment of TBMs paving the way to a more successful, or efficient, TBM attack.

V. Analysis of Responsive Threats

Analysis of responsive threats addresses responses of a TBM-operating enemy to the introduction of anti-TBM defense systems. The object of such responses is to negate the effect of the defense systems and preserve, to a greater or lesser degree, the effectiveness of the TBM force and its destructive power. In its broadest sense the responsive threat includes both a direct threat to the TBM defense elements in the form of their physical destruction, and employment of counter measures and deception means that decrease the effectiveness of the defense systems by reducing their kill probability.

As a first step, it is imperative to become familiar with the issue and come up with relevant questions that must guide information collection efforts. This information will support later analysis. Responsive threats can be devised and applied at all stages of the conflict, before TBM launch, during the boost phase, in the terminal TBM reentry phase, and even after the attack for concealment of activities preceding the next attack. Analysis of the "threat" and the "responsive threat" form one continuum that falls under the responsibility of the threat analyst and they must be treated as such.

A. Destruction

Physical destruction of TBMD elements, as one possible and expected responsive threat, does not differ, in principle, from destruction of any other target. Once the defense units and their equipment are included in the targets list, the means and methods are readily available. Survivability of TBMD units, and defense of its elements under direct attack, rely on a wide variety of means and tactics, most of which are outside the scope of the threat assessment topic.

On the other hand, there are in principle other means, such as electronic counter measures (ECM), directed against TBMD defense surveillance or fire control radar systems, decoys, or maneuvering reentry vehicles, for example. They might necessitate a special effort on the enemy's part, since procurement of suitable electronic gear or its development, as well as adjustment or calibration of available equipment, may be necessary.

B. Deception

Fielding of certain penetration aids, normally intended for deception or saturation of sensors and command and control functions, requires considerable preparation and testing and might take some time to accomplish. This time must be exploited by the various intelligence agencies to detect such developments and identify the main trends being adopted by the countermeasures developers.

The introduction of deception means and other penetration aids (PENAIDS), specially tailored to degrade the performance of TBM defense will probably not be implemented before the basic properties and at least some technical data regarding the target TBMs defense systems become known.

Responsive threat can also include special tactics and TBM launch strategies that put extra stress, during the critical phase of the interceptions, on the defense systems and the defense real-time decision-making process.

C. Technical Intelligence

Understanding of enemy force structure, chain of command, real-time command and control, operational planning and execution, etc., must be considered an important element in the responsive threat analysis, as it is in the basic threat analysis.

Technical intelligence and familiarization with the structure and properties of the various individual TBMs attract the attention of most people involved in development of TBM defense systems today. The whole field is relatively new, and interception of a single TBM by a single firing unit is not a battle-proven capability. The one-vs-one engagement solution therefore, at the present point in time, is a more urgent engineering task than the many-vs-many scenario, whereas the main effects of many types of responsive threats will be most acute in the many-vs-many scenarios. Consequently, the analysis of the many-vs-many situations is overdue. These situations introduce several important parameters that might, in time, present a most difficult challenge.

There are two possible approaches to analysis of enemy responses to the successful development of TBM defense systems:

1) Evaluation of possible developments and modifications, technically feasible at least on paper, before there is any indication that the TBM operator has even considered such modifications or upgrades. This approach might lead to a worst-case analysis of options that are far beyond what the enemy intends to do, or is capable of doing, in view of the enemy's technological or budgetary constraints. It is important to remember such constraints, which are especially applicable in the case of some of the rogue countries involved nowadays in development or procurement of TBMs. The advantage of this approach is that it enables study of the implications at an early stage and provides timely insight into the problems. Solution of the new problems will be easier and quicker once the decision is made to come up with effective answers, or counter-counter-measures.

2) The second approach advocates concentration of efforts to solving of specific challenges only when there are indications that new techniques, new hardware, or upgrades are being adopted by the enemy. This is a more economical approach but it has two weak points: The first is that there may not be the time to develop counter-counter-measures before the missiles will be used and the second is that the enemy's development effort may not be detected in time.

An early study of most feasible options, and a later, but much more profound, concentration on those devices and methods that the enemy appears to be implementing, seems to be a balanced compromise. Such an approach can yield timely answers for an affordable investment (in terms of both money and skilled personnel).

D. Decoys

Out of the many possible responsive threats, decoys can be taken as an example that illustrates the complexity of the issue and at the same time points out the options

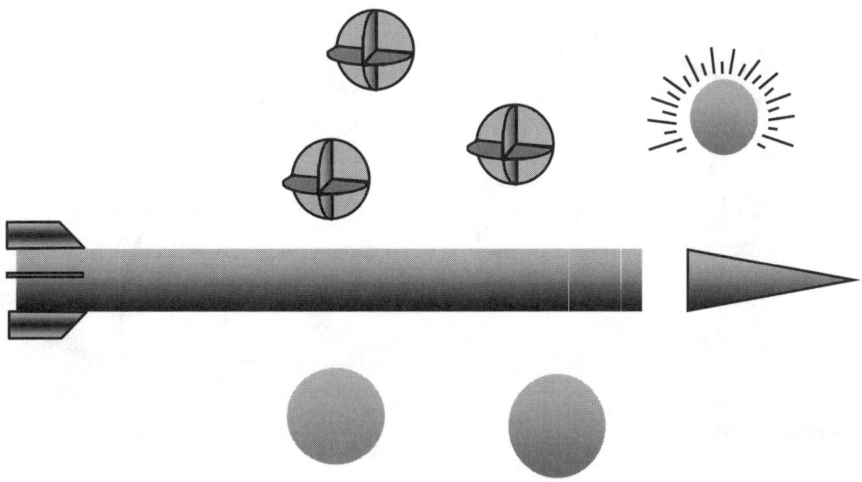

Fig. 5 Some examples of decoy types.

open to the analysts and system engineers in mapping the threat and producing satisfactory answers.

Figure 5 includes three types of decoys. The empty motor casing can be looked upon as an additional pseudo-decoy. The three identical objects above the missile represent corner reflectors made of metal-coated fabric supported by a flexible frame. These lightweight decoys remain folded inside the TBM until ejection and expand to their shown shape after ejection. Their size is determined by the wavelength of the radars they are required to deceive. Their radar cross section (RCS) should approximate the RCS of the conical RV shown on the right.

The two identical objects below the missile represent inflated, metal-coated balloons. Inflation takes place automatically after ejection so that the balloons occupy a minimum volume while inside the TBM The corner reflector and the metal-coated balloons are conceptual RF decoys. The "glowing" balloon above the missile on the right represents a heated, inflated decoy that emits infrared radiation, in addition to its radar reflecting properties. It is supposed to mimic the thermal properties of the RV at high altitude and at the same time serve as a radar decoy.

The empty, burned-out, cylindrical motor casing is not exactly a decoy but is a detectable object that behaves as the RV does at high altitude. It must be identified and eliminated as irrelevant for interception, in itself not a trivial undertaking. This also consumes a certain percentage of the radar resources. In a sense, the motor casing fulfills the task of a decoy in the exoatmospheric part of the trajectory.

Figure 5 illustrates schematically types of decoys that are feasible and relatively simple to implement. They need not necessarily all be used simultaneously. Nor does the figure indicate the optimal number of decoys any TBM should carry.

Such decoys, although relatively simple, necessitate engineering and technical solutions for a smooth, timely, and successful ejection and inflation, as well as for their packaging inside the TBM. Ejection velocity must also be closely controlled for successful deception. It must be high enough to let them appear as distinct targets at a relatively early stage along the trajectory. On the other hand, if their lateral velocity will be too high, most of them will have a trajectory that, when

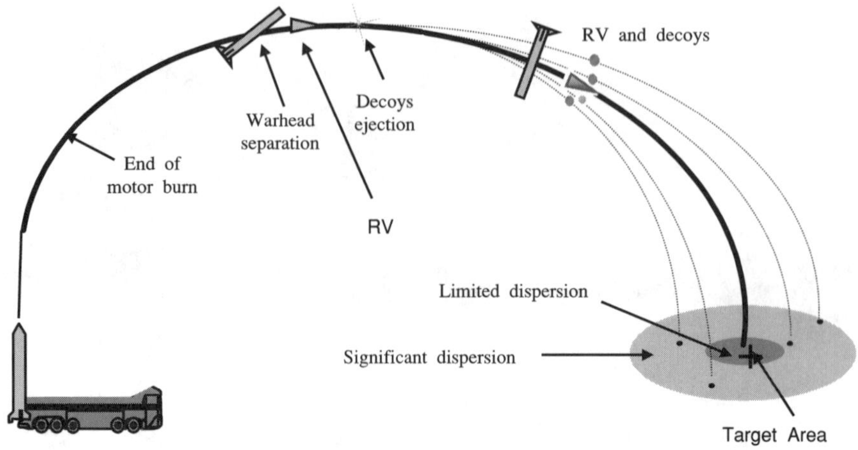

Fig. 6 Decoy ejection and trajectories.

extrapolated, will hit the ground far away from any identifiable target. Even if such a decoy is mistakenly identified as a real TBM, its trajectory will not justify an interception and thus it will not fulfill its role in the best possible manner.

The expected sky-view and a model of the various stages, or events, along the trajectory are illustrated in Fig. 6.

All decoys discussed here are light relative to their surface area, or in professional terms, they have a low ballistic coefficient, and therefore, compared with the real RV, they will be slowed down when they hit the upper layers of the atmosphere. Atmospheric discrimination will start at a certain altitude and thus identification of the real target will be possible below this point. In fact many of these decoys, for most practical purposes, will never reach the ground.

More sophisticated and exotic methods can be worked out for decoy discrimination, but it is also true that more sophisticated decoys can be developed and produced. The subject becomes a matter of a war of minds between the TBM operator and the defender (and their technical establishments), as in many other fields such as ECM/ECCM (electronic counter-counter measures). This is the point where intelligence and threat assessment and forecast come into the picture. Early detection of activities connected to counter-measure development, and the assessed nature of such counter measures, is part of the threat assessment that should serve as a trigger for system developers. Timely acquaintance with such counter measures is a precondition for defense systems upgrade, introduction of additional means that cannot easily be fooled, and development of modified procedures and algorithms that mitigate the problem. Optimization of interception height, and adjustment of other rules of engagement, such as number and preferred type of interceptors allocated for the task, in the new anticipated environment, are examples of only two possible answers to the decoys discussed.

E. Summary

Analysis of the preceding issues and study of their implications will contribute to formulation of the basic questions that must be asked and used as guidelines for prioritization of threat assessment topics. It should be noted that the required effort associated with responsive threat analysis has a significant technical component, but other aspects also play a key role. For example time of decoy introduction, rate of decoy introduction, mode of employment, other expected simultaneous activities, or means activated during employment of such decoys, etc.

VI. Threat Analysis for TBM Defense During Reentry

There are differences between the threat descriptions needed for interception in boost or ascent phase, midcourse interception, and interception in the terminal reentry phase. Midcourse interception is a very demanding task, the relevance of which to theater missile defense is questionable. It will not be discussed further here.

In reentry phase interceptions, two major points dominate the threat assessment:

1) The attacked target, on the ground, lies at the focal point of all defensive activities. In other words, if the target is hit the attack has succeeded, but if it is missed the attack has failed.

2) Successful defense depends on destruction of the TBM warhead only. The warhead is a small object that might appear on a cluttered background. It must be identified in time, engaged, and hit with adequate energy to ensure its destruction.

The relevant questions that derive from these two points include, among others, the following:

1) How many TBMs can reach the target and how many are assumed to do so within a given period of time (days, weeks)? That is, how many launchers are within range and how many TBMs is the enemy likely to allocate to the target?

2) From which TBM launch sites are the TBMs assumed to be launched, and how are these sites dispersed geographically?

3) What is the typical, or anticipated, launch distribution of the TBMs along the time axis, and what can be considered a "saturation" salvo profile?

4) What is the representative trajectory of each TBM type, and what is the velocity profile of the TBM along this trajectory?

5) What is a typical sky-view, TBMs and accompanying objects included, during TBM strikes, as seen from the target and its vicinity and by the detection and tracking sensors?

6) What are the typical signatures (radar, optical, thermal) of the reentering TBMs ?

7) What possible types of warheads could be carried by the various TBMs and what are their characteristics (high explosive, chemical, cluster)? In the case of cluster warheads, what is the dispensing altitude of the bomblets?

8) What is the structure of the warheads? What is the thickness of the structural material(s)?

9) What are the expected penetration aids and penetration enhancing tactics employed with the various TBMs?

It is quite obvious that a great deal of technical data and technical analysis are required to produce the answers to all of these questions. These data include TBM propulsion, weight, dimensions and shape (for aerodynamic coefficients evaluation), guidance systems and navigation accuracy, TBM stabilization, TBM staging data, etc. Regarding TBM salvos and concurrent reentries, distinction must be made between two important questions: 1) How many are aimed at any specific target, at any specific time? 2) How many TBMs take part in more or less simultaneous attacks against all targets in the whole country?

The answers to all of these questions are essential for defense strategy development and optimization of defense assets allocation under various possible conditions. They serve simulations and operations research studies in the development phase, and they are also inputs to both the operational and system engineering decision making processes. The interaction of intelligence producers and consumers results in a bidirectional flow of data and in views and observations that assist intelligence analysts no less than they assist the intelligence consumers.

Penetration aids, as implied by the name, are relevant to reentry-phase threat analysis and not to boost-phase threat analysis, which is discussed in Section VII.

Unfortunately, most assessments cannot be put to the test in peacetime, since no TBM salvos are fired, except in war. Good intelligence and analysis of isolated events in peacetime can produce partial answers to important issues or full answers to a limited set of questions. It is possible, in principle, to draw conclusions from massive TBM attacks by the enemy against another adversary, if such events take place and only if reliable data become available. Therefore, assessments will always, or in most cases, be fraught with uncertainty. The situation is even more severe regarding assessments concerned with boost-phase data.

One of the big advantages of terminal antitheater ballistic missile (ATBM) defense is that the defender does not have to disperse his defense assets all over the theater. He can keep them relatively close to the defended targets (to the extent made possible by footprint constraints) and expect the TBMs to come to him. In this respect his position is much more favorable than the position of a pilot engaged in strikes against TBM launchers, where *detection* and *identification* of the launcher is one of the main obstacles on the way to success. Target (launched TBM and/or the launcher itself) detection difficulty during TBM boost, or immediately after boost, is halfway between the two. The a priori intelligence needed for this type of ATBM activity is therefore different.

VII. Threat Analysis for Boost-Phase Interception

In boost-phase interception (BPI) or postboost TBM launcher strike, the focal point of all activities is around the actively deployed TBM unit and its launchers. Events during TBM reentry, several minutes later, are at best of secondary importance to the BPI setup, and serve mainly for early warning and cueing of terminal defense. For successful BPI, or post-boost launcher strike, many details regarding launcher sites and launcher deployment are needed. These are the main subjects, except technical intelligence, that determine the nature of the information the threat analyst is expected to provide.

A. Intelligence

In the boost phase the TBMs have a prominent and clear signature that cannot be mistaken and is very difficult to miss. Even in cloudy weather the TBM will break cloud ceiling at a relatively early point in its boosted trajectory. Exact figures depend on the type of TBM and weather conditions in the theater, but in typical conditions 60–80% of the boost will take place above the clouds.

Intelligence is required to obtain the approximate position of the launcher (before launch) accurately enough. This determination ensures that the weapon-carrying platform will be close enough to the TBM launcher at launch time to enable interception of the launched missile in the case of BPI or to strike against the launcher itself in the case of post-boost attack against TBM launchers.

Generally the engagement is between a small number of platforms, patrolling a specific area, and a TBM unit of several launchers deployed to that area. The complete ORBAT of the enemy's TBM forces does not play a role in the operational concept that governs the expected BPI engagement. The enemy's overall launcher ORBAT is an important factor in the sizing of the total defense system (number of platforms and kill weapons).

However, many questions must be answered in detail on the deployment of a specific TBM firing unit. These include the following:

1) What is the distance between adjacent launchers?

2) What is the typical number of launches in a salvo fired by a single unit?

3) What are the conceivable maximum and minimum intervals between first and last launch from a single unit?

4) How many launchers form a single firing unit?

5) What is the typical or minimum time that elapses from launch until the launcher vacates the launch site?

The responsive threat analysis with regard to BPI also addresses different questions than the ones asked in terminal defense. Decoys, for example, are a legitimate and valid topic, but in this case the decoy touches on different items. The TBM itself is very difficult to mimic in the boost phase, but camouflage, concealment, and deception can be applied easily to provide protection for the launchers, so these subjects are part of the responsive threat analysis.

B. Location and Mobility

Mobility of the launchers is a central issue together with the analysis of the topography and terrain properties that are a normal part of ground force intelligence analysis.

Potential threats to airborne platforms, manned or unmanned, become a main subject in responsive threat analysis. The subjects for study include: SAMs, interceptor aircraft, their technical performance and limitations, surveillance and tracking sensors, interceptor missiles, deployment of SAMs, and antiaircraft artillery (AAA) for TBM unit protection, defense doctrines, mobility of the protecting units, command and control practices and effectiveness, and many other similar questions. All of these can influence BPI tactics or attack tactics against TBM launchers detected as a result of the missiles they launched.

Because, as mentioned, the ability to locate the deployment of the single firing unit (battery, battalion, brigade) is a vital factor in the success of the defense system, TBM unit deployment practices are a major threat assessment issue. As evidenced in the 1991 Persian Gulf War, launcher survivability decrees that such a unit change position after each launch and redeploy to a new site within a fairly large area that serves it as a habitat within range from potential targets. The exact location of the launchers is normally not known but approximate area, or an "area of uncertainty," within which the unit can be expected to be when it next launches, can be designated. This area of uncertainty must be reassessed repeatedly after each engagement, and appropriate methods and procedures must be developed by the analysts to do so. The basic idea is depicted in Fig. 7.

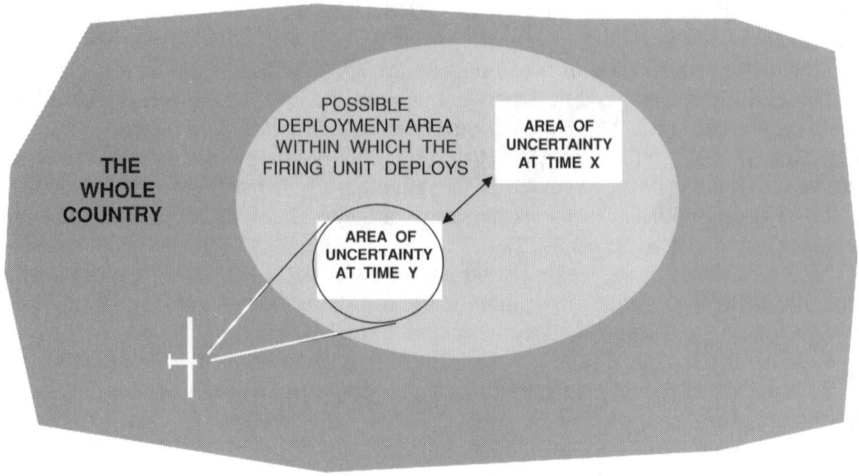

Fig. 7 Area of uncertainty.

C. Area of Uncertainty

The possible deployment area that serves a specific unit may contain more than one potential area of uncertainty, but only one area is occupied at a specific point in time until the unit deploys to another one. The uncertainty derives from the lack of accurate and comprehensive information available to the threat analyst. It is clear that the aim of the threat analyst is to reduce the area of uncertainty to the minimum possible dimensions. The allowed upper limit will be determined by the performance of the weapon and the reaction time of the patrolling air vehicles.

Assessment of the location and the dimensions of the uncertainty area, at any point in time, is a never ending and demanding task with which the analysts will be preoccupied throughout the conflict. A sound assumption regarding the dimensions and possible shapes of the area of uncertainty is a central element in the threat assessment, essential for the definition of the concept of operations of the defense system. Whenever TBMs are fired and detected the area of uncertainty is reduced (nominally) to zero since the exact location (theoretically) can be estimated within fairly accurate limits. However, from immediately after launch the area of uncertainty grows as a function of time. It reaches its maximum size just before the next TBM launch.

There is a functional relationship between the estimated size of the uncertainty area and the probability that the assessment is correct. The smaller the area the lower the probability, as shown in Fig. 8. The transition time between the curves in Fig. 8 is not dependent on the enemy only. It can be influenced to some extent by means of the activity of own forces in the area in suppressing the enemy and limiting his freedom of movement.

D. Other Factors

The subject will not be elaborated further, but this is the appropriate place to mention that intelligence–operations cooperation must not be characterized by

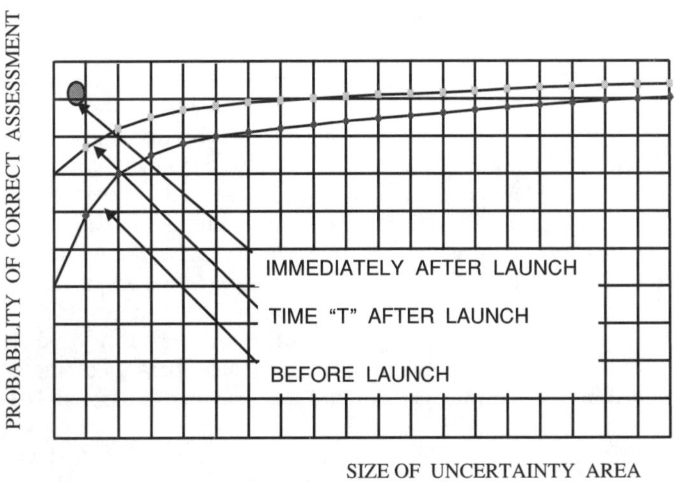

Fig. 8 Probability of correct uncertainty area assessment.

a unidirectional flow of data and services. In this example the direction can be reversed, by means of counter-force activities to limit the freedom of movement of enemy TBM units and thus enable a more accurate estimate of the area of uncertainty. Cultivation of such a relationship should be considered an additional task of the intelligence functions.

As the war progresses and TBM launchers are destroyed, another question comes up. Will the enemy merge depleted units and keep a reasonable number of launchers in a smaller number of full-strength units, or will depleted units continue to operate independently below full strength? The question is a difficult one to answer (as it depends on many factors) but it is an important one because the number of launch units (i.e., the number of areas of uncertainty) is more important than the number of launchers, in determining the concept of operations of the defense system.

VIII. Typical Mistakes and Assessment Errors

The main source for errors is the incompleteness and imperfection of the data on which threat assessments are based. This is the nature of intelligence work and it results because operational decisions usually must be taken before adequate, reliable and verified data is available. The obvious answers to this problem are 1) to enrich the variety and quality of intelligence sources, 2) to speed up the processing and improve the "quality control" in the intelligence production loop, and 3) to clarify to the commanders which parts of the assessment rely on solid data and which are derived from assumptions and guesstimates.

A common mistake made by analysts dealing with TBMD is that assessments and operational planning neglect the fact that TBMs are launched within the context of a war in which other military activities also take place. This might lead to wrong assumptions such as that all available air defense assets are dedicated to defense of TBMs only, that TBMs can move freely at all times, that the full industrial potential of the TBM operator can concentrate on crash program modifications of TBM-related equipment within days, that lessons regarding performance of TBMs can be learned and conclusions implemented within hours, and many similar assumptions that might be far from true.

For instance, one question is the TBM operator's capability to implement responsive threats *during* the course of a war. A simple study of lessons that can be learned about defense systems indicates that reliable and valuable conclusions cannot be reached within days and perhaps not even weeks unless special equipment, personnel, and procedures are established and practiced before the war. Orderly data regarding engagement of TBMs by defense systems can be collected mainly when single, or very few, missiles are launched in a specific time frame. Such data are not indicative of expected events and systems performance in a multiple TBM salvo. Collection of data and correct association of the various events in a crowded sky is a difficult and time consuming process that will probably yield results relevant only to a future war. Consequently, technical and operational implementation of the conclusions, in wartime, is a difficult exercise that will probably last till the end of the conflict, and much beyond.

It is important to highlight those changes that can be identified as important during the hostilities, and can be implemented within a short time, but at the same time one must be very careful not to attribute to the enemy capabilities that cannot be attained. Many scenarios can be run during TBMD system development and testing, and they can cover a wide variety of possible envisaged developments, but their number is finite and, probably, none of them truthfully duplicate the real battle. It is important to remember that the simulated scenarios are only representative of real life and that deviations from simulated battles are both possible and expected. Excursions from the nominal sequence of events and envisaged scripts are mandatory for sensitivity studies. The logical boundaries of such excursions must be carefully evaluated so that sensitivity beyond reasonable limits is not affected.

The uncertain nature of threat assessments makes it difficult to phrase them in terms that are unambiguous. If they are unambiguous, they might easily be interpreted as final verdicts that do not require a periodic revisit. Many intelligence consumers, who are not very experienced in interaction with intelligence analysts, might be misled easily by too specific and wrong interpretations, which results in hasty or wrong conclusions.

Threat assessment concerned with TBM defense is even more sensitive to this type of error since the discipline is new and there is little experience on which to base criticism of assessments or demands for clarifications whenever statements and recommendations do not conform with intuition.

Chapter 5

Defense Policies and Strategies

Ben-Zion Naveh*
WALES Ltd., Ramat-Gan, Israel

I. Introduction

AT THE beginning of the new millennium it is evident that a workable technical and operational answer must be found to the general problem of the ballistic missile threat. Ballistic missiles pose varied levels of threat to different targets, depending on the nature of the target and the type of warhead employed. Targets can be population centers, pure military targets of all types, transportation nodes, and various economic and infrastructure assets. Missile warheads can be conventional, chemical, biological, and even nuclear, and constructed as unitary, clustered, or even multiple independently targeted reentry vehicles (MIRVs). When designing a national defense architecture, all of the aforementioned points, including matches between various threats and their potential targets, must be considered. This process is to maximize the efficiency of the defense, minimize costs, and limit damage in case of a "leaker"—a missile that for one reason or another managed to penetrate through the different defense systems. In this chapter some of these considerations will be discussed. The focus of this discussion will be on defense against ballistic missiles, although some of the points pertaining to ballistic missile defense (BMD) may be relevant also to antiaircraft air defense, defense against cruise missiles, or other means of delivery that may pose similar threats. However, a discussion of defense against cruise missiles, for example, rates an extensive treatment in itself and should be the subject of another volume.

The different defense layers and the various options of handling the threat at each layer will be reviewed in this chapter. These technical and operational solutions are different for each defense layer, therefore policies for combinations of solutions are needed. One question however will remain: How effective can the proposed protection be, and what will be its cost for any level of protection? In other words, how to optimize the defense system architectures. Then, when the structure of a

Copyright © 2000 by the American Institute of Aeronautics and Astronautics, Inc. All rights reserved.

*Special Consultant and Chief Systems Architect. Senior Member AIAA.

proposed architecture is fixed, there will be more questions:

1) What will be the rules of engagements?
2) How robust is the architecture?
3) To what extent is it flexible?
4) What are the system's readiness requirements?

Later in the book these problems will be viewed from their operational and technical aspects, considering the range and accuracy (circular error probable) of the various extant ballistic missiles, rate of fire, and directions of incoming ballistic missiles. Also to be discussed is the reaction time of the various components of the ballistic missile defense system, system's reliability and sensitivity to component outages, requirements for redundancy and resupply, costs, and time to field. In the following chapters, analytical tools will be offered to the architecture planner to measure some of these properties.

One should realize, however, that even if a total, single valued, solution to such problems is not available, any improvement in the quality of any parts of the solution will materially reduce the threat's effect.

II. Operational Needs

The threats and their levels were previously defined, in Chapter 3. We will now define the underlying operational principles (antimissile warfare doctrine) that are essential to successfully counter the threat. It should be made clear from the outset that a total, hermetically sealed counter is not possible because of technical, operational, and probably economic reasons. So the question really is one of priorities so as to minimize damages.

For ballistic missiles carrying nonconventional warheads, the requirement is very simple: no penetration to the protected area from any direction at any time. The defense against such a threat has an absolute priority, even at the expense of other war-fighting missions. The cost of this task is also of a lesser importance. The main problem is that there is no way to predict (with 100% assurance) which missile is equipped with a nonconventional warhead. This will require the decision maker to err on the side of overcaution, with all the attendant problems involved.

For ballistic missiles carrying conventional warheads capable of causing limited damage, the basic requirement is to minimize the damages on the ground at a minimum cost, but coincident with military, economic, and political considerations. One should keep in mind that because of the limited accuracy of many of the ballistic missiles, in the past they were mostly aimed at civilian populations and intended as a terror weapon and thus as a political tool. Because of slow improvements in technology, this would not necessarily remain so in the future, and ballistic missiles may attain enough accuracy so as to make them militarily significant. In such a case the potential damage to various assets can be evaluated and serve as a criteria for setting of defense priorities, taking into account also war scenarios, ballistic missile data and quantities, geography, and climatic variables. This process is described in detail later in the book.

In our case the operational requirements were already adopted and the development or modification of certain systems to address these requirements was ordered. We will now proceed to examine the various layers of defense to better understand the various possibilities that can serve as the building blocks for any kind of

BMD system that can fulfill the basic requirements for defense at any worldwide location.

III. Deterrence and Retaliation

Deterrence is a significant concept and under certain circumstances can prove its value as the first of the defense layers. It's significance lies in the fact that, for the price of economic resources, and if handled properly, it can prevent actual wars that could prove to be much costlier, both in economic resources and in casualties. Deterrence became prominent during the Cold War when it prevented the outbreak of nuclear war between the Warsaw pact and NATO. However, during the Persian Gulf War of 1991, deterrence did not succeed in preventing conventional ballistic missiles attacks against Saudi Arabia and Israel, and only a full-scale war, and the virtual defeat of the Iraqi Armed Forces, stopped the missile attacks. Arguably, deterrence may have helped to prevent the Iraqi utilization of nonconventional (chemical) warheads.

An important basic premise of deterrence is that both the political will to retaliate and the retaliation itself are credible. Furthermore, it is not enough to (secretly) maintain a credible retaliatory capability. The "other side" has to be aware of this capability and of the political will to use it if necessary. There is another complication in the deterrence/retaliation game of wits. As already stated, the concept of deterrence became prominent and was extensively studied in the context of the Cold War. This was a competition between the two political blocs, but in which the gains and losses in an actual war were measured in similar terms. Furthermore, while the Soviet Union was a tough and dangerous competitor, few would have accused its leadership of rashness or impetuousness. This may not always be the situation in other parts of the world, with current and growing access to long-range missiles and weapons of mass destruction. Consequently deterrence and the usefulness of retaliation as a defense layer may prove difficult to maintain. It would also be very hard to predict their effectiveness in future wars because it may depend on transitory whims of local leaders. Nevertheless they should not be neglected because, as pointed out earlier, their potential to prevent wars from happening makes it an important component in any planning. Arguably this is the most important defense layer against nonconventional threats. However, the reliance on deterrence and retaliation as the sole defense layer is fraught with political and economic difficulties. Consequently, only rich, or desperate nations would choose this route. Other countries, like most of Europe during the Cold War, prefer to rely on superpower support. For other countries the logical outcome of this analysis is to strive to construct additional defense layers, that in their combination might prevent war or minimize damages if it did happen.

IV. Electronic Warfare

While the science fiction literature is full of descriptions of various "force fields" used to protect against all sorts of attacks, or destroy various electronic devices used by the adversary, the reality unfortunately is less promising. An electromagnetic pulse (EMP) conceivably could destroy electronic equipment and by its nature will be effective over wide areas.[1] However, such systems, even if they do exist as weapon systems, have never been used before and their real combat effectiveness is not known. There is another major complication in their possible use for defense. Small-sized EMP generators were tested but their range of operation is limited. An EMP that will be effective over a strategically significant area can be triggered only by a high-altitude nuclear explosion (in itself a dubious proposition), but it will not differentiate between friendly and hostile equipment. Furthermore, as a legacy of the Cold War, most advanced weapon systems are shielded to survive EMP effects, and the principal damage will be to civilian systems. All nonshielded electronics will be affected, probably destroyed. The havoc created in the wake of such an event, including the indirect loss of life, might compare with one resulting from a medium intensity conventionally armed missile attack. Furthermore, such a pulse is in essence very short lived, thus its triggering has to be precisely timed—but at what targets? Because of all of these considerations, EMP in essence is not a credible defensive system. In fact it could be better employed as an offensive one.

Consequently, one has to think about localized and more specific electronic warfare devices, which would be used primarily to jam various electronic equipment of the enemy. Such devices could be employed just before commencement of hostilities or during actual shooting wars, and a few words about them are in order. It is often argued that if we know how to jam an incoming ballistic missile we might as well kill it. There are, however, certain difficulties with this argument. It should be pointed out that today's state-of-the-art in missile defense essentially requires physical contact between the interceptor (or at least parts of it—fragments) and the target to achieve any kind of "hard kill." As the history of many such projects will show, this is a serious technological challenge. Jamming on the other hand is supposed to interfere with internal electronic systems of the attacking weapon. It is thus intended usually to interfere with its launch sequence, divert it from its target, or at best cause it to detonate at less than optimal altitude. All of this could conceivably be achieved even from large distances by some kind of radio frequency (RF) energy. This is called "soft kill." These kinds of electronic warfare solutions do exist for some war scenarios and enemy weapons, although not yet for ballistic missile defense. Thus they should be examined for their potential as part of the defense architectures. Furthermore, even if they would not provide a total solution, by essentially stopping or degrading the performance of the attacking force, they can be of enormous help before and after launch of the ballistic missile attack. Such systems are feasible but a detailed discussion of them is outside the scope of this book.

V. Destruction of Launching Systems

Destruction of launcher systems, if achieved, has many benefits.* For starters, it works against all kinds of missiles, carrying all types of warheads and, especially with the nonconventional warheads, carries this kind of war back to the attacker's territory. This kind of attack can be divided into two types, both with their peculiar political and technological problems. The first one is a preemptive attack, performed before an actual attack by the aggressor. While usually it has a better chance of catching the enemy unprepared, with some or all of his equipment in depots and equipment parks, it still requires extremely accurate and up-to-date intelligence information about the enemy's launcher locations. There is no point

*Because of methodological considerations, in this section we will not discuss ground operations against missile launchers.

after all of performing a preemptive attack and destroying only a small number of the launchers. Furthermore, in an environment where saber rattling is part of the diplomatic culture, such an attack could actually precipitate a war nobody really wanted, and without doubt cause the "defender" to be branded as the aggressor.

Another way to destroy the launchers is to attack them after the start of hostilities. While not burdened by political considerations, such an attack, by definition, will probably come after the first round of missiles was fired from these launchers. This in itself may limit the volume of the attack against the launchers, depending on initial damages to the retaliating force and the requirements of other missions that it will have to perform. There still remains the problem of real-time intelligence data. This concerns a large set of elusive targets that are mobile, simple, and easy to represent by decoys. To do this kind of work the United States has launched R&D programs to come up with a promising unmanned combat air vehicle (UCAV). In some scenarios the targets could still be attacked by manned aircraft. Finally, it is most likely that the enemy is equipped with large numbers of missiles in storage, and unless a very high percentage of the actual launchers were destroyed, these missiles still pose a tangible threat.

During the Gulf War the task of destroying the SCUD launchers was assigned to the allied air fleets but became one of the bigger failures of that war. Part of the failure stems no doubt from the fact that no special equipment or doctrine were developed for such missions. Today's technologies probably will enable us to design such equipment, and with the availability of dedicated equipment the proper doctrine can also be developed. In the future, this subject should be the focus of intensive development that might bring forth such antilauncher systems.

What are the technical obstacles to the design of such systems? 1) The launching sites are far away, in a hostile country, possibly (depending on the region) with other countries (some of them potentially hostile) in the way. 2) The launchers may be exposed for only a short time, on the order of minutes, during actual launch. 3) Launchers are simple and not expensive and it is easy to produce convincing dummy structures. 4) The potentially large number of launchers (and decoys) will require a large number of sorties to accomplish the mission, and a certain percentage of attacks against decoys has to be considered.

No doubt, even with proper equipment and doctrine for this kind of operation, it will not be an easy task. One of the main obstacles will be the necessity of having good, up-to-date intelligence on the location of the launchers. However, a successful campaign against launchers has many advantages and thus it is up to the decision-makers to decide how much should be invested in such a program. The fact that such a system may potentially be a very good answer to all kinds of long-range missiles and warheads may ameliorate the problems of the cost issues involved in such a program.

To sum up, the realization of this defense layer is attractive, but while technologically probably feasible the overall intelligence problem seems today to be one of the major stumbling blocks.

VI. Boost-Phase Interception

Boost-phase interception (BPI) is a generic name given to weapon systems intended to destroy the ascending missile during the first minute or two of its flight. It deals with the destruction of the missile at the time interval between the ignition of its rocket motors and the end of combustion in the motors—the boost phase of the missile. In many ways this defense layer is the most desirable one in which to kill the threat. The advantages of BPI are as follows.

1) At the earliest, the destruction of the missile occurs only after an actual attack was launched. All political constraints are thus removed.

2) The target has a big unmistakable signature and initially its velocity is very low.

3) The target's trajectory is known or predictable.

4) When the missile is destroyed it will probably happen over the aggressor's territory with all the attendant damage involved. This will be more so if nonconventional warheads are involved. Consequently, this type of defense, if credible, has an additional deterrence value.

5) The BPI system will also serve as an early warning system and it will be able to report and classify not-intercepted missiles (leakers), thus alerting and cueing the next defense layer.

A lot of attention has been given to the technical problems of this defense layer. Two different types of systems are known to be considered for this role: 1) Airborne laser systems (ABL), and 2) Airborne boost-phase interceptor (BPI).* An air-to-air missile launched either from an aircraft or from an unmanned air vehicle (UAV).

The ABL system is being developed by the U.S. Air Force, and has passed some feasibility tests. Basically it is an extremely long-range (several hundred kilometers) powerful laser that will track the target and damage and destroy it by its energy. It should be remembered that because of the loads imposed on the ballistic missile during high-speed long-range flight, almost any damage to its structure would result in its destruction somewhere along its trajectory. Furthermore, such ballistic missiles are jam-packed with very large amounts of sensitive fuel and delicate equipment, most of it mission-critical. This again makes the whole ballistic missile very vulnerable to any internal damage by high-energy beams.

There are still doubts whether the ABL system will work, and if it works will it be affordable. To start with, the technology of long-range high-power laser weapons is still being developed. While important advances are being made the likelihood of achieving the necessary long ranges (on the order of 400 km) is questioned by many in the technical community. Basically, this is a question of maintaining the coherence of the beam along variable atmospheric paths. Secondly, the size of the optical system of the laser (needed for the longer ranges) and the weight of the fuel necessary to power the laser require a large air platform, now satisfied only by a Boeing 747 aircraft. This is in itself an expensive platform and of course more than one will be required for any serious combat employment. Finally, at this stage and for the foreseeable future, this will be a manned platform. Combined with the fact that this is a (relatively) slow and cumbersome airplane this poses other problems that will be discussed later. In view of all these considerations the BPI (air-to-air missile concept) system seems to be technologically more mature and considerably less expensive.

---

*Some confusion might be caused by the fact that the concept as a whole, and including the ABL, is called BPI (boost-phase interception) and the air-to-air missile is also called BPI (boost-phase interceptor). Because these are the currently accepted terms we did not want to change them, and presumably with the evolution of the thinking on these systems the terms will later be better defined.

Basically the BPI system is very similar to an air-to-air missile system. It consists of a carrier UAV armed with self-homing missiles that will loiter above or near areas from which long-range missiles might be launched. This concept was looked at by a joint U.S.–Israeli team. While both the technologies of UAVs and of air-to-air missiles are well in hand, there are still many operational and technical questions to be resolved.

1) In the Middle East many of the potential target areas are far from friendly territory or from the sea, where UAVs may cruise without being attacked. This complicates the operational/logistical problem by necessitating long transit times. Furthermore, the route to the loiter area may be over hostile territory and the expected loiter area, by definition, will be over or near hostile territory.

2) The range from the UAV to the ascending missile. This will define the number of required UAVs and their combat loads and endurance.

3) The desirable and achievable performance characteristics of the interceptor missile.

4) Battle survivability of the air platform.

5) The battle management.

6) How to handle surprise attacks?

All of the components of such a system—UAVs, air-to-air missiles, and battle management—are within the state of the art, and except for the rather advanced battle management concept, were already proved in combat or in other operational scenarios. Consequently there is no real question whether such a system is technically feasible. There are two problems however that are really more within the purview of the political decision makers. First, finalizing design and development of the system will be a costly undertaking. Second, in certain countries there will always exist a knotty political/operational problem. The UAV will have to loiter, or even fly to its assigned area, over hostile territories that at best will view its operation with a jaundiced eye and will feel obliged to do something about it. Because the UAV is after all an aircraft, it is conceivable that it could be reached by other aircraft. This problem may not exist or may be of lesser magnitude in other parts of the world, but in the present political constellation in the Middle East it is a problem.

VII. Midcourse Interception

The midcourse segment of the trajectory of a ballistic missile is defined as that part of the flight path that lies above a certain altitude, usually pegged at about 200 km. This altitude is, for all practical purposes, above the atmosphere. With today's technology it is almost impossible to shoot down a ballistic missile in this, exoatmospheric, segment of the flight. Some thought was given to ideas to hit ballistic missiles with high-energy laser beams fired from satellites orbiting in outer space, but these concepts were not developed far enough. Another idea that was explored was the "pebbles" concept. The release of unguided or guided kinetic interceptors from a constellation of satellites. These interceptors will be placed in the way of a coasting missile or warhead and destroy it by impact. This idea too was not pursued into a practical system.

The only system to deal with the midcourse interception is the U.S. Navy's theater-wide tactical ballistic missile defense (NTW-TBMD). This "hit-to-kill" system is based on the standard missile family and is launched from a ship. Such a ship is a very flexible launching platform, being able to easily deploy to various globe wide regions. This geographical flexibility may enable the NTW-TBMD to perform interceptions in the ascent and descent (reentry) phases of the incoming threats.

Currently the development of high-altitude systems intended to hit a ballistic missile just before it reenters the atmosphere is being heavily supported. The other best known system is the THAAD (theater high-altitude air defense) developed by the U.S. Army. The program is faced with several technical challenges because of its high-velocity interception and hit-to-kill mode of destroying the threat. If the development program is brought to a successful conclusion it will add another defense layer, which will be effective against midrange ballistic missiles.

VIII. Reentry Interception

Because of its similarity to the traditional air-defense mission against conventional aircraft, the reentry defense layer got most of the initial attention when thinking turned to the problem of antimissile defense. This was enhanced by the fact that the first antimissile system was the Patriot, originally an antiaircraft air-defense system. Furthermore, compared with other antimissile defense concepts, endoatmospheric interception of ballistic missiles or their warheads seemed to be a relatively simple, straightforward problem, requiring only improvements in performance of existing systems and not a new way of thinking. Such a defense system was to be deployed in a known territory and sit there waiting for the ballistic missiles to come to it. Most such proposed systems are expected to be reasonably priced (including cost of development) and thus affordable by less than major powers. It was also said that such an antimissile system could support the conventional air-defense forces. Although admittedly antimissile systems probably could be successful in this role because of their improved performance, the higher price of the active part of the system, the missiles, will probably militate against such use, except under extreme circumstances.

Currently, the most known reentry-interception system is the Arrow, developed by Israel with the support of the United States. The Arrow system has successfully concluded most of its development tests and is entering the fielding phase. The system is able to engage certain types of ballistic missiles at the initial phase of reentry and if the interception fails still has time to perform a second interception attempt at a lower altitude, the so called shoot-look-shoot mode. At the time of this publication, the Arrow system is the only dedicated weapon system being fielded against tactical ballistic missiles.

After the Persian Gulf War, and as a result of lessons from that war, the Patriot (Pac-2) has undergone an extensive upgrading program, and today it is thought to be able to perform better as a point defense system intended to engage short-range ballistic missiles. We would like to add that a combined system of Arrow and one of the versions of the Patriot (Pac-2 or Pac-3) working together may prove quite successful as an overall integrated air-defense system.

Another system is operated from sea and is based on the U.S. Navy's surface-to-air missiles (SAMs), which comprise the Navy's lower tier. Because of the high mobility and flexibility of ships, this system can be most helpful in defending a country with an approachable shoreline.

All in all it is almost certain that different systems, sometimes operated by various national forces, will have to operate in harmony, and because of the nature of ballistic missile warfare, the pace of such operations will be very brisk. This brings up the problem of interoperability. These issues range from sharing information obtained from different sources or systems to a "division of labor" so to speak, in handling different threats, some of them arriving simultaneously.

There are two problems associated with all reentry-phase defense systems. The first one is one of residual time. At this phase the time for observation and decision-making is very short, increasing workloads and the potential for mistakes by human operators in the loop or less-than-optimal solutions by automated systems. Second, because even a successful interception will be carried out over the defender's territory, all sorts of debris will fall in this area with potential for damage to the defender's assets. This in fact may have happened during the 1991 war when it was claimed that there was extensive damage from debris of the Patriot missiles. This problem will be compounded in the case of a nonconventional warhead, where any less-than-total destruction of the warhead may still cause substantial casualties.

It should be clear that the real success of any of the proposed defense layers and the systems involved in creating them cannot be totally proved, except in real combat. In the meantime, the next best way to test the effectiveness of the system and its architecture is by constant practice, simulation, and the use of analytical tools.

IX. Passive Defense

Unfortunately the expected leakage rate (penetration of warheads that for some reason or other were not destroyed) is not, and probably will never be, zero. Any responsible defense planner has to consider this possibility and employ means to reduce damage and casualties in the case of a successful penetration. During the 1991 Persian Gulf War, the Israeli population was alerted about incoming missiles and most of it was sheltered. The damage caused by the Iraqi missiles was limited mostly to property, and only two deaths can be attributed directly to a missile attack. Much of the population however was in near panic and some died because of it (from heart attacks and mishandling of safety equipment). Obviously the civilian population can be prepared for such an eventuality, both psychologically and physically, by shelters and other emergency measures.

There are now two questions that require an immediate answer. Should the main effort be directed at providing various kinds of protection for the civilian population and the hardening of essential facilities, or should bigger slice of the pie go to weapons for deterrence and active defense systems. This issue is complicated by several factors. First, this is not a purely technical problem but a question of the tradeoffs between resources to be invested in the various methods of defense. Second, nobody can present definite numbers on the efficacy of shelters or interception systems. Whereas the question of shelters against conventional warheads is fairly well understood, there are no data about the success of chemical attacks against urban populations and no hard data at all about protection against biological weapons. Consequently, providing an assumed 100% protection against these threats will be extremely expensive. The same will be true about any kind of protection (even partial) against even a limited nuclear attack, or in bolstering retaliation and active defense to such a level that nonconventional attack will cease to be a viable option for the aggressor. In any case the planner of the total architecture, in conjunction with political decision makers, will have to make these determinations.

X. Defense Strategy

Antimissile defense planning is as yet an unusual, little-practiced, and difficult task. Although operational systems to best take care of the situation are being developed in several countries, as of now, and in the near future, they will provide only partial answers. Therefore, to maximize the return on the investment, one should define a strategy for long-range planning to deal with the problem of an enemy equipped with long-range missiles, possibly armed with WMD warheads. For a small country, such a plan may include the following steps:

1) Analyze the political situation and the potential threats.

2) Define your own assets and the desirable levels of protection.

3) Educate your population to cope with potential threats and with their actual materialization.

4) Analyze the capabilities of potential temporary or permanent allies while considering problems of entanglement with their agendas.

5) Form an alliance or a coalition with other politically acceptable nations that may possess useful components of a defense system.

6) Together with such ally or allies define a deterrence, retaliation, and defense plan.

All of this can be achieved by means of long-range planning but must be subjected to periodic revisions and modifications. This book is meant to educate the reader on such issues based on the Israeli experience and know-how.

XI. Robustness and Flexibility

The only good thing about the enemy's ballistic missiles is that their technical and kinematic characteristics are predictable. Given a certain missile one can find out the spectrum of potential reentry velocities, warhead sizes, and ranges that the missile can attain. On the basis of this information one can design a defense architecture that will be able to handle current and possibly also future threats that might evolve from this system. If the architecture is well-designed in all respects and able to address new threats and new rates of attack, it is considered robust. If only minor changes are needed to upgrade a given defense architecture to meet new threat situations, then it is deemed flexible. The architecture designer should be continuously aware of threat evolution (capabilities and numbers) and of future possible war scenarios, so that the defense architecture can be adjusted (and possibly changes in hardware can be affected) in time to the evolving threat and will not become suddenly obsolete. These issues are discussed in detail in Chapter 14.

Finally, it may happen that in some instances all of the defense layers discussed herein will not be enough to handle potential threats, and other means will be needed to rectify such a situation. Such war scenarios are out of the scope of this book.

Reference

[1]Glasstone, S., and Dolan, P., "The Electromagnetic Pulse and its Effects," *The Effects of Nuclear Weapons*, U.S. Dept. of Defense and U.S. Dept. of Energy, Washington, DC, 1977, Chap. 11.

Chapter 6

Theater Ballistic Missile Defense Architecture Development

Ben-Zion Naveh,* Elie Levy,† and Dror Cohen‡
WALES, Ltd., Ramat-Gan, Israel

I. Introduction

THE tactical ballistic missile defense (TBMD) architecture is defined as the aggregate of all defense systems operationally deployed to meet the ballistic missile threat in a certain country/region, together with their command and control structure, and associated concepts of operations. A TBMD architecture may be composed of one or several types of weapon systems (e.g., higher and lower tier systems, boost-phase interception system), sensors (e.g., forward-deployed radars, early warning satellites), and associated command, control, and communication centers (either distributed at each weapon system location or centralized over the entire architecture). From this definition, it is clear that the qualities of an architecture depend heavily on the qualities of the various systems and sensors of which it is comprised. Our goal in this chapter is to focus on the ways in which these different systems are combined to address a common goal and on the methods to select the proper combination of systems, sensors, and rules of engagement (ROE) to achieve efficient defense. The methods for evaluating specific system qualities and performance are presented and discussed in other chapters of this book. (See, for instance, the chapters dealing with defense process, interoperability, and external cueing.)

Let us, at the outset, attempt to clarify the nature of the problem with which this chapter deals. A defense planner is supposed to construct a TBMD architecture to defend a specific geographical entity (country/region). To achieve this goal, the architecture planner should take into account 1) a statement, by policy makers, of the specific goals to be achieved, 2) intelligence assessments of the threat facing the architecture, 3) several defense systems and sensors, and their associated qualities

---

Copyright © 2000 by the American Institute of Aeronautics and Astronautics, Inc. All rights reserved.

*Special Consultant and Chief Systems Architect. Senior Member AIAA.

†Vice President for Systems Engineering. Member AIAA.

‡President. Member AIAA.

and 4) constraints: budget wise, time wise (e.g., production constraints), available deployment sites, and others.

In the following sections, we will discuss each one of these elements and the possible ways in which it may be expressed and used in defining a TBMD architecture. We will then address, through a simple example, several possible methodologies for building the architecture based on a specific set of data. We will conclude this chapter with a discussion of the ways in which different candidate architectures could be compared and a word on the iterative nature of architecture planning.

II. Defended Assets and Defense Policy

A major factor in the process of constructing an architecture is the definition and selection of assets to be defended. It is one thing to know the enemy's intentions in general and against what targets he is aiming his weapons, but it is another thing to define the type of protection to be given to the different defended assets. Some of these assets are point assets (military targets) and others are large areas (cities); some require more protection and some need less. In the established procedure, each defended asset will be assigned a figure of merit that will define to what level that target is going to be defended against each kind of threat (e.g., conventionally armed TBMs, or TBMs suspected of carrying weapons of mass destruction).

The level of defense required is usually related to the damage level (in its broad definition) and to the risk the defender is ready to accept in various assets. This measure of effectiveness (MOE) is difficult to implement so that usually, in the initial phases of architecture sizing, a fixed leakage rate per asset and type of threat is used as an MOE for testing the compliance of the architecture. Other MOEs could be used later to refine the architecture and enable selection between candidate architectures meeting the basic defense level requirement (robustness, cost effectiveness, etc).

The required defense level per defended asset (DA) and per threat type will later be used to select the ROE of the weapon systems participating in the architecture, and thus, through consideration of the foreseen threat, dictate the architecture sizing. A simple example to illustrate this point is the case of one system defending a single defended asset against a single TBM type. The relationship between the leakage rate and the number of interceptors launched is given by Eq. (1), where we assume a shoot-shoot policy, without kill assessment:

$$\mathrm{LR} = (1 - P_k)^n \tag{1}$$

where P_k is the single-shot-probability of kill ($\mathrm{SSP_k}$) of the interceptor, and n is the number of interceptors launched against each TBM. Thus, if the P_k of the weapon system is known, dictating leakage rate (LR) will in turn dictate n by Eq. (1), and if we anticipate an enemy attack of m TBMs, will dictate a sizing of nm interceptors.

We will now define an example that will be used throughout this chapter to illustrate the process of architecture development and assessment. In our example, country D (for defender) has six assets that it needs to defend, as depicted on a generic map in Fig. 1. The DAs are scattered throughout the country. Some of them are large urban areas (DAs 1, 2, 4) and some are small military bases (DAs 3, 5, 6). The defense goals decided upon by country D are presented in Table 1.

As can be seen in the table, country D's decision makers have opted to favor the defense of population (and possibly infrastructure sites located in cities) over

Table 1 Country D's defense goals

DA	Defense level, DL	Allowed LR (100% − DL)
1	97.5%	2.5%
2, 4	99%	1%
3, 5, 6	85%	15%

defense of its military assets. In the following sections of this chapter, we shall see how the architecture planners of country D may act to achieve these goals.

III. Threat Scenario

The second consideration with regard to the construction of a TBMD architecture concerns the threat and war scenarios. The many facets of the threat were discussed in Chapter 4, and in the real world serve as inputs to the defense weapon system designers. However, the building of a TBMD architecture requires more information, such as 1) the enemy (allies, foreign suppliers, and advisors), 2) the enemy's intentions (political and military considerations), 3) the war's possible duration and launch-time distribution, 4) the enemy's doctrine (preferred targets, capability of saturation attacks), 5) threat size (quantities of TBMs) and warhead types, 6) the enemy's real-time flexibility and potential for responsive threats, and 7) the enemy system's serviceability and attrition due to potential counter-force operations. All of these items, together with the known or estimated technical parameters of the enemy's ballistic missiles serve in building the required defense architecture.

The war's different scenarios have to be examined as early as possible but (for obvious reasons) the real picture is often very much unknown to the decision makers: the old dilemma of the commanders vs the intelligence providers.

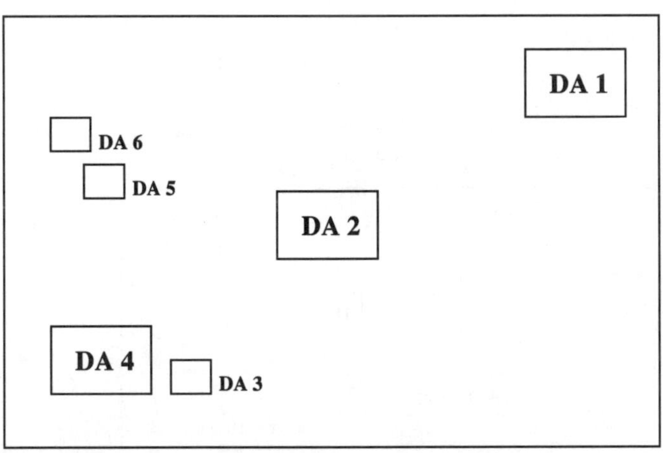

Fig. 1 Country D's defended assets.

A. Approaches to Scenario Definition

Several approaches exist, as to how the threat can be represented, varying in complexity, as well as in their impact on the resulting architecture. Three representative approaches that will be demonstrated in this chapter are as follows.

1) *Definition of a worst-case scenario.* In this approach the most severe intelligence assessment regarding enemy order of battle (ORBAT) is assumed to hold, both in terms of the number of TBMs and that of the launchers available. Because no knowledge of enemy intentions is postulated, each TBM is considered a threat to each DA within its range.

2) *Most probable scenario.* In this approach some knowledge of enemy intentions is postulated, leading to several possible attenuating factors over the worst-case scenario, such as the following: a) Assuming a certain weight assigned to different DAs by the enemy leads to the assumption that not all TBMs capable of reaching a certain asset will be fired on it. b) The enemy is not operating the TBM forces in isolation from the overall war effort. Considerations such as the need to support long-duration hostilities will limit the available number of TBMs for any given salvo. c) If the defender is likely to respond to TBM attacks with counter-force operations, some attrition and suppression of TBM launchers may be assumed.

3) *Creating a family of scenarios.* The process involves using several assumptions to create different scenarios starting from the most severe and making several sets of attenuating assumptions or starting from the most probable scenario and making several sets of either lighter or more severe assumptions. This approach may be implemented manually, creating a small "family" of scenarios, or by computerized models, creating almost an unlimited number of scenarios.

B. Scenario Definition Example

Let us now return to our example of country D, which wishes to defend itself against ballistic missiles. The enemy of country D is country A (attacker), which borders it. Country A possesses two kinds of TBMs: short-range and medium-range (designated, from here on as SR and MR, accordingly), deployed in four launch sites, as depicted in Fig. 2. Each launch site has five launchers, and each

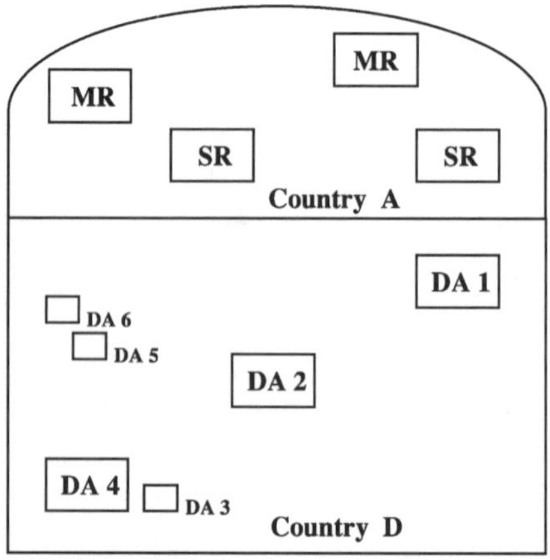

Fig. 2 Country A vs country D.

Table 2 Possible attack scenarios

	Saturation attack	Full attack 1st day	Full attack 2nd day	Total attack
Worst case	20	40	40	80
Most probable (20% attrition)	20	40	32	72
10% attrition	20	40	36	76
5% attrition	20	40	38	78

site is capable of launching no more than twice a day, because of logistic and operational constraints. There is no limit on the number of TBMs of each type.

We will now create the possible scenarios, based on the three approaches to be discussed, assuming a two-day war (which means that country D's policymakers either assume that, in a war of more than two days, they will be able to force country A to cease launching TBMs and have therefore decided to plan a defense architecture for only two days, or that the resources of country D will not permit it to plan an architecture for more than that.)

First, we shall assess the absolute number of TBMs aimed at country D during these two days of war. Because there are four sites with five launchers in each site, the worst-case saturation scenario, where all of them launch simultaneously, is of 20 TBMs. Because each site is capable of launching twice a day, the worst-case scenario is of 40 TBMs in the first day, and 80 TBMs during two days.

For the most-probable scenario we will make an attenuating assumption, which is that because there is a common border between country A and country D, country D's defense forces are able to respond in time against country A's launch sites, inflicting a 20% attrition on the launchers before the second day. The second day attack in this scenario consists, therefore, of only 32 TBMs, and the entire two day scenario consists of 72 TBMs.

The third approach already suggested is to create a family of scenarios to increase the robustness of the architecture developed. We will use the most-probable scenario as a starting point and, as an example, create two more scenarios between it and the worst-case scenario, using again the attrition assumption: 10% and 5% attrition. Table 2 presents all of the attack scenarios generated.

For this example, we have alternated one scenario parameter only. Applying the same process to other parameters, and generating logical combinations of parameters, will lead to a large and diverse set of possible scenarios. (See further discussion of these topics in the chapters dealing with threat assessment and analytical methods and simulations.)

If country D possessed a weapon system that is capable of defending all of the DAs from a single deployment site, this characterization of the threat would suffice to calculate the size of the required defense architecture. Otherwise, we now have to look at the number of TBMs threatening each defended asset on its own.

Because of the relatively short distance between the launch sites and the DAs in our example, no range problems are seen to exist, and each TBM is capable of reaching every DA. In the worst-case scenario, we do not assume anything about country A's intentions and thus we have to contend with the possibility that any one of the DAs will have to withstand the entire 80 TBMs attack. On the most-probable scenario, we assume certain knowledge by country D's intelligence analysts regarding the nature of country A's TBM forces and their

Table 3 TBMs threatening each defended asset

DA	Worst-case saturation	Most-probable saturation	Worst-case total (2 days)	Most-probable total (2 days)
1	20	8	80	29
2, 4	20 (each)	15 (each)	80 (each)	54 (each)
3, 5, 6	20 (each)	10 (each)	80 (each)	36 (each)

intentions as part of the overall war effort. Specifically, we assume that because the medium-range TBMs are inaccurate, they will not be used against the small area military targets. We furthermore assume that country A attaches more importance to DAs 2 and 4 than to DA 1, which is a smaller city, without any large infrastructure facilities. Thus, we assume the enemy will not, under any circumstances, launch more than 40% of its missiles against DA 1 and no more than 75% on DAs 2 and/or 4. Table 3 shows the scenarios resulting from these assumptions. Note that the number of missiles the defense has to counter is much larger than the actual size of the attack, because of the need to defend against all of the possible combinations of TBMs to different targets. The same consideration can be applied to the other two scenarios already defined, with similar results.

IV. Defense System Qualities

Once we know what the defense goals are, and what is the threat to be countered, the next step is understanding the qualities of the weapon systems and sensors available to the architecture planner. From the point of view of the architecture planner, the two most important qualities of the candidate weapon systems are the footprint and the SSP_k.

The footprint of a defense system is the area on the ground into which any TBM launched by the enemy could be countered. There are any number of variants to this definition: the area for which defense is provided against a specific TBM, from a specific launch site, at a given SSP_k, at a given interception altitude, etc. All of these carry different meanings from the point of view of the defense planner. (More information on footprints, how they are calculated and what are their uses, can be found in the chapter dealing with the defense process.)

In case the defense system is capable of shoot-look-shoot (i.e., it has the ability to obtain reliable data on target destruction and thus perform kill assessment), the footprint at the second layer is important. This footprint is calculated taking into account the first layer interception altitude as well as the time required to perform the kill assessment process.

The SSP_k of the defense system is important for determining the number of shots required to achieve a desired defense goal, as is shown in Eq. (1). Usually, this is not a single number but a continuum of different values, depending on such factors as TBM type and interception geometry.

Footprint size and shape, as well as interception geometry parameters that affect the SSP_k, are determined by the combination of a defense system's sensor, launcher, interceptor, and ROE (rules of engagement) parameters, as well as by the direction and type of the incoming threat. Other factors, such as the load-handling capability of the system, also come into play in determining the defense capability. All of these issues are covered extensively in other chapters of this book, and we therefore chose not to discuss them at any length here.

In the field of theater missile defense (TMD), where most systems are still in various stages of development, and where actual testing and combat experience is meager, it is especially hazardous to take measures such as footprint size and SSP_k at face value. These attributes of the weapon systems are mostly estimates, and therefore sensitivity analysis is required to properly define an architecture based on them. Throughout the rest of this section, we shall give an example of one method for dealing with the uncertainty regarding weapon system performance.

Let us continue to develop our ongoing example by introducing the weapon systems on which country D will have to base its architecture. Country D's defense planners have a choice of two weapon systems. The first system, designated system 1, is an area defense (higher tier and large footprint) system. System 1 has a shoot-look-shoot capability with very good (for our purposes, perfect) kill assessment. Each launcher of system 1 carries four missiles. A representative deployment of system 1 is depicted in Fig. 3. In this figure, continuous lines represent first-layer footprint, and broken lines depict the second layer. This deployment allows for defense of all defended assets in one layer, and all except DAs 5 and 6 in two layers, using three deployment sites (batteries). The second system, system 2, has only single-layer defense capability, and a deployment covering all DAs requires four batteries, as shown in Fig. 4. Each launcher of system 2 carries six missiles. The SSP_k of the two defense systems against the different types of threatening TBMs are provided in Table 4. For the sake of simplicity we have assumed that SSP_k is constant throughout the interception envelope of each system, and the same SSP_k holds both in the first and second layers. Notice that the point defense system (system 2) has trouble dealing with the faster, longer range TBMs (MR), and thus has a lower P_k against them. This fact will become significant later on in defining the architecture size required to meet a specific attack scenario.

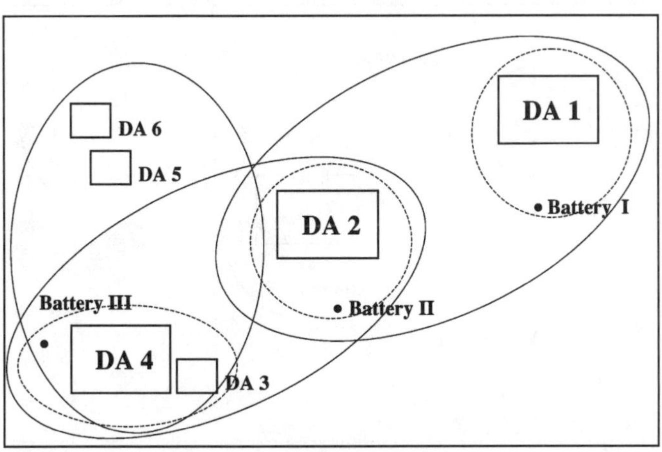

Fig. 3 System 1 deployment.

Table 4 Single shot probability of kill of systems 1 and 2

	TBM	
Defense system	SR	MR
System 1	0.85	0.85
System 2	0.85	0.8

V. Constraints

Defense architectures are defined to meet a certain set of requirements, against a specified threat, and at a given time. However, they are not being planned in empty space. The architecture planners may always expect to encounter constraints imposed by the country's decision makers, and even some technical constraints.

Constraints on architecture planning may take the form of political considerations (the country cannot equip itself with systems manufactured by a certain company/state, a specific ability of one defense system or another violates arms control agreements, etc.), budget considerations (cannot spend more than a certain amount at a given period of time), or even technological and industry considerations (e.g., a specific system will not be available in large quantities at the desired time because of manufacturing capability thresholds).

In our example, country D's budget authorities have declared that the country will not be able to afford more than 200 interceptors of the area defense (system 1) type, and not more than 450 interceptors of the point defense (system 2) type. We shall see at a later stage how these constraints affect the structure of the architecture.

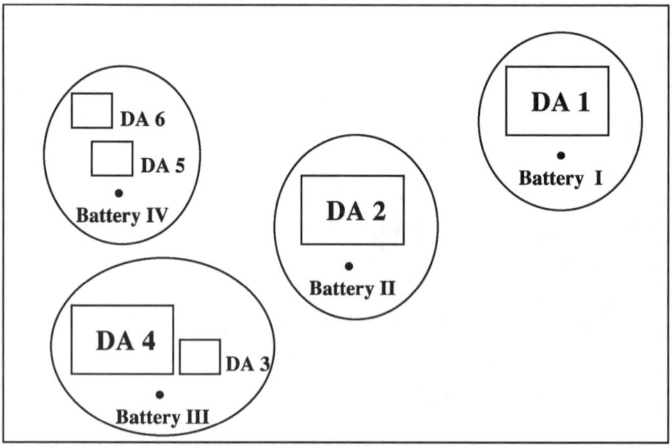

Fig. 4 System 2 deployment.

VI. Constructing the Defense Architectures

We now have at our disposal all of the relevant information required to assess the sizing of the defense architecture and to compare between several architecture options. The first step we will take is to define single-system architectures, based on systems 1 or 2, and then discuss the issue of combining defense systems.

A. Architectures Based on System 1

Let us start with system 1, the area defense system. The first step in constructing the architecture is to decide upon the ROE for each DA against each threat. From Tables 1 and 4, we can see that a ROE of one interceptor per TBM, in a single layer, will suffice to defend DAs 3, 5, and 6 (because the defense level required equals the probability of kill of a single interceptor). DAs 1, 2, and 4 will require a two-layer defense. To calculate the number of interceptors required, we need a formula for the combined probability of kill of a two-layer engagement. Such a formula is given in Eq. (2). (An elaboration of the kill assessment mechanism and its implications can be found in Chapter 7 dealing with the defense process.)

$$\text{LR} = (1 - P_{k1})^{n1}(1 - P_{k2})^{n2} \tag{2}$$

If we fire $n1$ interceptors in the first layer, we get a combined LR of $(1 - P_{k1})^{n1}$, where P_{k1} is the SSP_k of each interceptor in layer one. Only those TBMs that survive the first-layer interceptors will be intercepted in the second layer, and thus Eq. (2) may be obtained [we assume absolute accuracy of the kill assessment (KA) process]. In our example, taking the required LR from Table 1, the reader may easily ascertain that a ROE of one interceptor in the first layer and one in the second layer is good enough for defense of DA 1, whereas two interceptors in the second layer are required for defense of DAs 2 and 4. The ROE of system 1 is summarized in Table 5.

Now that we have the basic deployment of defense assets, and the ROEs for the defense of each DA, we may calculate the number of launchers and interceptors required, thus completing the architecture description. We will create two distinct architectures: one designed to counter the worst-case scenario, and one designed against the most-probable scenario. It should also be mentioned, that because system 1 batteries have large overlapping footprint areas, extensive deconfliction capabilities are required to make sure that interceptors are not wasted by double interceptions. This means that a centralized command and control structure will probably be required.

Table 5 System 1 rules of engagement

DA	ROE	LR, %
1	One interceptor in first layer One interceptor in second layer	2.5
2, 4	One interceptor in first layer Two interceptors in second layer	1
3, 5, 6	One interceptor in a single layer	15

1. *System 1 Architecture Against the Worst-Case Scenario*

The first thing we need to do is look at the number of missiles required to counter the saturation part of the scenario. Because the TBMs launched in a saturation attack reach their destination more or less concurrently, no reloading of launchers is possible, and therefore the number of launchers in each battery is dictated by this calculation.

Battery I (see Fig. 3) provides defense to DA 1 in both layers, and may provide defense to DA 2 in the first layer. To do this, it needs 20 interceptors (in the worst case the saturation attack is of 20 TBMs, and each of the two assets defended by Battery I may encounter the entire attack). Battery I also needs to supply second-layer defense to DA 1. If 20 TBMs are launched at DA 1, three of them will leak through the first layer (on average, since the SSP_k is 0.85). The ROE for the defense of DA 1 calls for one interceptor per TBM in the second layer, therefore we need three more interceptors, which brings us to 23 interceptors. Each launcher of system 1 carries four interceptors, thus six launchers are needed in Battery I. Let us skip, for the moment, Battery II, and continue our calculation at Battery III. This battery may supply first-layer defense to DAs 3, 4, 5, and 6 and second-layer defense to DA 3 and 4. Once again, each DA may encounter the full 20 TBM saturation attack; this battery requires 20 interceptors for the first layer. The only asset requiring second-layer defense, in battery III's footprint, is DA 4 (see Table 5). The number of leakers through the first layer to DA 4, if the full attack is aimed at it, is again three. For DA 4 we require two interceptors per TBM in the second layer, this entails a requirement of six additional interceptors, bringing us to 26 interceptors and 7 launchers.

Let us return now to Battery II. This battery provides first-layer defense to DAs 1 and 2. However, both assets are already covered by Battery I, and need not be counted again. The only additional interceptors required at Battery II are those required for second-layer defense of DA 2. Because DA 2 is identical in all parameters to DA 4, this means six interceptors and two launchers. All in all, the architecture we have just defined requires $6 + 7 + 2 = 15$ launchers. To counter the saturation attack we need $23 + 26 + 6 = 55$ interceptors. Because the full worst-case scenario consists of two saturation attacks per day for two days, a total of $55 \times 4 = 220$ interceptors are required. Note that the architecture we just defined is not well balanced, because Battery II has too few assets. For reasons of redundancy, interceptors and launchers might need to be added to Battery II, at an additional cost. Table 6 presents the resulting architecture.

2. *System 1 Architecture Against the Most-Probable Scenario*

In performing the same process already outlined for the most probable scenario, we may see that the size of the saturation attack on DA 1 is 8 TBMs, and on DA 2,

Table 6 System 1 architecture vs worst-case scenario

	No. of interceptors	No. of launchers
Battery I	92	6
Battery II	24	2
Battery III	104	7
Total	220	15

Table 7 System 1 architecture vs most-probable scenario

	No. of interceptors	No. of launchers
Battery I	80	6
Battery II	22	2
Battery III	94	7
Total	196	15

15 TBMs (from Table 3). To counter the saturation attack, we need in Battery I, 20 interceptors for the first layer (the full saturation scenario), plus two interceptors for the second layer, and six launchers. Using the same principles, the reader may easily ascertain that Battery III will require 26 interceptors and 7 launchers, and Battery II will require six interceptors and two launchers, to deal with the saturation scenario. This brings us to a total of 15 launchers and 54 interceptors for the saturation attack, Note that these numbers are hardly different from those of the worst-case scenario, because the overall size of the saturation attack remains the same.

In calculating the total number of interceptors required, we should take into account the 20% attrition expected in this scenario on the second day. For the first day (two attacks) we need 108 interceptors and for the second day we need only 87 interceptors, which brings the total to 195 interceptors. Table 7 presents the resulting architecture. (Note that while the theoretical calculation requires 195 interceptors, having to divide them between the batteries brings us to 196.)

B. Architecture Based on System 2

With the deployment of system 2 from Fig. 4, the defense requirements from Table 1, and system 2 qualities from Table 4, we may now deduce the ROE required for defense by system 2 on each DA. Two points have to be remembered to conduct this calculation. First, we need to acknowledge that, because system 2 defends in a single layer, the number of interceptors required per interception may be calculated directly from Eq. (1). Second, the fact that system 2 SSP_k is different for the short- and medium-range TBMs means that there should be different ROEs for these two cases.

Taking all of these factors into account, we may arrive at the ROE described in Table 8. Each cell in this matrix contains the number of interceptors required under a specific set of circumstances. Note, that the command and control structure of an architecture based on system 2 will be simpler than for system 1, because there are no overlaps between batteries.

1. System 2 Architecture vs Worst-Case Scenario

For calculating the required architecture size, we repeat the process already used for system 1. The saturation scenario has 20 TBMs that may be aimed at DA 1. We have to assume the worst possibility—that all TBMs launched will be of the MR type (in system 2, the ROE against MR requires more interceptors than for SR). Therefore, we need 60 (20×3) interceptors, and 10 launchers (each launcher of system 2 carries six interceptors) at Battery I. The same holds true for Battery II, defending DA 2.

Table 8 Number of interceptors per TBMs required by system 2

DA	SR	MR
1	2	3
2, 4	3	3
3, 5, 6	1	2

Battery III defends DAs 3 and 4. Each of these may be facing the full attack, and thus again we need $20 \times 3 = 60$ interceptors (preparation for the worst case—that all of the TBMs are aimed at DA 4) and 10 launchers. Battery IV defends DAs 5 and 6. Again, we have to assume the worst, i.e., that all of the TBMs threatening DAs 5 and 6 will be of the MR type, and thus require 40 interceptors and seven launchers.

Thus we find that a total of $10+10+10+7 = 37$ launchers and $60+60+60+40 = 220$ interceptors are needed to counter the saturation scenario. The two-day scenario includes 80 TBMs, 40 of which are of the MR type. Therefore, each DA has to be defended against this mixture of TBMs, which brings us to a total of 800 interceptors. The resulting architecture is presented in Table 9.

Notice the marked difference between the size of the architecture required by an area defense system (220 interceptors, 15 launchers) and the size required for a point defense system. This is mostly the result of the overlap between batteries in the area defense system, which allowed us to group together DAs and thus defend against each TBM fewer times (we defend against a TBM in each *distinct* asset that it may threaten). Another factor that affects this difference is the shoot-look-shoot capability of system 1.

2. *System 2 Architecture vs Most-Probable Scenario*

Using the same process for the most probable scenario, some changes are evident. We start again at Battery I. The number of TBMs aimed at DA 1 in the saturation portion of this scenario is eight. To counter them we need 24 interceptors and four launchers. For Battery II the maximum number of TBMs to be countered is 15, requiring 45 interceptors and eight launchers. Battery III defends two assets, one that may encounter up to 15 TBMs, and one that may encounter only 10. Together, they cannot encounter more than the total size of the attack, which is 20 TBMs. The worst possible distribution between these TBMs is 15

Table 9 System 2 architecture vs worst-case scenario

	No. of interceptors	No. of launchers
Battery I	200	10
Battery II	240	10
Battery III	240	10
Battery IV	120	7
Total	800	37

Table 10 System 2 architecture vs most-probable scenario

	No. of interceptors	No. of launchers
Battery I	87	4
Battery II	162	8
Battery III	180	9
Battery IV	36	2
Total	465	23

aimed at DA 4 (each requiring three interceptors) and five SR TBMs aimed at DA 3 (we have assumed in the most probable scenario that only SR missiles will be aimed at point targets). Thus $45 + 5 = 50$ interceptors are required, along with nine launchers.

Battery IV defends DAs 5 and 6, each of which may expect up to 10 SR missiles to arrive. Considering that the saturation attack contains only 10 such missiles, we need to count them only once, giving a total of 10 interceptors and two launchers. Taking once again into account the 20% attrition in the second day, we may arrive at the architecture described in Table 10.

Comparing Tables 9 and 10, one can see a very marked difference, in contrast to the modest difference between Tables 6 and 7. This is because the point defense system is much more sensitive to changes in the inner distribution of the attack salvo, because of its lack of any overlap between batteries.

C. Combined Architectures

Having looked at single-system architectures, we may now examine the possibility of combining the two defense systems in a single architecture. There are a number of obvious benefits to such an architecture in the area of redundancy and flexibility in countering different situations. The resulting architecture will also be less dependent on the performance parameters of any one system (which is of particular importance when we consider, as previously mentioned, that the performance parameters attributed to most TMD systems are doubtful). There are also drawbacks, stemming from the added complexity in defense planning, and in command and control. However, it is the authors' view that given the immense uncertainties involved in TMD, and the wide range of possible threats, multisystem architectures are preferred in order to provide efficient and reliable defense.

The range of possible combinations in creating multisystem architectures is enormous, even in our simple example. Candidate combinations have to be evaluated based on cost-effectiveness principles. We will present two examples to demonstrate the thought processes involved. Our examples will center on the most probable attack scenario.

Let us look at the architecture based on system 1, for the most-probable scenario (Table 7). One point that comes to mind immediately is that we have a full battery (Battery II) that is there only to provide second-layer defense for DA 2. It does not make sense to acquire a full battery of an expensive area defense system for this purpose. Our first example, therefore, calls for replacing Battery II with a system 2 battery.

Let us calculate the number of interceptors and launchers required for this architecture. We assume that the first-layer defense of DA 2 will still be provided (as in the original architecture) by Battery I, which is of the area defense type. This means that we are postulating either a central command and control structure capable of operating two-layer interceptions with two different systems, or a very good coordination ability between these systems. (This issue is covered in more detail in Chapter 8.)

In the saturation scenario, 15 TBMs attack DA 2. As we are unable to determine which type of TBM is attacking DA 2, we will assume they are all MR type TBMs (the worst-case from the point of view of system 2). The ROE against such TBMs [from Table 1 and Eq. (2)] will be one system 1 interceptor in the first layer, and two system 2 interceptors in the second layer. This means that for second-layer defense of DA 2 against the saturation attack, we need six system 2 interceptors (3 out of 15 TBMs leak through the first layer), and one launcher. The full threat to DA 2 in the most-probable scenario consists of two full-saturation attacks followed by a TBM force, weakened by 20% on the second day, requiring a total of 22 interceptors, the same as the number required by Battery II in our original architecture. Clearly, using system 2 together with system 1 in this case brings us to a more cost-effective architecture (replacing expensive area defense interceptors with the same number of point defense interceptors). Of course, the cost of connecting the systems should also be taken into account.

Our second example concentrates on a different possibility. Looking at Figs. 3 and 4, one can see that DA 1 is an isolated target. We may consider defending DA 1 by system 2, thus freeing system 1 to deal with defense of all other assets in a two-battery formation. Let us calculate the number of assets needed in this architecture. For the battery of system 2 defending DA 1, we need 58 interceptors and three launchers (from Table 10, because system 2 has now to counter the full threat to DA 1). For the battery of system 1 defending DA 2, we need $15 + 6 = 21$ interceptors and six launchers for the saturation attack. Looking at the entire scenario, this battery requires 76 interceptors. The third battery is unaffected by these changes and remains the same as in Table 7. Comparing these results to Table 7 we see that by replacing the original Battery I with a point defense battery, we saved 26 interceptors (the original architecture had 102 interceptors in Batteries I and II—80 in Battery I and 22 in Battery II—whereas our new architecture has 76 interceptors at Battery II), and two launchers of the area defense type, at the price of adding 58 interceptors and three launchers of the point defense type. This is a smaller contribution compared with what was achieved in our previous example. The difference stems from the fact that in our first example, we made use of system 1's shoot-look-shoot capability, where in the second example we gave up the option of using it (for DA 1). We will thus, from now on, deal only with the first option already presented as a viable architecture.

D. Constructing Defense Architectures—Summary

Let us summarize the process of constructing a defense architecture as we have defined it up to this point. The process starts with the selection of defended assets and assignment of defense requirements to be met by the architecture (usually in terms of allowed LR over each DA).

Then we consider the threat. An architecture is designed to counter only a specific portion of the possible threat scenario (in our examples we used only two

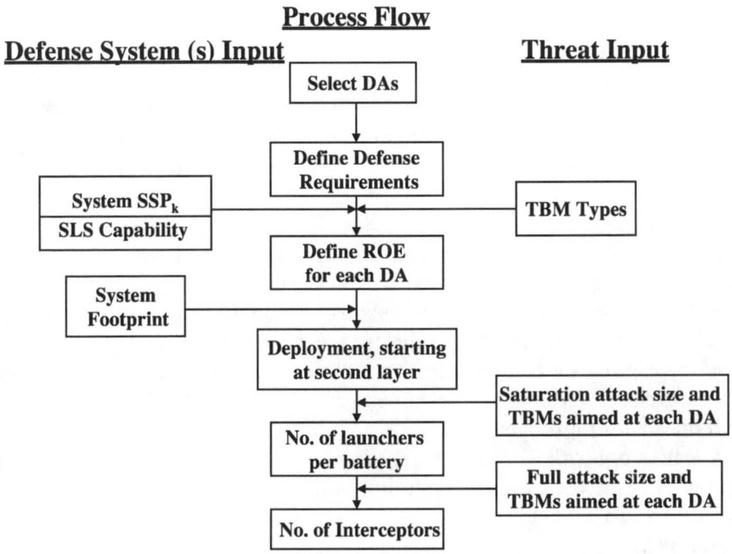

Fig. 5 Architecture definition process.

scenarios). We have seen that there may be a significant difference between the resulting architectures, based on relatively simple assumptions made regarding the threat scenario.

Our next phase is to deploy the defense systems. In the case that the systems have shoot-look-shoot capability, the deployment is mostly affected by the need to cover the DAs for which two tiered defense is required. Then we calculate the size of the architecture. The saturation attack size determines the number of launchers needed at each battery, while the overall number of TBMs threatening each DA, and the mutual backup capabilities, determine the required number of interceptors. The process is described in Fig. 5. In this figure, the main process flow is depicted in the middle column, whereas the inputs to the process are presented on the two sides (defense system parameters are seen on the left side, threat parameters on the right). This is, obviously, a very simplified description. A lot of issues that need to be brought into these calculations, such as the level of connectivity between various defense systems, the existence of external cueing devices, or the actual nature and quality of the defense planning and KA algorithms used, are not included. However, we believe that the figure covers the most important attributes of the architecture definition process. The other issues of concern are dealt with extensively in other chapters of this book.

VII. Comparing Defense Architectures

In the previous section, we presented a number of candidate defense architectures, using different weapon systems and characterizations of the threat. The time has now come for country D's architecture planners to make a choice—which is the best way to defend their country?

To make this choice, one needs to define a measure by which to compare the various optional architectures at hand. In constructing such a measure, the following considerations have to be taken into account:

1) The first thing that differentiates between various architectures is the cost. Obviously, an architecture that achieves the same results at a significantly reduced cost is preferred. Cost, in our view, should be treated as a driving function rather than as a yardstick to measure architectures by. If both architectures compared are feasible in terms of the budget allocation, we must first find out what is the added benefit of one over the other in terms of actual performance, and only then decide whether the difference in performance justifies a specific difference in cost.

2) The performance of an architecture against the threat that it was designed to counter is not an adequate yardstick. Unless we made significant errors in planning the architecture options, they will all perform adequately against the threat scenario around which they were built. The difference in performance ought to be marginal.

3) Also, it must be remembered that the chosen architecture has to meet any attack scenario, and the actual war scenario is bound to be different from the one used in the planning process.

4) Another point that must be kept in mind is the fact mentioned earlier that our knowledge of the defense system's performance parameters is very limited. We would like to have a measure that tests the architecture's dependence on these assumptions.

From the preceding observations, it is clear that what is needed is some process of sensitivity analysis. We will demonstrate one such process, leading to the definition of a measure for comparing architectures that we term the "risk" measure. Other processes can, of course, be defined, but the underlying principles will remain unchanged regardless of the chosen application. Let us first deal with the architecture constraints. Looking at country D's constraints (defined previously in Sec. V), the reader may easily ascertain that the architectures defined to meet the worst-case scenario are unaffordable. Therefore, country D's decision makers have opted to prepare an architecture for defense against the most probable scenario. This leaves us with three architectures, one based on each system and one of a mixed configuration. For convenience, we will term these architectures "area," "point," and "mix." The basic quantities of launchers and interceptors in each architecture are provided in Table 11.

In Sec. III we created two excursions from the most probable scenario, changing one of the basic assumptions—that of the attrition inflicted on country A's launching capability on the second day. These excursions will now be used to define our measure for comparing the architectures. The same sort of treatment may be given to parameters of the weapons systems involved in the architecture. To give an example, we will take a single parameter—SSP_k of the defense system—and create two excursions from this value one being a 20% degradation of P_k from our

Table 11 Architecture options vs most-probable threat

Architecture	System 1 launchers	System 1 interceptors	System 2 launchers	System 2 interceptors
Area	15	196	—	—
Point	—	—	22	436
Mix	13	174	1	22

Table 12 Parameter excursions

Parameters	Most-probable scenario	First excursion	Second excursion
Attrition of launchers at second day	20%	10%	5%
Weapon system SSP_k	System 1: 0.85 System 2: 0.85 SR 0.8 MR	−20%	−30%

original estimated values and the other, a 30% degradation. Table 12 summarizes the excursion cases we have defined.

The excursions in each parameter represent different levels of confidence. The probability that the original value is the one that will materialize during the actual war is deemed the highest, and the probability of occurrence of each excursion is lower as the parameter moves farther from the baseline.

We are now ready to define the "risk" measure. This measure is based on the defense goals defined by country D's policy makers (in Table 1). Clearly, because the architecture planners decided to create architectures for defense against the most-probable scenario, any architecture that fails to achieve these defense goals against the original set of parameter values (for this scenario) is unacceptable from the point of view of the architecture planners. An architecture that succeeds in reaching the goals under the original set of parameters, but fails to do so if one parameter slips only slightly from its intended value (1st excursion), is deemed to present a high "risk," since it fails in relatively high probability cases, and so forth.

Table 13 describes the level of risk attributed to each combination of parameters. The risk of the architecture is determined according to the first set of parameters that cause it to fail in reaching the defense goals. Notice also that we assume that the combination of two parameters deviating from the baseline at the same time is of lower probability than deviation in only one parameter and therefore we assign to the combined excursion a lower risk value.

Based on Table 13, we may now calculate the risk associated with each of our three architectures. To do this, we need to run the attack scenario vs each architecture, at each possible excursion level. However, we still have one more degree of freedom to deal with, and that is the fact that the most-probable scenario defines only the overall number of TBMs launched, but not their distribution between the various DAs. In principle, any such distribution is possible. For our purpose we

Table 13 Risk level per parameter combination

	Parameter 1		
Parameter 2	Baseline	Excursion 1	Excursion 2
Baseline	Unacceptable	High	Medium
Excursion 1	High	Medium	Medium
Excursion 2	Medium	Medium	Low

Table 14 TBMs launched at each defended asset—most-probable scenario

DA	SR	MR
1	—	12
2	—	14
3	10	—
4	1	10
5	12	—
6	13	—
Total	36	36

will define only one such possibility, as presented in Table 14. We assume that the proportion of TBMs launched at each DA remains the same regardless of excursion combination.

As an example, let us look at our point architecture. Looking at Battery IV of this architecture we see that if the SSP_k against SR-type TBMs was lower by 20% (a first excursion), two interceptors per TBMs would be required to reach the desired defense goal. Because such a number of interceptors is not available at Battery IV, it would fail to achieve the desired result. Thus, the point architecture carries a high risk. From similar considerations, as previously presented, the reader may ascertain that the area and mix architectures both carry medium risk. The risk of all candidate architectures is presented in Table 15. Our crude version of the risk measure (we have only used two parameters) cannot differentiate between the area and mix architectures, although it quite clearly favors them over the point architecture. The obvious path for continuation of the analysis is to test more excursion parameters and more values for each parameter. However, there may be cases in which at the end of the process several architectures remain undistinguishable from each other. In such a case, considerations of budget come into play ("mix" is slightly less costly than "area" because it replaces area defense assets with point defense assets). Other, more refined MOEs, measure different attributes of the architectures being compared. For a more systematic discussion of MOEs, the reader is referred to Chapter 14, dealing with analytic methods.

Before we leave the subject of the risk measure, a few words regarding real-life application are needed. The example we gave is, of course, simplistic. No one will compare two architectures based on a single-attack scenario and two parameters in the sensitivity analysis. In a real-life application, computerized models have to be used to keep track of results achieved over a large number of scenarios and excursions from the baseline system parameters. One must also keep in mind that for any

Table 15 Architecture risk level

Architecture	Risk
Area	Medium
Point	High
Mix	Medium

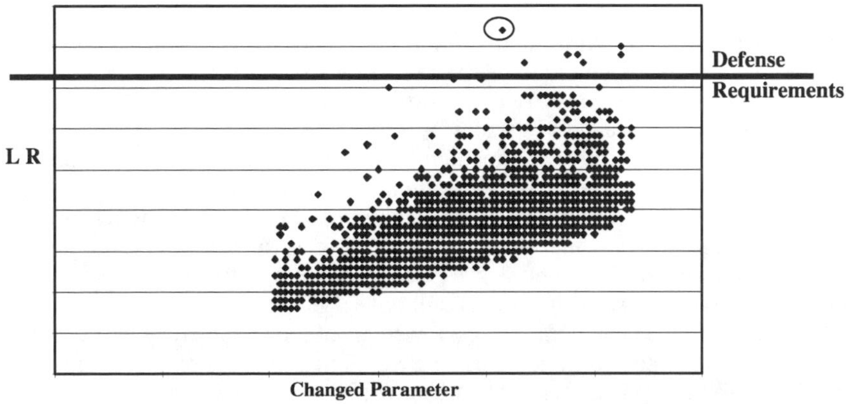

Fig. 6 Risk measure example.

given set of parameter values, a large number of attack scenarios exist. (Think, for example, of how many different attack scenarios we could generate by alternating the distribution of TBMs to DAs, while still maintaining the basic assumptions of the most probable threat.) Out of these myriad scenarios, it is quite probable that a few will include a particular set of circumstances that will cause an architecture to fail, even if it performs well in the majority of cases. Of course, we would like the risk measure to reflect this possibility and not "punish" an architecture for extremely rare failures. To do this, a threshold value must be inserted in the calculation. The measure will allow up to a specified percentage of failures to occur, and will declare that the architecture failed at a certain risk level if the percentage of scenarios for which it does not meet the defense goals is over this threshold.

To clarify these points, let us look at Fig. 6. This figure plots the results of a specific architecture vs 1000 different attack scenarios. The chart was obtained by running a computerized scenario generation tool in conjunction with a simulation of the war. One can see that, as the selected parameter is increased, the LR also increases. There are rare cases (like the one marked with a circle) where the architecture cannot meet the requirements even at lower parameter values. The line across the chart indicates the level of defense requirements. If the number of dots above this line exceeds a predefined threshold, the architecture ceases to be viable at this level and a certain risk is associated with it.

VIII. Iterative Nature of Architecture Development

The process of architecture definition is by nature an iterative one. There are a number of reasons for this, including, among others, the following:

1) The threat is continuously changing. This is true when we look at the threat by itself, but is particularly true when we consider the possible developments following the successful deployment of a TBMD architecture and the fact that the adversary may take steps to negate the usefulness of a given architecture (responsive threat).

2) Defense system development is constantly advancing. As the development progresses, more data are accumulated with regard to the system's performance, and assumptions made at earlier stages may be revisited and changed.

3) In most cases, comparing the defense requirements and available systems to the full spectrum of the threat, both existing and responsive (i.e., which may exist in the future), leaves something to be desired. A full-blown architecture assessment, based on the principles we have demonstrated in this chapter, will almost always wind up with a list of unsolved issues.

There are a number of ways in which limitations found in the architecture can be amended. One of them, maybe the simplest, is to increase the budget and buy more defense assets. Unfortunately, this solution, even if within the resources of the defending country, cannot cope with all of the problems. For example, if a certain defense system cannot deal with long-range TBMs because they are too fast for it, buying more such systems will not solve the problem. A second possibility is to continue developing the core systems of the architecture. The unsolved issues list points the way to a list of "growth paths," which are improvements to the core systems. When these are implemented, the planning process has to be performed again to arrive at the best way of incorporating these new features into the architecture.

Another way to circumvent the limitations found in any architecture is through interoperability with other weapon systems and sensors in the possession of the defending country's allies. This solution is complex to define and implement. The principles underlying it are treated in separate chapters of this book.

IX. Summary

Let us summarize, therefore, the architecture definition and development process described in this chapter. Figure 7 presents the full process. The threat scenarios, defense goals selected, and available systems drive the creation of architecture options, as was shown in Fig. 5. These options are filtered through the various

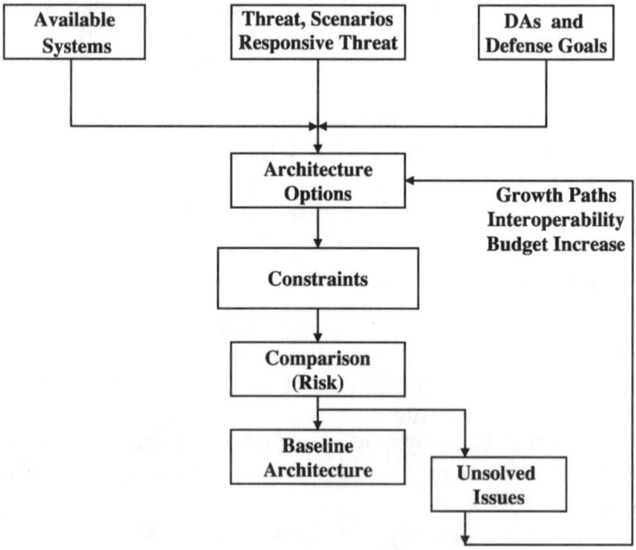

Fig. 7 Architecture development process.

constraints imposed by decision makers, and the remaining options are compared based on selected MOEs. This process leads to the definition of a baseline architecture and a list of unsolved issues that trigger a set of changes in the architecture, and then the process is repeated. We tried, through the use of a simplified example, to describe some of the principles underlying this complex process, and some of the techniques used in its various stages.

This chapter concentrated on the theory and analytical processes of architecture development. We chose to omit any discussion of the technical questions involved in each one of the topics discussed. For a more technical treatment of some of the issues discussed in this chapter, the reader is referred to other chapters in this book, notably, Chapters 4, 7, 8, 9 and 14.

Chapter 7

Antitheater Ballistic Missile Defense Process

Ayala Gur,* Eli Levy,† and Nathan Farber‡
WALES Ltd., Ramat-Gan, Israel

I. Introduction

THE defense against the theater ballistic missile (TBM) threat is a complex undertaking involving a large number of interacting elements, each contributing to the defense process. The defense process starts with the deployment of the defense system and involves several steps. Among them, defining the correct deployment (based on the assessed threat and system performance), continually maintaining the operational availability of the system (both technically and in terms of operator capabilities), using the system in combat and finally (and as necessary) upgrading or replacing it. Various aspects of this process are presented in other chapters in this book.

Because the goal of the defense process is to prevent or neutralize TBM attacks, there are a number of options during the various stages of the TBM attack. Figure 1 illustrates the various stages, which include the following.

1) *Counter-force:* Attacking the TBM development and production infrastructure or the launch facilities, either mobile or in fixed bases.

2) *Active defense:* Attacking the TBMs in flight, during their boost, midcourse, or reentry phases.

3) *Passive defense:* Minimizing damage on the ground, mostly by sheltering people and equipment.

In this chapter we will concentrate on the characteristics of the midcourse/reentry defense option. Boost-phase defense, in which the TBMs are intercepted during motor operation, essentially belongs in the same category.

The main stages of the defense process for a single TBM are shown in Fig. 2. It starts with the detection of a TBM in flight. The TBM is tracked and classified, and a defense plan is generated and executed. The execution of the defense plan may involve launching a number of interceptors and can include target-kill assessment.

Copyright © 2000 by the American Institute of Aeronautics and Astronautics, Inc. All rights reserved.

*Senior Systems Analyst. Member AIAA.
†Vice President for Systems Engineering. Member AIAA.
‡Senior Systems Engineer. Member AIAA.

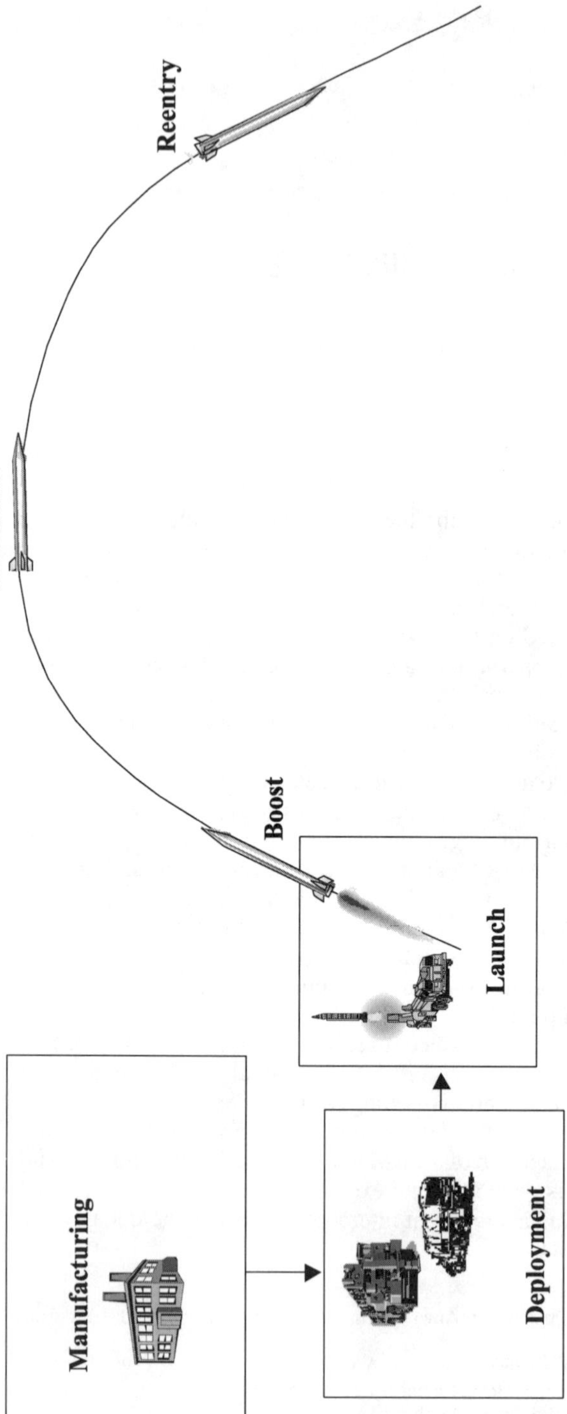

Fig. 1 Possible stages to eliminate TBM attacks.

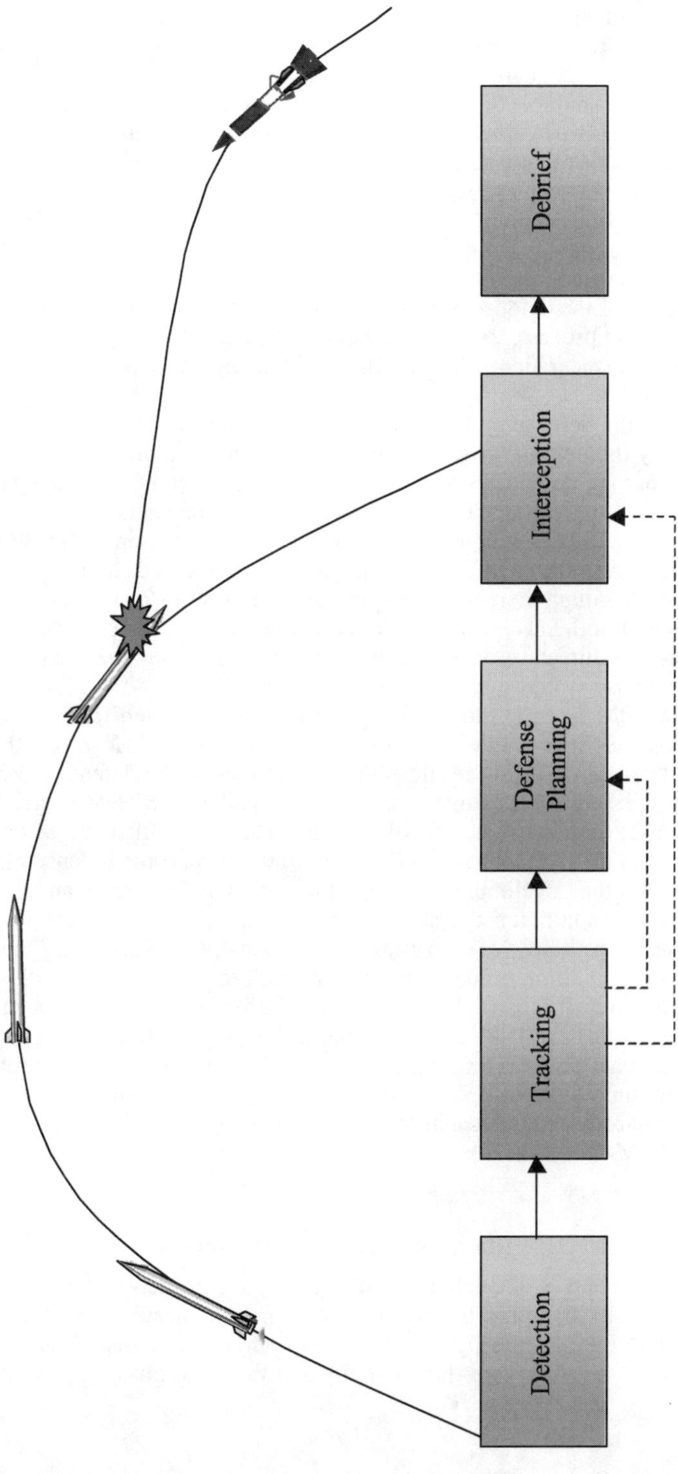

Fig. 2 Defense process stages.

The final stage of the defense process that is included in this chapter is the data gathering and debriefing process necessary to enable improved performance during the next attack and adequate response to enemy actions.

When there are a number of simultaneous attackers, the issue of limited resources and interaction between interceptions complicates the defense process. In this case it is necessary to consider prioritization of threats, resource handling, and interdependence between events.

The purpose of this chapter is to present the basic terminology of TMD as well as provide an overview of the descent phase defense process and "rules of thumb" as to how to determine the main relevant parameters. This chapter will describe the main stages of the defense process, including 1) the impact each stage has on the entire defense process, 2) the contribution of each defense system element to each stage, and 3) the tradeoffs between the various system elements' performance parameters.

In addition, the defense system's measures of performance (MOP), which are determined by the defense process, will be described. The principal MOP per a single TBM are the defender's weapon system footprint and battlespace volume. The MOP for an entire attack is the defense system's total capacity.

This chapter will deal with ground- or sea-based interception systems that use missiles to perform the "kill." Additional systems (air-based, high-energy) will not be assessed, though there are many similar aspects in the management of their operation within a defense system. The issues related to the performance of an entire defense architecture over a long time, which includes the operation of a number of defense systems, are discussed in Chapter 6.

The basic TBM defense process has been basically adopted from air defense against aircraft as many aspects of the threats are similar. However, the specific characteristics of TBMs result in unique features of the defense. TBMs are launched from relatively long distances. Also, the path of the TBM (trajectory) is fully predictable for a long part of its flight—it performs a ballistic trajectory. This feature provides the defense system the opportunity to start the defense planning process early in the development of the attack, though this drives an additional requirement from the defense system, to be able to acquire and track targets at long distances. The TBMs are very fast and physically small, making them difficult targets. In addition, unlike a manned aircraft, the mission of which will be aborted if the aircraft is partially damaged, a TBM will never abort a mission. The defense options available include either destroying the warhead or diverting the TBM's impact point. The first, the so-called hard-kill option, is preferable because it is impossible to predict where a damaged (diverted) TBM will fall. However the hard kill requires a high-energy interception within a small, specific area of the TBM (its warhead).

II. Main Defense System Elements

The main elements of the defense system are 1) search, acquisition, and tracking sensors (SAT), 2) battle management command, control, communications, computers, and intelligence (BMC^4I), and 3) intercept systems. These are presented in Fig. 3 together with their functions in the main phases of the defense process.

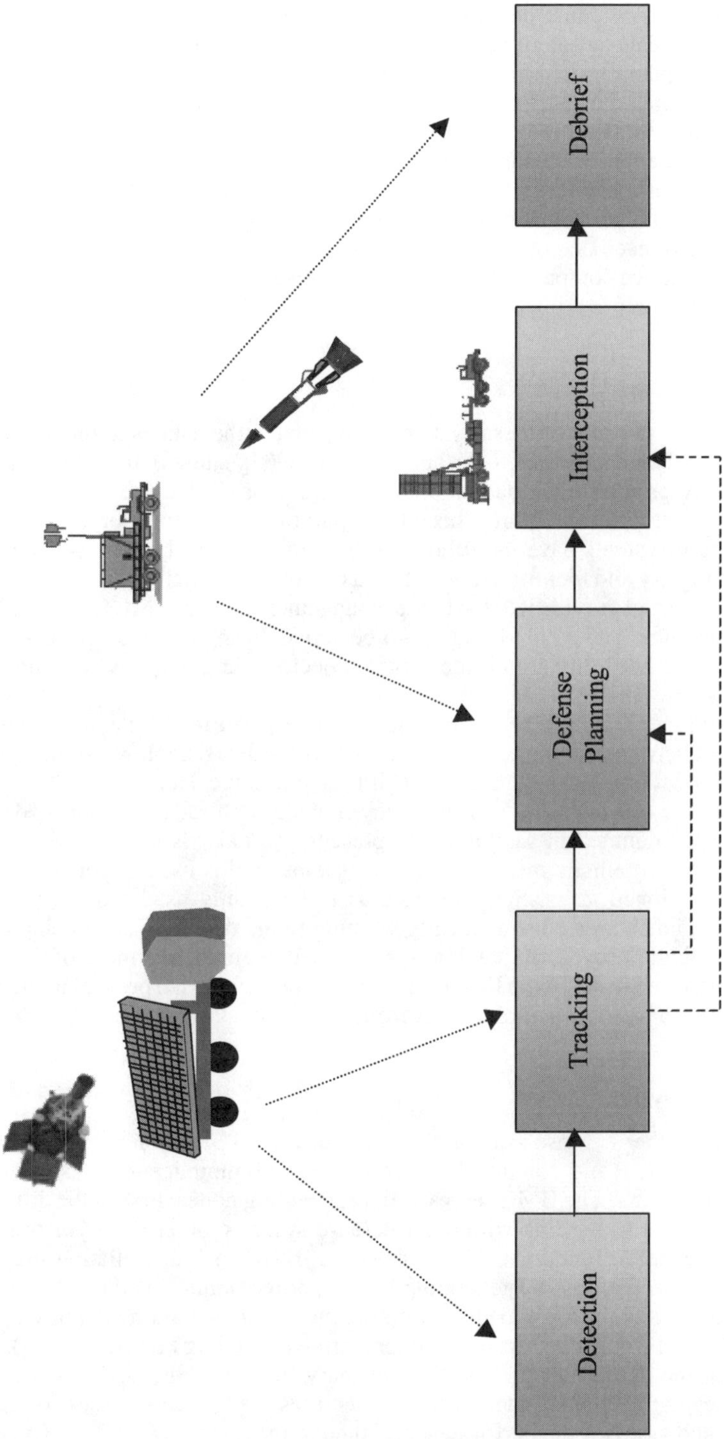

Fig. 3 Defense system elements.

The *SAT systems* must be capable of detecting the TBM threats, identifying the relevant threats out of all detected objects, and providing sufficiently accurate track data for planning and fire control. The *BMC⁴I system* chooses and prioritizes targets, generates defense plans, manages the interception process, handles the interaction between the defense system elements, manages and distributes available resources, and enables human intervention in the defense process. The *intercept system* performs the actual interception of the threat to achieve the desired result of TBM kill. The performance of the entire defense system is determined by the performance of each one of its elements and the interrelations between them. It is possible to achieve comparable results by tradeoffs between the capabilities of the various elements.

A. SAT Systems

The primary mission of these systems is to provide the data as to the existence of a threat, its behavior (trajectory), and appearance (signatures). In addition, these systems may provide track data about the interceptors in those cases where the specific defense system requires this data as part of the guidance logic.

Thus these systems have the following three main tasks: 1) search—to detect objects in the sky and identify relevant threats, 2) track—to generate the necessary trajectory data and provide it to the battle management center (BMC) to be used for defense planning, and 3) fire control—to be active during the interceptor's flight and to process both threat and interceptor trajectory data, required to guide the interceptor.

In a complete architecture these tasks could be performed by a single sensor type or split between a number of different types of sensors, deployed as necessary to fulfill the defense tasks with the capability to exchange data.

Relevant (to our purpose) sensors today include both radar and infrared (IR) sensors (e.g., mounted in satellites). At present, the radar is the main sensor of most antitheater ballistic missile (ATBM) systems, and is used to perform all of the aforementioned tasks. Satellite systems are currently used only to provide continuous launch area coverage, early warning to the defender, and cueing data. As technology improves, the satellite systems will begin to take more of the SAT tasks from the radar. Airborne IR sensors also can be included to provide additional data, mainly for discrimination (target from decoy) and kill assessment.

B. BMC⁴I System

As in any other defense system, the BMC of the ATBM system performs the battle management and command and control and communications tasks within the defense process. The BMC serves as the connecting node between the different elements as well as the link with other defense systems, other deployment sites, and higher echelon functions. The tasks of the BMC include collating the data from the various sensors and generating a sky-picture, monitoring the defense system resources, identifying and characterizing the threat, generating defense plans, monitoring and controlling the actual interception (including kill assessment), and controlling the debriefing process. The primary impact of the BMC is the way it processes the available data, correctly identifies the target, assesses its future behavior, and assesses the performance of the interceptor.

There are several options for the configuration of the BMC and the specific algorithms and functions performed. Chapter 10 presents a detailed analysis of the BMC options and modes of operation.

C. Intercept System

The intercept system includes the interceptors and their launch systems. Its task is to perform the actual kill of the TBM. Current interceptors (in existence and those being developed) are similar to antiaircraft missiles but with unique characteristics in terms of improved lethality against small, hard-to-kill targets, long-range, high-altitude (exoatmospheric) coverage, and rapid response to high-velocity targets.

III. TBM Defense Process and Time Line

As stated before, the main stages of the defense process are search and acquisition, tracking, target identification, defense planning, interception flyout, interception (including kill assessment), and debriefing. The mission for which this process is developed is to provide a given level of defense over a specified territory and/or specified assets. The actual performance of a given defense system is dependent on the performance of each of its elements and on the interaction between them. In this paragraph we will provide an overview of the flow of the defense process. In the following sections we will discuss each phase in detail including the relevant parameters involved, the problems to be solved and the possible tradeoffs between these parameters.

To successfully intercept an approaching TBM, the defense system must be able to accurately send an interceptor to meet that TBM at an appropriate location. This problem needs to be solved by providing the necessary information to the pertinent elements at the appropriate times and correctly processing this information. The technical capabilities of the defense system elements (mainly the radar and interceptor) will determine the battlespace of the defense system: the volume of interception operations with a reasonable level of success against the various threats.

For example, the detection capability and accuracy of the radar (as a function of range) will determine the range at which the TBMs are detected and the achievable track accuracy. The velocity of the interceptor will determine the time required for flyout, and therefore inversely, the time available for tracking. The capability and onboard sensor coverage of the interceptor will determine the required tracking accuracy of the radar (and similarly, radar limitations may drive onboard sensor requirements and maneuverability) at different stages of the flight.

Figure 4 presents the basic time dependence of the interception process. If we look at the defense process "backwards," the desired interception point is determined according to interceptor parameters—the range and altitude at which the interceptor is best capable of killing the TBM. The interception time t_i is determined by the trajectory of the TBM. The first requirement is the fly-out time of the interceptor. This is the time it will take the interceptor to reach the interception point from its launch location. This determines the interceptor launch time t_l and the location of the TBM at this time. The performance parameters of the interceptor (mostly trajectory-correction capability) define the required accuracy of the assessed TBM trajectory and interception point prediction, before launch

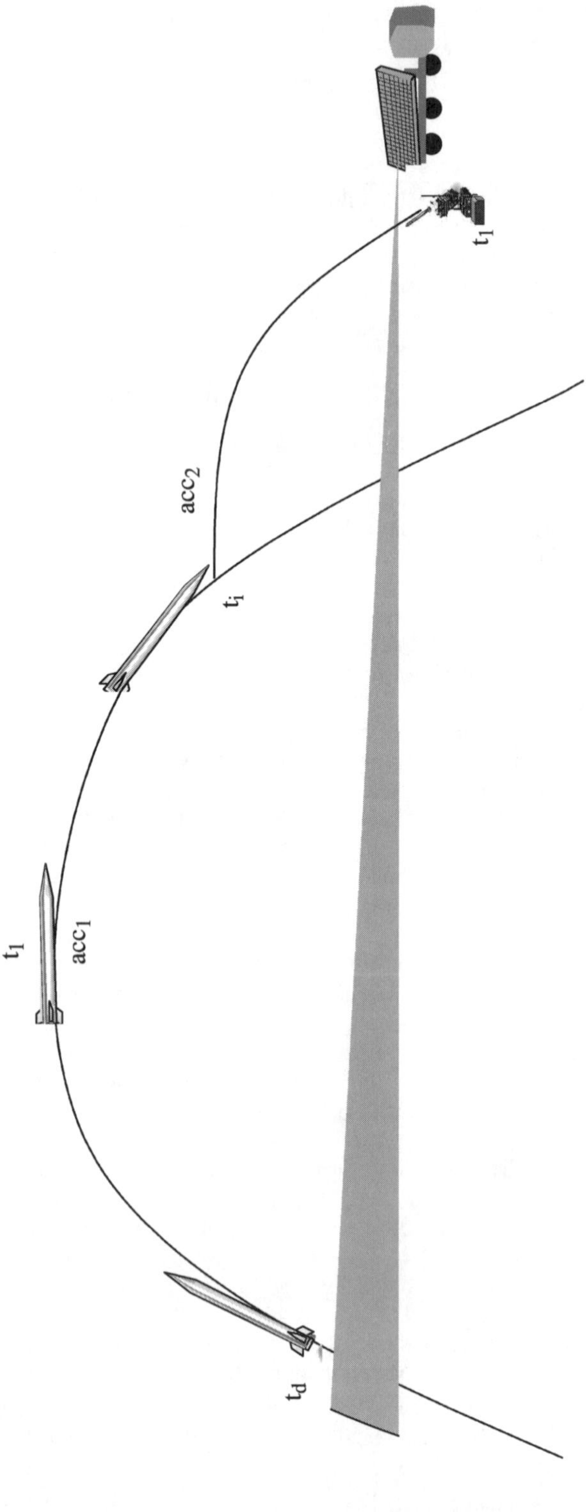

Fig. 4 Basic defense process time line.

Table 1 Results of a numerical example for different range interceptions

	Interception point	
	100 km	150 km
t_i	0	0
t_l	40 s	60 s
TBM's range at interceptor launch	209 km	300 km
TBM tracking time	10 s	15 s
Required TBM detection range	225 km	335 km

t_l and at different stages of the fly-out. The accuracy of the TBM's trajectory prediction is mainly a function of the accuracy of the estimation of the ballistic trajectory (state vector) and available knowledge of the target's performance. In turn this accuracy is a function of the various sensors' capabilities and the quality of data processing at the BMC.

For a given sensor with a certain accuracy as a function of range, the required accuracy of the trajectory's parameters can be achieved either by tracking for a long time or by concentrating the tracking effort for a short time. The required TBM acquisition time t_d (and acquisition range) will determine the required accuracy at various stages of the process, the sensor accuracy as a function of range, and the necessary resources. The detection time and TBM velocity determine the required detection range.

This process is explained in the following numerical example. An interceptor with an average velocity of 2500 m/s is used to intercept a long range TBM. Two interception options, at ranges of 100 and 150 km are compared. The required interception point prediction accuracy is the same in both cases. The TBM's range at the interceptor's launch is greater for the longer-range interception. This results in a higher accuracy requirement (longer extrapolation time of the interception point) and lower sensor accuracy (increased tracking range). To achieve the required accuracy at interceptor launch, it is necessary to track for a longer time. To secure this longer tracking time, detection of the TBM must be achieved at greater ranges. Table 1 illustrates this fact numerically.

It is clear from the previous discussion, that there is a certain amount of tradeoff between the performance of the elements. Up to a certain level, a faster, more maneuverable interceptor can compensate for a less accurate, less powerful radar, or a better radar can compensate for a less agile interceptor.

The defense process presented up to now is very simple. Two additional issues can, however, affect the effectiveness of the defense system. These are the attacker's counter measures and penetration aids (PENAIDS) against the defense system, and the impact of a multi-TBM attack.

Among the attacker's range of responses to the defense system are maneuvering reentry bodies and warheads, electronic counter measures (ECM), and decoys. The defense system has to be capable of handling these additional complications. Specific requirements include advanced data gathering and processing to enable "learning" about the attacker's potential responses. TBM's terminal maneuvering requires improved track accuracy, tracking that identifies and assesses the maneuvers, and/or highly maneuverable interceptors. The decoys' option drives requirements for more detailed processing of the sky-picture, multiple sensor tracking, and data fusion. Additional responses such as ECM and physical attacks against the defense system elements are handled by improved robustness of the defense system elements or defense architecture.

When the issue of multiple TBMs is included in the defense process, additional factors are the problem of radar resources and interceptor interactions. Increasing either the tracking accuracy (or rate) or the detection range requires more radar resources resulting in a limit on the number of TBMs that can be handled. Launch limitations and debris from previous kills can result in interference between one interception and the next in a salvo attack by TBMs. The following section will describe each of the stages of the defense process in detail.

IV. Defense Process Stages

A. Search, Acquisition, and Track

The initial task in the defense process is to identify that a TBM attack is in fact occurring, and then to gather enough data about the incoming threat to plan and execute a suitable defense. This task has two main stages: 1) search and acquisition, the purpose of which is to detect and identify possible attacks as soon as possible, and 2) tracking, the purpose of which is to collect sufficient and accurate data throughout the process, to perform the following defense process tasks and provide early warning to the defender.

The main parameters that affect these stages are the size of the area from which the threat can originate, requirements for data accuracy as a function of time, and the capabilities and available resources of the sensors used for the tasks. If only a single sensor is available, it is necessary to shift the quantity of resources, between the two main tasks, to achieve the required level of performance. If additional sensors are available, it is possible to better optimize the use of the resources by assigning specific tasks per sensor and using the BMC to collate, compare, and fuse the data from the various sources, to provide a complete and accurate sky-picture.

1. Sensor Types

Theoretically, both radar and electro-optical (EO) sensors can perform the aforementioned tasks. At present, in most cases, EO sensors are used only for search and acquisition whereas tracking is performed by radar. The main parameters of the sensors are 1) detection range: the range from the sensor at which the target can be detected with a sufficient probability, 2) detection coverage: the footprint size of the defender's radar at the potential TBM launch area, 3) accuracy: the accuracy in measuring the immediate position and velocity of the target, and 4) resolution: the capability of the sensor to differentiate between close objects.

The main characteristics of each of the sensor types and the considerations to be taken into account in the use of each are presented in the following sections.

a. Electro-optical sensors. The relevant EO sensors are passive detectors based on IR signature. The main characteristics of these sensors are as follows.

1) A passive EO sensor measures angular location only. To calculate the three-dimensional location of the target it is necessary to either make assumptions about

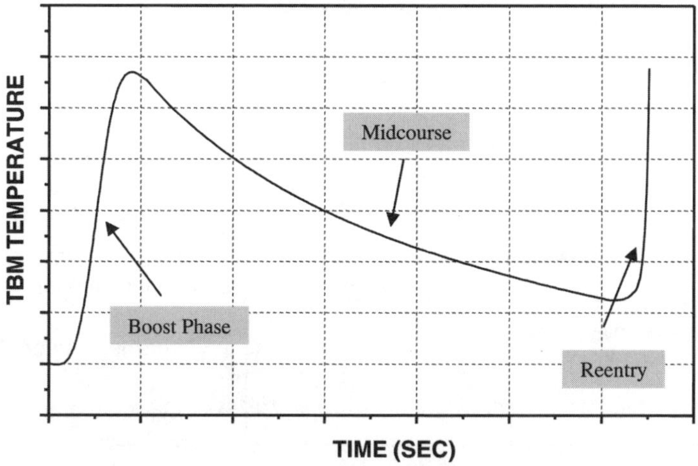

Fig. 5 Generic TBM temperature profile.

the target and its behavior based on preexisting data or to triangulate the position using two or more sensors.

2) Detection range is a function of array sensitivity and signature intensity.

3) Target EO signature is a function of temperature, emissivity, and surface areas. The temperature (and resulting signature) of a TBM are large during the boost phase, while the rocket motors are operating. The temperature lessens during the midcourse flight stage and increases drastically at reentry, as a result of air friction. Figure 5 presents a generic TBM EO temperature profile as a function of time.

These characteristics of the signature make the EO sensors useful mainly during the boost phase and the reentry stage. The former occurs at a great distance from the defense system deployment sites. Consequently, the use of ground-based and airborne sensors is limited as a result of physical and deployment limitations. Figure 6 presents the line-of-sight range for a ground sensor or an airborne sensor (at 10-km altitude), assuming 10-km altitude cloud cover over the target. The end-of-boost location (range and altitude) of representative minimum energy trajectory TBMs is also indicated. To detect the TBMs in boost, these sensor-carrying platforms must be deployed relatively near the launch site, which usually is not possible. In addition, ground-based sensors are very limited as a result of atmospheric effects (attenuation losses, clouds).

As a result, ground-based sensors mainly can be used to assist in data gathering during the descent and reentry phases of the TBM flight for discrimination and kill assessment (see later section) and this necessitates physical proximity to the area of reentry. For the primary early warning, search and track tasks satellite-borne sensors are used.

In all cases the range (from the sensor to the TBM) is large. The present technology limits the use of large starring arrays. Therefore, to achieve sufficient accuracy and detection capability, the coverage by a given array is limited, and scanning is used to increase the monitored area. Accuracy is determined by the following parameters: pixel size of the elements in the array, the characteristics of the optical

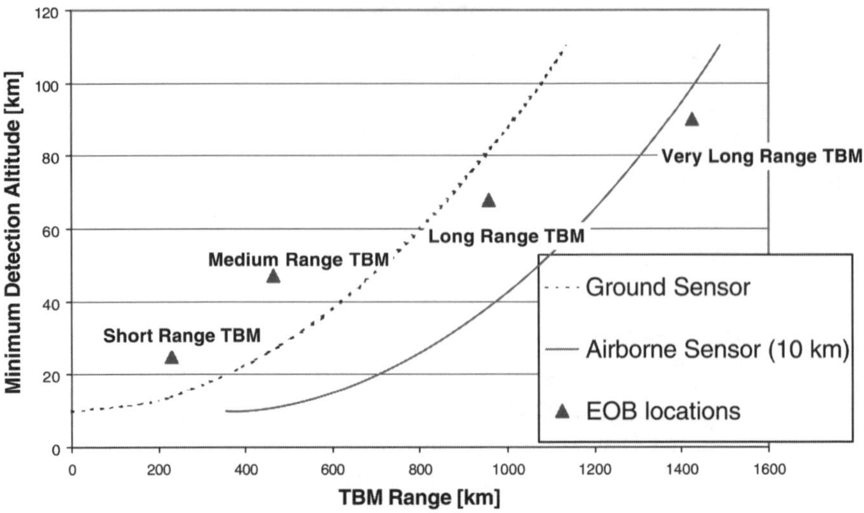

Fig. 6 Representative line-of-sight ranges.

telescope, and the accuracy of the platform's location and attitude. Target position accuracy can be improved by triangulation by a number of platforms.

b. Radar sensors. The main characteristics of a radar sensor are the following.

1) Measurement of angular position, range, and radial velocity.

2) Detection range is a function of the transmission power of the radar, the reception sensitivity, noise, and the target's cross section.

3) Target's radar cross section (RCS) widely varies, depending on the angle at which the target is seen at different stages of its trajectory.

4) The radar operates by sending a beam in a certain direction and determining the target's location within the beam according to the pointing angle and the range of the detected object within the beam.

5) The covered area per beam is determined by the angular spread of the beam. Angular accuracy and resolution are increased when the beam's width is decreased by an increase in antenna gain. However, the area covered by a single beam is reduced. To cover large areas with sufficient accuracy, a scanning pattern is necessary either electronically (in phased array radars) or mechanically.

6) Range accuracy per measurement is dependent on the radar range gates, the beam width, and processing of the return signals.

7) Radar resolution is dependent on bandwidth and processing methods.

2. *Process of Search and Acquisition*

The first stage of providing an adequate defense is to acquire the TBM at the appropriate range and time. Similar to many other threats, the time and direction of a TBM attack are not accurately known, therefore it is necessary to maintain constant surveillance of suspected launch sites to guarantee that ascending TBMs will be acquired. The main requirement from the surveillance system is constant availability, looking toward the possible regions from which the threat can originate.

Once an object has been detected, it is necessary to identify it quickly and reliably and determine if it is really a threat. For the theater missile defense (TMD), a threat is a TBM that is flying toward any defended region. Therefore the initial identification process should include both identifying the object as a TBM and assessing its trajectory to predict its impact point. The main requirement from the surveillance system for this stage is sufficient tracking accuracy as early as possible. In both stages, the main limitation are the sensor resources available.

As explained previously, to intercept a TBM at a given location (altitude and range), it is necessary to achieve a certain accuracy for the trajectory assessment. To achieve the required accuracy it is possible to either acquire the TBMs at long ranges and track them for a long time at a low sampling rate or to acquire the TBM at shorter ranges and to achieve the required accuracy by tracking at a high rate. In most cases it is much less "expensive" (in radar resources) to track for a longer period of time at a lower rate. Figure 7 compares the total and average radar resources (relative) required for three different detection ranges. The graph presents the results of a simplified radar simulation. The basic radar parameters were defined and the plot accuracy (target signal-to-noise ratio S/N) as a function of range and dwell time (resources) was determined. Track accuracy was calculated by accumulating the radar plots in a root-mean-square (RMS) filter. For each case, the interceptor launch time and required accuracy at launch were the same, and accuracy was achieved at the required time by varying the track rate. The graph presents the total resources required for tracking in order to achieve the required accuracy at exactly the correct time. It is clearly seen that for these conditions it is preferable to acquire at long range and track at low rates. Additional advantages in acquiring the TBM at longer ranges include additional prioritization flexibility by providing a more complete battle picture and more time for the discrimination tasks and dealing with unexpected problems.

Even though it is preferable from the considerations of tracking load to acquire the TBM at long ranges, we should remember that searching at long ranges with a reasonable probability of detection (Pd) requires much more energy from the radar. In addition, because the accuracy of the measurement is also a function of the S/N, beyond a certain range the radar does not have enough energy resulting in a degradation in tracking accuracy.

Figure 8 presents the same detection cases as in Fig. 7 with the addition of the required search resources (fixed Pd) and degraded accuracy in tracking at long ranges. To determine the required search resources, it was assumed that the exact TBM trajectory will be known, but not the launch time. As a result, the search pattern selected scans a specific limited location at the minimal revisit rate required to guarantee that the TBM is detected successfully as it passes through the search area. In this case, there is clearly a "break-even" point where long-range detection no longer saves resources. In addition, at long ranges, the Pd (assuming a maximum resource level per dwell) will reach a value that is no longer useful, and the TBMs simply cannot be detected even if their location is provided by external sources.

The previous analysis was performed under the assumption that the TBM trajectory is known, therefore it was possible to limit the search to a specific volume in space. In an actual defense situation, the launch locations, impact locations, and exact trajectory parameters are not known. If the TBM attack can originate at various launch sites at different ranges, the radar must provide coverage for a wide range of trajectories at different locations and ranges, resulting in a need to define and execute a search pattern.

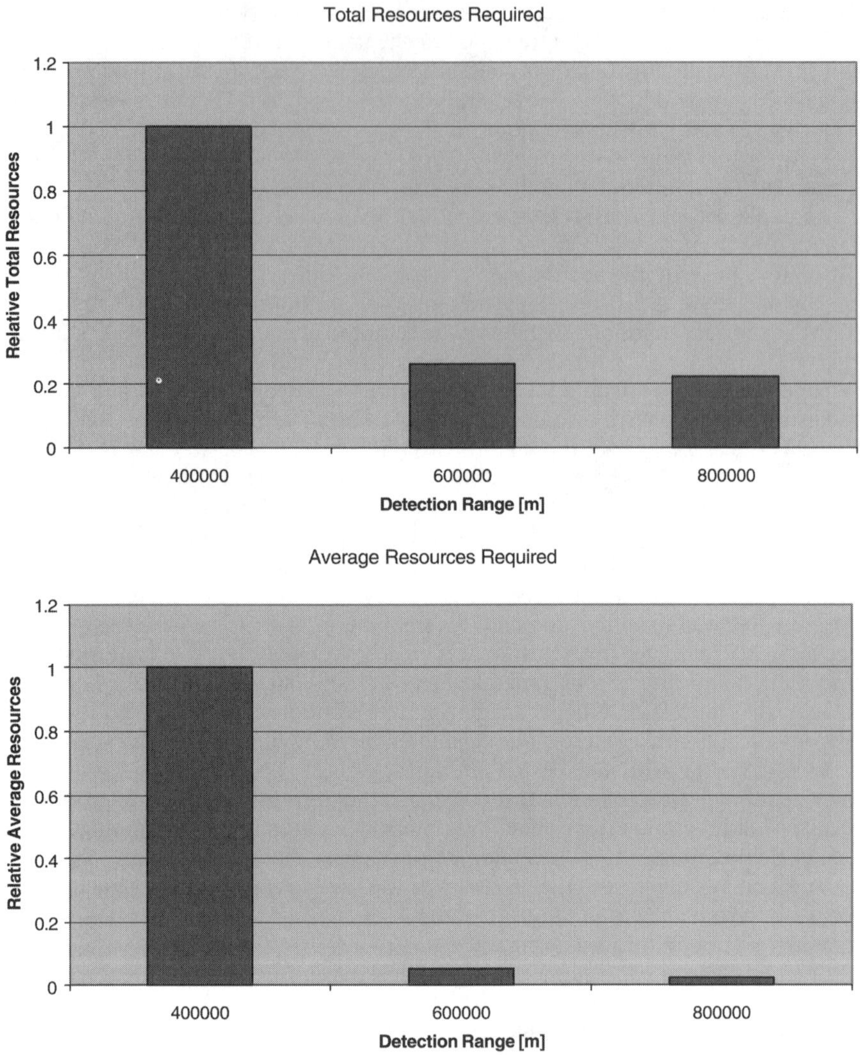

Fig. 7 Required radar resource comparison (track).

One important advantage of tactical missile defense lies in the fact that TBMs execute relatively well-defined *ballistic* trajectories. By limiting the possible launch and impact areas, and using intelligence data and task assignment, it is possible to define a more limited search coverage, and in this way to provide full defense, while still conserving radar resources.

The radar search pattern is defined according to the angular coverage in azimuth and elevation, the coverage in range (minimal and maximal), and the revisit rate. The angular coverage determines the area that will be covered, which must include a sufficiently long segment of each possible trajectory. The maximum range is determined by the quantity of resources provided and the required detection time

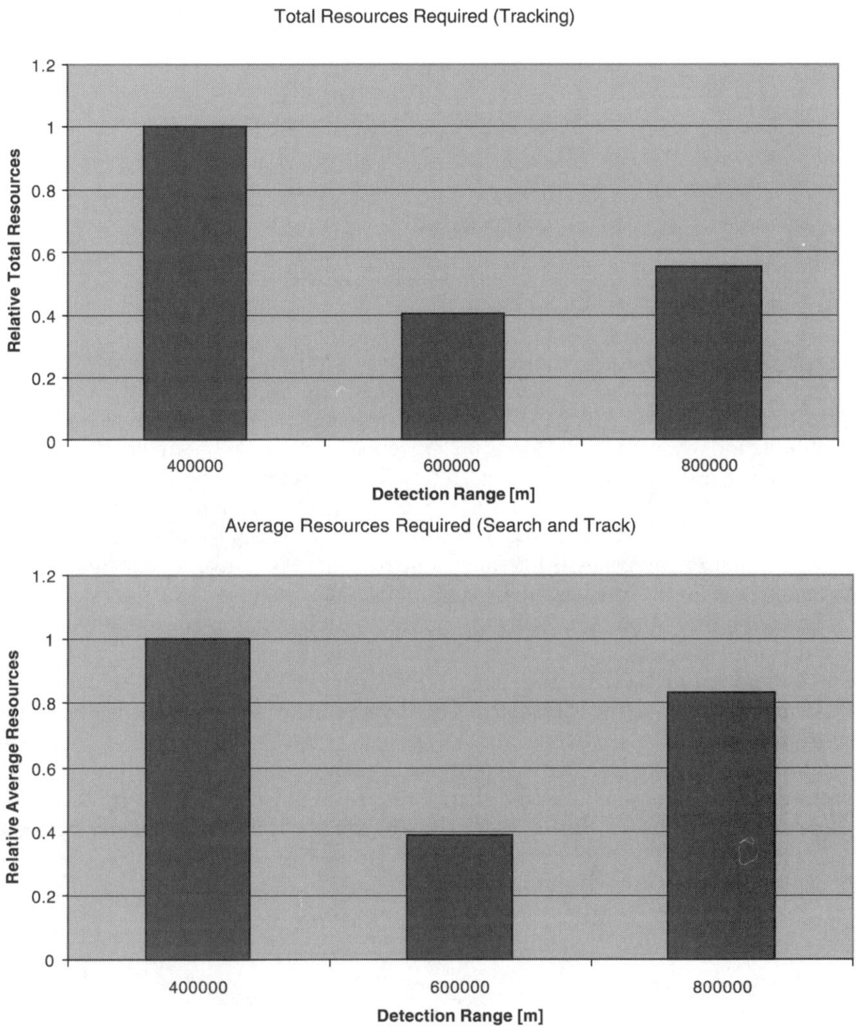

Fig. 8 Required radar resource comparison (search and track).

before the impact. A minimum range can be defined to avoid acquiring targets that are too close to interception. The revisit time should enable sufficient illumination of each TBM during its flight to guarantee its detection. It is possible to define a more optimal search pattern to save resources while dealing with the entire set of relevant trajectories by 1) determining the desired detection time for interception, 2) determining the trajectory location at the relevant times, and 3) finding the minimal search pattern that covers all the desired detection points while providing a sufficient number of detection attempts.

As an example, a possible threat scenario with three different TBM trajectories (short, medium, and long) was defined. The defense requirement is to provide coverage to all assets as far as 200 km in front of the defense system deployment.

Table 2 Required radar resources for search

Option	Sector	Resources (relative to option 1)
1		1
2	Short	0.12
2	Medium	0.16
2	Long	0.25

Figure 9 presents two possible search logics. Option 1 shows a single search sector coverage option. The elevation and revisit rate were set to enable successful detection of the shorter-range targets at the correct time, while its range was set to detect the long-range targets. Option 2 presents an "optimal" search pattern based on detecting each TBM at the required time for interception, based on interceptor capabilities. It is clearly seen that the longest search beam (fence) is less then half the range of the search fence of option 1. Because the energy required to maintain an equivalent Pd increases as the range squared, there is an overall savings of 50% in resources. Table 2 presents the required resources relative to Option 1.

The main limitation in defining an optimal search pattern is the dependence on intelligence. Longer-range TBMs or those with lofted trajectories could fly beyond the defined search pattern, whereas shorter-range TBMs or those with depressed trajectories can fly below the pattern. TBMs also can be launched outside the edges of the coverage.

The preceding analysis defines a minimal search pattern that still provides the required coverage for all TBMs. If this pattern is not performable by the radar as a result of a lack of resources, there still are a number of available options,

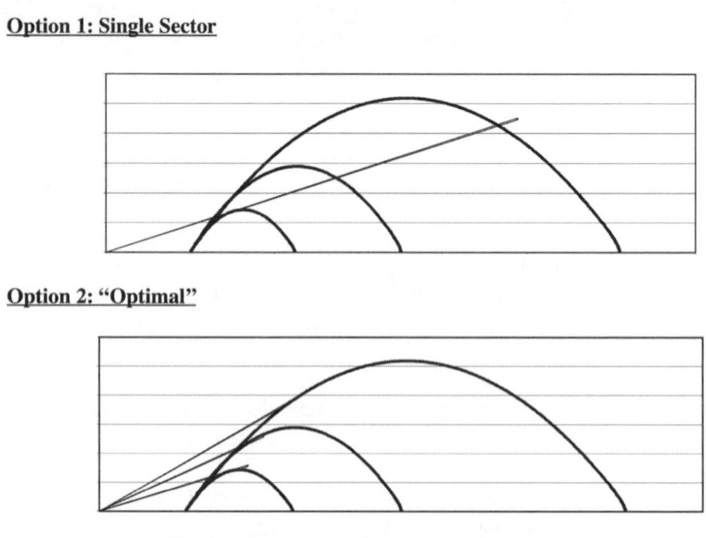

Fig. 9 Radar search pattern options.

including reducing the defended area, increasing tracking rate (reducing interception capacity), or receiving TBM data from additional sensors (including external cues).

The use of external cue data, and in particular of satellite IR systems, is analyzed in detail in Chapter 9. The main contributions of external cues (XQ) are in providing data as to the occurrence of a launch and an assessed trajectory. Even if the assessment is relatively inaccurate it still can be used for initial filtering (relevant TBM vs "not" TBM or not relevant one) and acquisition. The availability of XQ can enable the planning of a search pattern that does not include the longest range threats. If the XQ data is also included in the trajectory assessment, it is possible to delay acquisition, using the external data for trajectory initialization.

3. Process of Tracking

As stated before, to perform the interception process it is necessary to be able to estimate the trajectory of the TBM with sufficient accuracy. Two types of data are required. First, the ground-impact point needs to be assessed to determine whether the TBM should be intercepted. Second, the location of the TBM, as a function of time, needs to be available to plan and perform the interception.

The tracking process is what gathers data about the TBM's trajectory. It enables the calculation of the entire trajectory with sufficient accuracy, to provide the means for the defense system to operate in the allotted time with limited resources.

The purpose of ground-impact point assessment is to determine whether the TBM should be intercepted. The accuracy required is dependent on the size of the defended assets of the system. The physics of the TBM flight result in limitations on the accuracy achievable. Even if the trajectory of the TBM is known perfectly during its midcourse phase, reentry effects will result in uncertainties. These include lack of knowledge of exact ballistic coefficients of the specific TBM,* reentry maneuvers caused by stabilization and their impact on ballistic coefficients, and atmospheric conditions including wind. There is no reason to try and achieve prediction accuracy that is better than one achieved under the influence of these values. A second limiting parameter is that it is necessary to determine whether or not to intercept a TBM while it is still at a great distance from the impact point. Track accuracy is defined in terms of position and velocity. The accuracy of the prediction of the impact point is determined mainly by the velocity accuracy together with the time until impact.

The requirement for trajectory assessment comes from the need to generate a successful defense plan and execute it. The requirement is that the interceptor reach the target with a sufficiently small miss distance (see subsequent sections), therefore the inaccuracy of the tracking prediction must be no greater than the capability of the interceptor to correct as a function of time.

Early in the defense process, before interceptor launch, this correction limitation is affected by limitations in launch capability. For any point on the TBM trajectory within range of the interceptor, there is a single launch time that is defined by the interceptor time of flight. Clearly, at any given time the range of possible launch times (interception points) is limited. The interceptor must be effective (maneuver

*The ballistic coefficient equals the ratio of mass/aerodynamic drag, and it determines the deceleration and thus the trajectory of bodies in the atmosphere.

wise) at the interception point and there must be enough time to prepare the interceptor for launch, this of course being a parameter of the specific system.

Once an interceptor is in the air, the capability to significantly change the interception point is seriously limited. As the interceptor approaches the interception point, its correction capability becomes more limited. The relationship between interceptor divert capability and the required tracking accuracy is presented in more detail in Sec. IV.A.4.c dealing with the interception stage of the defense process.

As described in Sec. IV.A.2, along with achieving the required accuracy, an additional goal is using minimal radar resources. Because radar resources are used for tracking, and it is expected that TBM attacks will occur in salvos, it is desirable to use minimal resources per TBM, thereby increasing the capability of the defense system. If the various measurements have a constant accuracy, it is "cheaper" in resources to track the target at a low rate for a longer period of time. However for a radar it is very expensive to achieve a high accuracy at long ranges because the S/N degrades as a function of range.

4. *Multiple Sensors*

The previous discussion considered the case of a single sensor, mainly radar. If more than one sensor is available, it is possible to greatly increase the defense capability. To gain the maximum benefit from this situation, specific functions must be provided to the defense system elements.

In general, in the case of multiple sensors, the BMC^4I provides the monitoring and control that enables the required teamwork. It collects the data from all of the sensors, identifies the relevant threats, generates a uniform sky-picture, generates defense plans based on all available data, and distributes the data back to the sensors as required. The possible benefits include assigned search patterns, mutual cueing, improved track accuracy, improved resource assignment, and improved discrimination capability. To achieve these capabilities the requirements from the system include data and track fusion-algorithms, well-developed defense planning, and resource planning.

a. Shared search. As stated before, for a given radar the achievable probability of target detection is a function of the range searched and the energy used. In addition, a phased array radar has the best performance in the center of its coverage (as a result of off-broadside effects), therefore if a large area needs to be covered, significantly improved performance will be achieved by deploying each radar to cover a specific sector. Figures 10 and 11 show schematically two search options that can be used in a set-up that includes two defense systems providing defense to a large defended area against three possible launch sites. The two options are two radar systems working independently and two radar systems with mutual cueing. In the mutual case, overlap of search is avoided so that the resources used for search are less than the sum of the resources of the two radars in the individual case.

b. Improved resource assignment. If the attacks become too massive the radar may be unable to provide resources for all of the required tasks. This is particularly true when the radar performs both search and acquisition tasks, as well as tracking and fire control tasks. If more than one radar is available, then when one radar is overloaded, it is possible to transfer some of its tasks to the other radar. This is particularly useful if there are load prediction functions that enable assessing

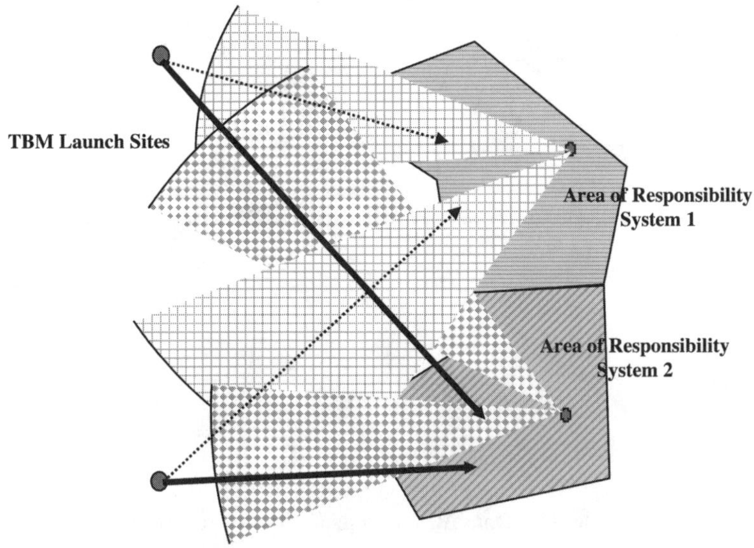

Fig. 10 Search coverage: independent systems.

when each radar will be overloaded and thereby reassigning interceptions and switching search patterns as appropriate.

c. Improved tracking accuracy. There are several ways to merge data from two (or more) sensors to improve tracking accuracy. First, it is possible to take tracks generated by two different sensors, to synchronize them with reference to

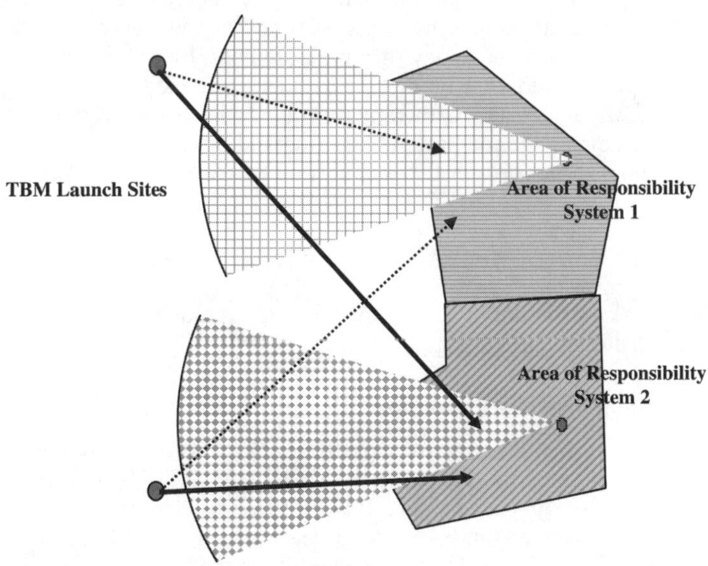

Fig. 11 Search coverage: mutual cueing.

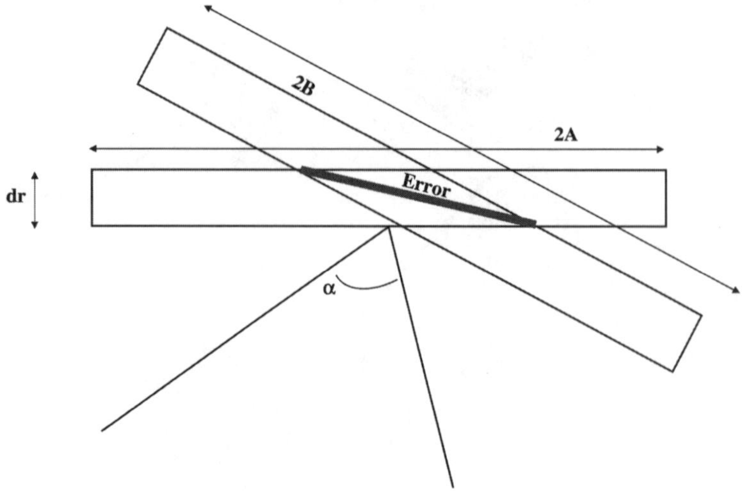

Fig. 12 Data fusion accuracy improvement.

time, and to combine them. This can be done either by some method of data averaging or by choosing the best out of the two. In most cases, choosing the best is preferable because it is a simpler method, and the added benefit of data fusion is limited. A second method to improve track accuracy is to combine the measurements of each sensor. The simplest realization is to add measurements from each sensor to the tracking filter as they are generated. This is equivalent to increasing the tracking rate. However, with appropriate deployment it is possible to have the added benefit of compensating for the "shape" of the error of each sensor. In general, a radar sensor has highly accurate range measurement and less accurate angular measurements. Figure 12 shows how it is possible to significantly improve the accuracy of a measurement, by triangulating the measurements from two radars. The error per radar is defined as a rectangle with angular error $2A$ or $2B$ and with range error dr. Because the target is within both of the rectangles the maximum error (marked by the heavy line) is defined as the maximum dimension in the intersection of the two areas. Geometrically this is

$$\text{Error} = \text{Min}\{2A, 2B, 2dr \times [\cos(a/2)/\sin(a)]\}$$

To achieve this contribution it is necessary to limit as much as possible the biases between the radar, in particular time biases.

5. *Classification and Discrimination*

To perform an effective defense against a single TBM, all that is necessary is acquisition and tracking. However, in a real attack, TBMs will probably be accompanied by closely spaced objects (CSO). These will include various remnants (of TBMs and interceptors) and other "junk," as well as PENAIDS of various sorts, including intentional decoys. Therefore, identifying the correct target is one of the important tasks of the defense system, mainly during the tracking stage. This includes three main steps.

1) Discrimination: Separating between the various objects in the sky-picture.

2) Classification: Classifying each of the objects seen.

3) Identification: Identifying the relevant threats to be intercepted including either whole TBMs or warheads.

The most common objects that can be present within the sensors' sky-picture are 1) TBMs: whole TBMs that include a warhead connected to a motor or other parts of casings, 2) RVs: reentry vehicles that constitute a warhead separated from a motor, 3) spent motors: motor casings that have separated from the RV, 4) missile debris: various objects that were generated or broken off during the separation process or during flight (missile breakup at reentry), 5) motor debris: pieces of fuel and other material that is released from the motors during the postboost phase, 6) multiple TBMs or RVs: from a salvo attack or from an advanced warhead, and 7) decoys: see Chapter 4.

Clearly, interceptor divert capability is an important parameter in defining the requirements from the discrimination task. Because the interceptor is maneuver-limited after launch, the target chosen must be the relevant target or close to it physically. Since the incorrect object may be chosen before launch, the discrimination process continues during interceptor flight. The interceptor guidance logic must be informed of the correct object when correction is still possible. The interceptor onboard sensors are an important part of the discrimination process.

The identification process is performed by measuring various characteristics of the detected objects and comparing them to what is expected from a potential threat. The use of multiple characteristics, preferably from multiple sensors of one type, or various types of sensors, increases the reliability of the identification process. Possible characteristics include trajectory characteristics such as trajectory shape and relative trajectories within a group of objects, both of which are dependent on the ballistic coefficient, and radar or IR signature parameters such as form, peak, and median values, a range of values, and rate and behavior of changes in the signature. Because the behavior of these parameters over time, and in particular during reentry, is very important to the process, the identification operation is performed continuously throughout the defense process.

B. Defense Planning

Defense planning is the process of determining, for a given TBM, whether or not to launch interceptors, which sensors to use for fire control, which interceptors to launch, when to launch them, and toward what interception point. The goal is to achieve the desired level of defense in terms of the acceptable leakage rate—the number of functional TBMs that reach defended assets. This goal can include different (required) levels of defense for different assets (military, civilian, infrastructure) or for different TBM payloads (conventional vs unconventional).

For a single TBM, defense planning generates the best possible plan based on available data. The quality of the data is limited by intelligence about the enemy, understanding of the defense system's capabilities and achievable tracking accuracy (as a function of time). Intelligence limitations include information about the type of payload in the TBM's warhead including possible PENAIDS and decoys, physical characteristics (construction) of the TBM, and how it will behave in flight (intended maneuvers or erratic flight path). The limitations in knowledge about the defense system may stem from limited testing of the system and from its reliability, in particular in "real" environments and from the efficiency of the personnel, particularly under real battle conditions. The limitations of accuracy (as discussed earlier) include both the inaccuracy of the assessed trajectory that can result in an incorrect interceptor trajectory as well as incorrect or insufficient discrimination of the target out of a set of objects.

In an attack scenario including a number of TBMs, it is necessary to take into account the interaction between the interception attempts as well as the data about each specific TBM. These include the availability of resources (radars and interceptors) at any given time, problems of interceptors interfering with each other, and previous kill debris confusing the picture.

With the availability of a number of defense systems it is possible to provide improved defense by use of advanced interoperability. This comes at the cost of a more complex defense planning and coordination process, with a greater sensitivity to timing and lack of information. The benefits and limitations of interoperability are presented in Chapter 8. In the present chapter we will focus on the method of defense planning within a single defense system.

1. Single TBM Defense Planning

Preparing a defense plan is in most cases an automatic process performed according to predefined rules. A human operator (in the case of a single system) will be involved mainly in those cases where there are problems such as 1) limited resources and 2) changes in the value (priority) of a threat. The defense plan takes into account both previously available data and data about the TBMs as collected, in real time, by the sensors. The defense planning process then chooses the most appropriate rule of engagement (ROE) that achieves the required level of defense within the immediate capabilities of the defense system.

a. Rules of engagement. A ROE is a possible set of interceptor launch options against a TBM and includes which interceptors to launch and to what location to direct them. The basic options are 1) shoot: launching a single interceptor against a target, 2) shoot-shoot: launching a salvo of interceptors (at least two) against a target; a variation of this ROE is shoot-wait-shoot in which there is some time between the launches of the two interceptors, and 3) shoot-look-shoot: launching a single interceptor, performing kill assessment, and if necessary launching an additional interceptor.

If more than two interceptors are planned to be launched, the additional ones are launched in variations of the shoot-shoot or shoot-look-shoot ROE. An actual ROE could include a combination of the two, for example a high altitude salvo followed by kill assessment and then a low altitude salvo.

The defense system chooses the ROE per TBM to achieve its goal of defending effectively against all threatening TBMs. It is desirable to achieve this goal using a minimal number of interceptors because it is necessary to take into account future attacks. The shoot-look-shoot ROE is a method by which interceptor consumption is reduced while still maintaining the required level of defense. For the shoot-look-shoot ROE to be effective, the defense system must possess certain essential characteristics:

1) Intercept capability at sufficiently high altitude. This ability provides, in the case of a "no kill" assessment, for a second interception attempt at a lower altitude (above the minimal interception altitude).

2) Ground capability (with appropriate confidence level) of assessing a "kill/no kill" at minimum time after the first interception attempt. This characteristic requires appropriate sensors and sophisticated algorithms (to be described later in this chapter).

b. Defense planning considerations. To generate the defense plan, the assessed capability is compared with the required capability. The main parameters are the following.

1) Required leakage rate (LR): The goal of the defense system is to provide a level of defense such that the percentage of leakers (TBM that effectively deploy their payload) is no greater than the predefined leakage rate. This is achieved by intercepting each TBM with a sufficient number of interceptors of different types and capabilities so that the probability of kill against the TBM will be at the level of the required leakage rate ($P_k = 1 - \text{LR}$).

2) Single shot probability of kill (SSP_k): The probability of kill by a single interceptor, SSP_k, is a function of the interceptor (performance and reliability) and its interaction with the target, and it is strongly affected by the location of the interception. These parameters are known, with a certain level of confidence, before the commencement of an active conflict. Sets of probability of kill tables are generated by simulations and tests. The level of detail of the tables (density of the parameters) is a function of the available information as well as the sensitivity of the interceptor. If, for example, a change of 1 km in the interception point significantly changes the performance of the system, this must be included in the planning considerations.

3) Probability of kill (P_k): This parameter assesses the probability of kill by the entire set of interceptors to be launched against the TBM, including the impact of kill assessment on the results.

In general, preparing a defense plan for a certain attack scenario means finding the best ROE from a previously prepared set of ROE. These ROE are graded and ordered according to number of interceptors used. The best ROE, the one that provides a sufficiently high P_k (above the requirement) using minimal interceptors is chosen.

It is not always possible to achieve the level of the permitted LR. This may be a result of either a lack of resources or of limited sensor and interceptor capability. Lack of resources includes a shortage of available interceptors (e.g., if all of the in-range, ready interceptors have been used or already committed to a previous defense plan) and a shortage of radar resources (e.g., if the appropriate radar is participating in other interceptions or has failed). Lack of capability includes low P_k of the interceptor at the assigned interception points and evolving a requirement that exceeds the maximum interceptor rate of fire or falls below the minimum time between intercepts (for shoot-shoot ROE).

2. *Multiple TBM*

Multiple-TBM attack scenarios have two types of impact on defense planning. First, because the TBM conflict is expected to include many launches, some of them even simultaneous, it is necessary to define a defense planning algorithm that considers interceptor inventory. Second, in a specific attack the defense plan against one TBM can influence the defense plan of the next. Possible results include a lack of radar tracking resources to achieve the required accuracy at the required time; an inability to launch consecutively from the same launcher, or depletion of interceptors on launchers; and debris from one interception interfering with the next.

The way to deal with this problem is to modify the defense plan. The modification options include the following: 1) Identifying a ROE that will fulfill the mission but that will consume more interceptors. This is possible when interceptors' stocks are not a problem or if a very high level of defense is necessary. 2) Using fewer interceptors or intercepting at different locations, along the trajectory, with a lower P_k, accepting the possibility of a TBM leaking through. 3) Using other launch sites or other defense systems. This requires a centralized control of the available defense assets. 4) Knowingly allowing a certain number of TBMs to leak.

To perform a modification process, the defense system must include a logic to choose which defense plans to modify and must have access to relevant information for this purpose. The two main categories of modification processes are "first-come, first-served" and prioritization.

The first-come, first-served method is simple and does not require any additional information. However, it will not be applicable if there are threats (TBM types) that may require a higher level of defense. For example, if a low-priority TBM is identified first, it may cause resources to be earmarked, or even consumed, which may prove short later if a higher priority TBM were to be engaged.

In the TBM priority method, each identified TBM is assigned a value according to certain parameters that include potential defended assets that might be attacked by it, TBM type (warhead), and launch site. This is an ongoing, dynamic process, dependent on available information. Obviously, when information is short, the number of possible modifications during an engagement is limited. If a defense plan is generated and priorities change, or a higher priority TBM is unexpectedly identified, these events may necessitate the cancellation of the interception of lower-value TBMs. A successful prioritization method would result in providing the desired level of defense (permitted leakage rate) over all defended assets for all TBMs. The relevant information for prioritized defense planning requires constant monitoring, including the state of each interceptor (free, earmarked, optional), the available radar resources (present load, future load for interceptions, predicted load from interception debris), and the enemy's capabilities, successes, and failures. Early arrival of "quality" TBM information at the defense system enables a more detailed level of prioritization. This is an important use of good external cue data, and is further discussed in Chapter 9.

If more than one defense system is available, defense planning optimization can also take into account the capabilities and status of the other systems. Defense planning methods that optimize the ROE over a set of defense systems based on the status of the various resources (radar, interceptors) are described in Chapter 8.

C. Defense Execution

The defense execution stage starts with the "launch" of a first interceptor and continues until either the target is killed, the TBM impacted or, for this or that reason the defense effort was stopped. This phase can include a number of interceptors launched from different locations at different times, according to the defense plan.

This phase can also include kill assessment, if a shoot-look-shoot defense plan was executed. The main operations performed in the defense execution stage are interceptor flight, TBM kill (lethality) and kill assessment (KA).

The main player in this phase is the *interceptor* that flies toward the target according to best available data on target's location. The *BMC* generates the defense plan at the interceptor level and provides the relevant information to both the radar and interceptor. In addition it generates and sends the various commands and event flags to the subsystems, such as launch, intercept, and kill. The execution of the BMC's tasks is system dependent. Possible relevant parameters include types of interceptor guidance (command to line of sight, semiactive, active, or passive*) or methods of target track-generation (single sensor, linked sensors, and data fusion). Figure 13 presents the main phases of the interceptor flight. In most defense systems that are being considered today, and in all of the new MDAPs, the *radar* tracks the TBM to provide the interceptor with more updated track data during the phases of its flight before self-acquisition. At the end-game phase, the interceptor acquires the target using onboard sensors and performs active guidance to the target. To enable communication between the interceptor, and the ground and to improve the accuracy of the interceptor's guidance, the interceptor itself may be tracked from the ground. In the case of a multiobject sky-picture, the discrimination process (target/nontarget) may continue after the interceptor has been launched and, if found justified, a change of target will be performed. For the interceptor to successfully integrate the radar discrimination information, it may be necessary for the radar to provide the interceptor with the entire set of tracked objects (in the relevant location), to enable correct identification of the target. To perform the kill assessment, the radar maps the sky-picture immediately before and after the interception.

1. *Interceptor Flight and Guidance*

The unique characteristics of the TBM target drive specific requirements that have a bearing on the interceptor flight process. Compared with "standard" aerial targets the TBM target is relatively small and very fast, and it has the capability of continually performing violent maneuvers. These include both unplanned ones caused by end-of-boost and reentry effects as well as planned aerodynamic and powered maneuvers. Because the target is small and requires a large energy transfer to result in an effective kill, the final miss distance must be very small. The resulting missile solutions available today include an initial command guidance phase followed by a self-acquisition (by the interceptor) and closed loop guidance end-game phase. Various guidance solutions, in particular those dealing with the end-game problem, are described in detail in Chapters 11–13 of this volume.

During the command guidance phase of the flight, the interceptor flies toward the predicted interception point, according to an external sensor's (mainly radar) tracking of the target. This point can be updated during fight. At handover, when the interceptor switches from command to self-guidance, its path and attitude must enable it to acquire the target and close the handover error. This is the error between the location toward which the interceptor is flying and the actual position of the target.

---

*In some cases the latter two can render a missile a "fire and forget" system.

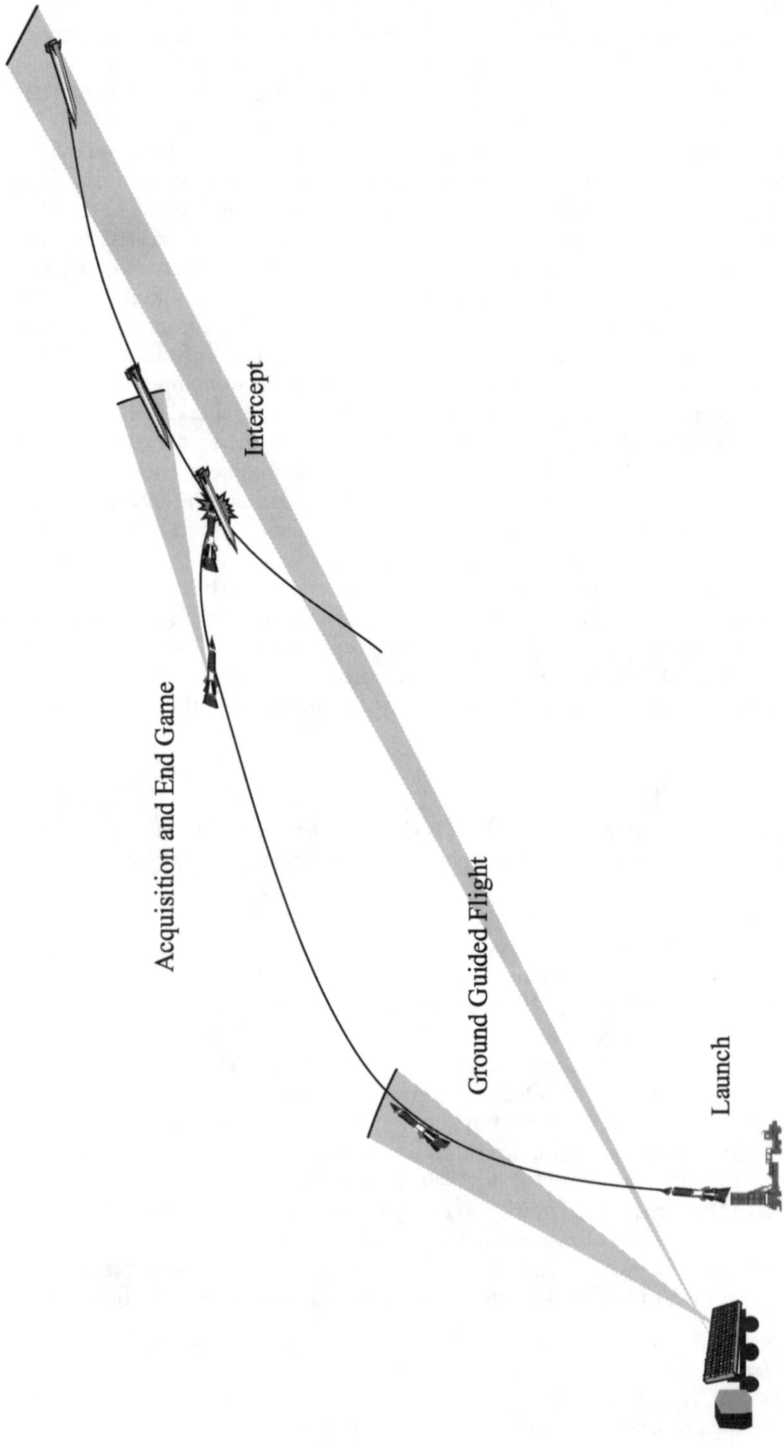

Fig. 13 Interceptor flight phases.

Throughout its flight, the interceptor has a finite correction capability that is dependent on its available energy, maneuvering capability, and the time available to perform the corrections. The total error at a given time must be less than the total correction capability from that time until intercept, as well as potential target maneuvers during the end game. The error sources include both errors in the estimated trajectory of the target and errors in the actual trajectory (location and velocity) of the interceptor.

The sources for the target's estimated trajectory errors are measurement errors by the ground sensor and unknowns or unexpected variations in the behavior of the target. The sources for interceptor trajectory errors are drift and inaccuracies in the internal measurement of the interceptor's trajectory and limited correction capability of known errors in earlier stages of the flight.

The only parameter that can be controlled by the defense process is the influence of ground-sensor measurements, in terms of resources, on the target's assessed trajectory. The required tracking accuracy must be defined, in all stages of the defense process, taking into account both interceptor capabilities and reasonable values for all other parameters. Available tradeoffs include reducing either the accuracy requirement or the time requirement. It is possible to reduce the requirements of accuracy from the external sensor by increasing the maneuverability of the interceptor or increasing its allowable miss distance. In addition, it is possible to set the time of trajectory assessment convergence (as required for interceptor launch) to a later time relative to the TBM time of flight by increasing the velocity of the interceptor thereby delaying the launch.

2. *Lethality*

The final goal of the defense process is to neutralize the TBM warhead. This is the lethality phase of the process. The important parameters in this phase are the construction of the TBM warhead and the type of interceptor kill mechanism.

a. Kill mechanisms. The potential threat's warhead payloads, as described in Chapter 4, are high explosive (HE) payloads or unconventional ones, such as chemical, biological, or nuclear. The payload can be configured either as a unitary (bulk) warhead or as a cluster warhead from which submunitions (high explosives, chemical, or biological, or, to some extent, even nuclear) are released at a certain stage of the TBM's flight. In this chapter we will discuss the kill mechanisms against conventional (high explosive) and chemical payloads.

There are various ways to neutralize or "kill" a TBM so that it can no longer perform its mission. Table 3 summarizes the various options according to level of effectiveness and warhead type. The main characteristic of a *mission kill* (occasionally called mission denial or soft kill) is that the TBM's payload still operates as intended and impacts the ground, but at a location that does not require defense, like in the sea or in an unpopulated area. In a *hard kill* the TBM payload is rendered ineffective.

Mission denial is characterized by damage to fins, control surfaces, guidance and control system, or altering missile aerodynamics to such an extent as to cause the missile or the warhead to miss intended its target. The main hard kill methods are payload destruction, dismemberment, or dudding. Payload destruction is the elimination of the effective payload while still in flight and at such an altitude that no residual effects can be observed. This includes the initiation or deflagration of high explosive or the neutralization/pyrolyzation of chemical payload. Payload dismemberment involves payload ejection and/or breakup caused by massive

Table 3 TBM "kill" options

Kill type	Threat warhead type	Damage mechanisms
Mission kill	All	Trajectory perturbation or vehicle breakup
	Submunitions	Premature submunitions dispersal
Hard kill	Conventional	Violent reaction of high explosives Payload dismemberment Payload dudding
	Chemical bulk	Neutralization/pyrolization Agent container's breakup and dispersal Payload dudding
	Chemical submunitions	Neutralization/pyrolization of contents of all submunitions Premature dispersal of agent from all submunitions Payload dudding

structural damage, again, in a manner that will render it ineffective at its target. Payload dudding is destruction of critical functional components that will result in the payload's failure to operate as required. This includes damage to fuses, sensors, and gas generators.

b. Interceptor lethality mechanisms. The main effective lethality mechanisms against TBM's are 1) kinetic energy (KE) or hit to kill (HTK), 2) fragmentation warhead (FWH), 3) blast warhead , and 4) directed energy. The first two mechanisms are the most commonly used in TMD at present and will be discussed in more detail in this chapter.

The key question regarding the choice between KE and FWH is related to the predicted kill capability that is a result of the achievable miss distance (MD). If the guidance system is accurate enough to achieve a MD in the neighborhood of 10–15 in. against warheads of all targets, then body-to-body contact with the TBM's warhead is guaranteed. Under these circumstances KE is probably the best answer since this method will impart a significant amount of energy to the warhead, totally destroying it. However, if achieving a minimal MD is problematic, a fragmentation warhead will be a better overall solution because in this way it is possible to significantly increase the likelihood that sufficient energy will impact the TBM's warhead.

Within the defense systems that are being developed and deployed at present, the theater high-altitude area defense (THAAD) and PAC3 extended range interceptor (ERINT) are typical examples of a KE kill systems. The Arrow, PAC2, and AEGIS area defense systems are examples of a FWH systems.

We will now discuss in more detail how the two interceptor kill mechanisms execute the kill options, in particular payload destruction, which is the goal of the current defense systems.

c. High explosive unitary warheads. To perform payload destruction, it is necessary to impact the TBM's warhead with sufficient energy. For a KE (interceptor) warhead, the energy that is transferred to the target at impact, if the impact occurs in the area of the payload, will cause a shock-to-detonation transition or deflagration-to-detonation transition.

For a fragment kill, it is also necessary to transfer sufficient energy. However, because the mass per fragment is small, this requires either high fragment velocities or a large number of fragments. In addition, for fragments, the penetration process itself may cause the loss of significant mass and velocity in certain impact geometries. This makes the fragmentation warhead much more sensitive to intercept geometry, though less sensitive to miss distance. An additional possible kill mechanism for the HE warhead is that a hot fragment becomes embedded in the high explosive causing a thermal initiation.

d. Chemical bulk (CB) warheads. Against a CB warhead, the goal is to disperse or pyrolize the chemical payload. Dispersal occurs if the warhead envelope is destroyed or ripped sufficiently. Pyrolization occurs if the sufficient energy is transferred to the payload.

The KE warhead is highly effective against the CB if it impacts the relevant area. In this case the payload will be completely destroyed.

The fragmentation warhead is highly effective against CB warheads if it produces the hydraulic ram effect, as a result of very fast and sufficiently massive fragments ejected from the warhead. To understand the high efficiency of a FWH against a bulk warhead as compared with its limitations against a submunitions warhead (see next section), one has to understand the role of ram effect in the kill mechanism.

The hydraulic ram occurs when an impacting fragment, penetrating into a container full of liquid, generates an intense shock wave that is localized in a small area. This shock wave moves toward the opposite wall with a wake behind it and eventually ruptures it with explosive pressure. This is described in Fig. 14. Such a rupture will enable the release of the payload within a minimal time. A large portion of the payload will be destroyed, the rest will be dispersed and will not

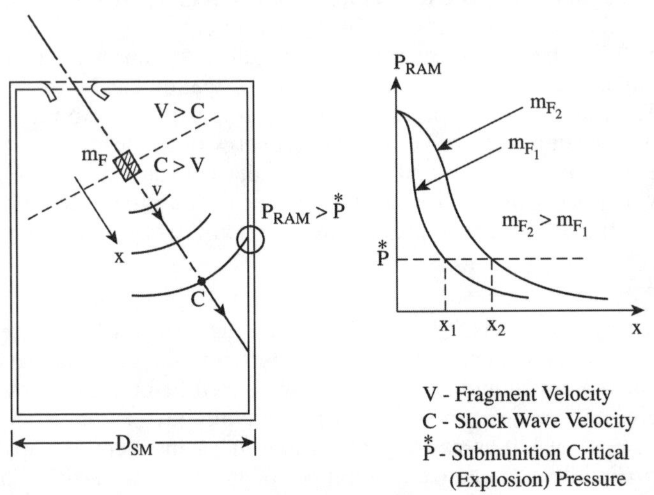

Fig. 14 Ram effect description.

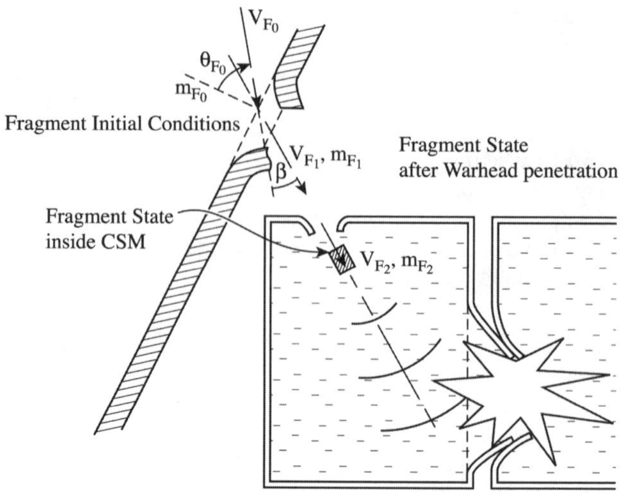

Fig. 15 Submunition kill process.

be effective upon reaching the ground. When multiple impacts occur, the result is more dramatic, completely destroying the warhead's envelope. Only a few high velocity fragments are needed to destroy a bulk warhead.

e. Cluster submunitions (CSM) warheads. The submunitions warhead is the most difficult to kill of the three types discussed. In this type of warhead, the payload is packed in small amounts in individual canisters. To perform a sufficiently effective hard kill, it is necessary to destroy a large portion of the canisters.

As in the other payload types, if a KE warhead impacts in the correct location, it will destroy the CSM. However, in this case, if the warhead is sufficiently large, then even a slight miss by the KE vehicle will result in a partial destruction of the CSM and enable some level of effective operation of the threat.

For the FWH, the number of fragments required to impact the target is high, driving a small miss distance requirement. The situation can be explained using Fig. 15. The ram energy released by a single fragment is more than enough to destroy a single submunition. The explosive energy of the destroyed submunition is capable of destroying a limited number of adjacent submunitions. However, if only a few fragments hit the TBM warhead it may not be possible to kill a sufficient portion the submunitions or to prevent an (even partial) effective deployment.

3. *Kill Assessment*

Kill assessment (KA) is the capability of the defense system to determine the success or failure of an interception and to determine whether or not an additional interception attempt should be performed. As stated before, kill assessment is a requirement in those defense systems where saving interceptors is an important goal. By the use of kill assessment and a multilayer interception capability it is possible to significantly reduce the number of interceptors used by the defense system. We will now describe the impact that KA has on the defense system effectiveness, what are the requirements from an effective KA algorithm, and possible KA methods.

Table 4 Kill assessment results

Reality	Assessment	Results
Kill	Kill	Correct—saves interceptors
Kill	Miss	False—wastes interceptors
Miss	Miss	Correct—launch another interceptor
Miss	Kill	False—a leaking TBM

a. Effectiveness calculation. Kill assessment accuracy is composed of two different values: the probability of correctly identifying a "no kill" and the probability of identifying a "kill." The two probabilities can result in two different errors. A P_{miss} error (identifying a "no kill" as a "kill") will result in not launching an additional interceptor(s) against a TBM that has not been killed, automatically resulting in a leaker. This can occur if a TBM motor is hit instead of the warhead and kill remnants are generated. A P_{fa} error (incorrectly identifying a "kill" as a "no kill") will result in the wastage of interceptors. Table 4 summarizes the possible KA results and their impact.

For a given KA error level, the following equations enable the calculation of LR and interceptor consumption (IC) in the case of a single TBM (under a given set of ROE) and with the assumption that the SSP_k is constant, where i is the layer number and n_i is the number of interceptors in layer i.

Shoot-shoot:

$$\text{LR} = (1 - \text{SSP}_\text{k})^n$$

$$\text{IC} = n$$

Shoot-look-shoot:

$$\text{LR} = (1 - P_k)^{n_1} P_{\text{miss}} + (1 - P_k)^{n_1}(1 - P_k)^{n_2}$$

$$\text{IC} = n_1 + (1 - \text{SSP}_\text{k})^{n_1}(1 - P_{\text{miss}})n_2 + [1 - (1 - \text{SSP}_\text{k})^{n_1}]P_{fa} \times n_2$$

Table 5 presents a number of examples demonstrating the savings in interceptors resulting from using kill assessment for a number of kill assessment levels. In each case, the ROE was determined so as to achieve the permitted overall leakage rate. The basic tested parameters are TBM attack size = 100, interceptor $P_k = 0.8$, and permitted LR = 1%. The cases tested were 1) no kill assessment, 2) perfect kill assessment in which the result was always correct, 3) 10% false alarm and no miss errors, and 0.5% miss and no false alarm errors.

Table 5 Kill assessment's impact on defense system effectiveness

KA level	ROE (first, second)	Total interceptor consumption	Achieved leakage rate
None	3	300	0.008
Perfect (no errors)	1, 2	140	0.008
$P_{fa} = 10\%$	1, 2	160	0.008
$P_{\text{miss}} = 0.5\%$	2, 1	219	0.0082

In each case, the ROE was chosen under the assumption that all relevant parameters (SSP_k, KA errors) were known and the best ROE (the one that gives the required defense level with the minimal interceptor consumption) was performed.

The table shows that the savings in interceptors, if a multilevel KA ROE is used, can be very significant. This saving is very sensitive to the number of missiles launched at first layer, which is fixed by the ROE.

The possible savings and appropriateness of using KA is dependent on kill assessment accuracies. From the results it is seen that the defense system is much more sensitive to P_{miss}, since it is the probability to assess a failed interception as a success, resulting in an automatic leaker. If the product P_{miss} times P_k (first layer) is greater than the allowable P_k (permitted leakage rate), KA is not a relevant option. In the limit of P_{fa}, more interceptors may be launched in the shoot-look-shoot case than in the shoot-shoot (salvo) case. This is because a large number of interceptors are launched in the second layer at TBM mistakenly assessed as "not killed" during the first engagement. In the previous example, this limit is $P_{fa} > 70\%$.

b. Kill assessment algorithm. Assuming that sufficiently accurate assessment can be performed, the defense system must have a KA algorithm. The purpose of this algorithm is to determine whether the interception was successful as well as to identify any remaining viable targets. The decision of whether or not to launch an additional interceptor is based on the confidence level of the kill assessment and on defense planning considerations. Because the purpose of the defense systems is to prevent TBM leakers, the defense system is much more sensitive to miss errors, and this results in a requirement for a very low P_{miss}. Consequently, in most cases, the default decision will be "launch," whereas a "stop launch" command is sent if the probability of having performed a successful interception according to the KA, is above a specified threshold, relative to the required defense level. It is also possible to have a defense logic where interceptor savings is the primary consideration. In this case the default decision if the interception results are unclear will be "no second layer." A second launch is performed only if it is obvious that the interceptor has failed.

The KA algorithm is based on data received from the interceptor (via downlink) or remote sensing (radars or EO/IR sensors). The components of the decision algorithm are shown in Fig. 16. The main calculation is the determination of the success of the interception based on two types of data: $P_{KA}pre$ is the preinterception estimation of interception success based on intercept parameters and lethality assessment. $P_{KA}post$ is the postinterception KA based on kill remnant assessment.

Both of the required interception conditions for a successful kill and the types of remnants generated in the kill are dependent on the TBM warhead type. Therefore the probability of destroying any type of warhead is determined based on existing intelligence data and sensor data if available. The final P_{KA} is a combination of the two values. The method of combining the two elements is a function of the relative reliability that the system designer places on each. Though P_{KA}post is based on actual postinterception data and should be more reliable, if a very limited time is available for data collection, the relative weights of the two could vary. The P_{KA} is first calculated at interception and is based on P_{KA}pre. As the results of the kill develop and more data are collected, P_{KA} is continually updated and compared to two thresholds: α, the "kill" threshold (if P_{KA} is greater than this value the

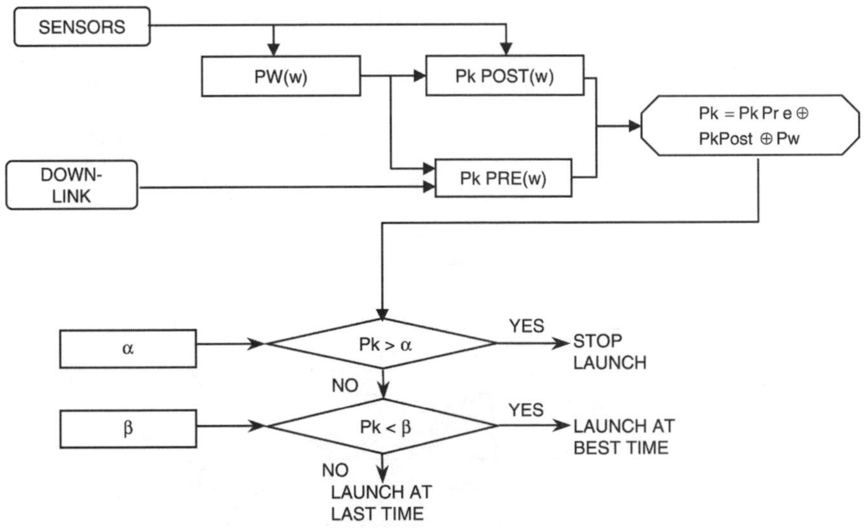

Fig. 16 Kill assessment algorithm.

interception is assessed as a success), and β, the "miss" threshold (if P_{KA} is less than this value, the interception is assessed as a failure and a second interception layer is activated).

The sensitivity of the algorithm to the two types of errors is tuned according to the values of the thresholds, the behavior of the system when results are not clear, and the method used to calculate P_{KA}pre and P_{KA}post. In the algorithm presented in the figure, preference has been given to avoidance of leakers. Therefore, if no clear decision is made within a sufficient time an additional interceptor will be launched.

P_{KA}pre—kill probability estimation: The parameters that impact the SSP_k are the interception geometry and the TBM warhead. Based on the parameters received from the fire control center and from the guidance and control of the interceptor, transmitted via the downlink, the miss distance and other end-game parameters can be estimated. These can be used to calculate the various probabilities of the kill process and to provide a value for an on-line P_{KA}, including a confidence level.

P_{KA}post: P_{KA}post is an assessment of probability of kill based on the sky-picture as generated by the available sensors immediately after the intercept. The KA decision needs to be performed in a very short time and automatically sent to the launching system. Figure 17 presents the available KA time for two different ROEs against a TBM aimed 10 km in front of the interceptor launcher. In ROE 1, both the first and second layers are performed at higher altitudes than in ROE 2. In addition, the altitude difference is greater in ROE 1. For shorter range TBMs there is sufficient time to perform detailed kill assessment and reach an accurate conclusion in both cases. For the longer TBM, the available time and the resulting available data is very limited. In the example given ROE1 is preferable. The actual result is dependent on the specific characteristics of interceptor (time of flight, available intercept altitudes) and TBM (reenty velocity, drag).

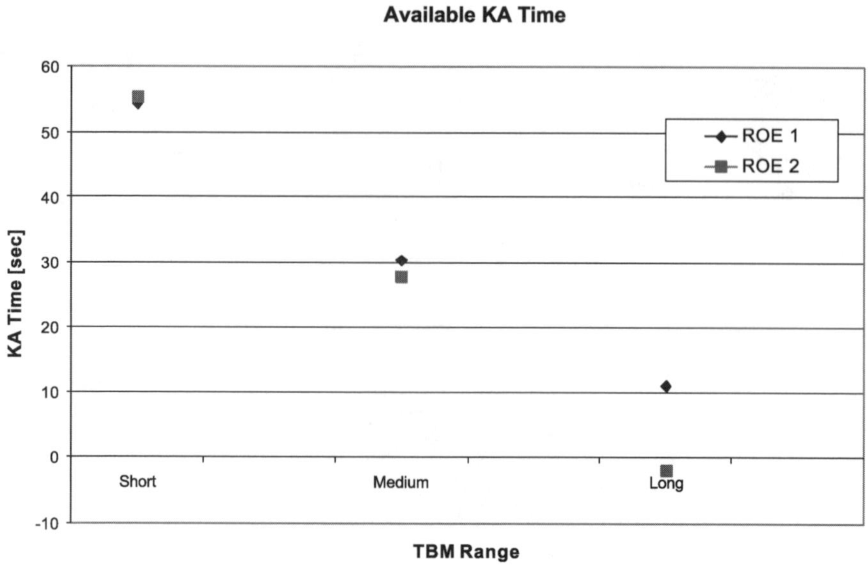

Fig. 17 Available kill assessment time.

The algorithm is mainly based on correlating the observed sky-picture of the kill (explosion, disintegration, change in trajectory and aerodynamic coefficients, appearance of new objects/debris, etc.) to a reference database of kill pictures.

c. Kill pictures. It is clear that for each specific threat warhead type and interceptor kill vehicle the kill picture and criteria are different. The following section will discuss the parameters of the kill picture for the bulk and cluster submunition warheads as well as some "no kill" cases that cause difficulties in the kill assessment process.

No-kill: To successfully identify a kill situation it is necessary to differentiate it from a no-kill situation. The obvious no-kill situation, in which the interceptor warhead is a KE vehicle, is not initiated or does not reach the TBM, is clear because, unlike all kill situations, no debris is generated.

The problematic no-kill cases are those in which debris are generated. In this case it is necessary to identify the unique characteristics of no-kill debris and, in particular, what are the identifying characteristics of a still viable target (payload) out of the debris.

The two main types of TBMs (separating warhead and nonseparating warhead) also constitute two different no-kill cases. A reasonable assumption for a separating-warhead TBM is that an interaction between the interceptor and the RV, which causes changes to the RV, will in effect destroy it. Therefore an undamaged RV will continue on its nominal trajectory. A hit on the accompanying motor will generate debris that could appear to be debris from a kill of a warhead, which of course it was not. For the nonseparating TBM, the case of no-kill develops if the interceptor impacts or damages the TBM's body, behind the warhead. This could result in either breaking off of small parts from the TBM or the total breakup of the TBM. In this case the warhead continues, in or near its original trajectory, possibly with parts of the TBM's body attached to it, while other body parts continue separately. From this assessment it is clear that the existence of debris is not sufficient to provide a definite kill result. It is necessary to identify additional unique characteristics.

Bulk high explosive: A bulk HE warhead consists of an explosive charge within a metal casing. The warhead's casing may constitute the outer envelope of the warhead or may be installed within an RV container made from thin metal. In either case, the outer envelope is (usually) coated with ablative material as thermal protection. The two main types of warhead kill are detonation or deflagration of the warhead.

If the HE warhead is initiated, the warhead and casing become a cloud of small fragments of various sizes and velocities. If at interception the warhead is still attached to the rest of the missile, the explosion will damage the other stages, ripping them apart and releasing additional debris. In addition, there will be a clear explosion. The main parameters that can be measured, to be used for kill assessment are 1) relative velocities and trajectories of the various fragments, 2) size, shape, and RCS of dispersed casing fragments/debris, and 3) explosion "fire ball" characteristics.

The dispersal of the casing (and housing) fragments and debris is dependent on the energy of the explosion. Many of the fragments are very small and will be released at high velocity radially from the warhead. In addition the body of the TBM will be significantly damaged and its trajectory will change depending on its mass and the force of the explosion. The direct change in velocity for the large debris (those that could be mistaken for a viable target) is limited. The significant effect is the change in ballistic parameters. This will be apparent only at lower altitudes because such phenomena depend on air density. Figure 18 presents the variation of the velocity of a damaged compared to an undamaged TBM (ratio of ballistic coefficients) as a function of the available time for both a separating and nonseparating TBM. At high altitudes (because of the lower air density) only very damaged remnants (ratio of ballistic coefficients of 0.01–0.02) will be detectable in a short time by their change in velocity. We will remind the reader that ballistic coefficient is the ratio of mass to aerodynamic drag, and drag depends, among other things, on the air density. It is thus clear that at high altitudes the various trajectories will

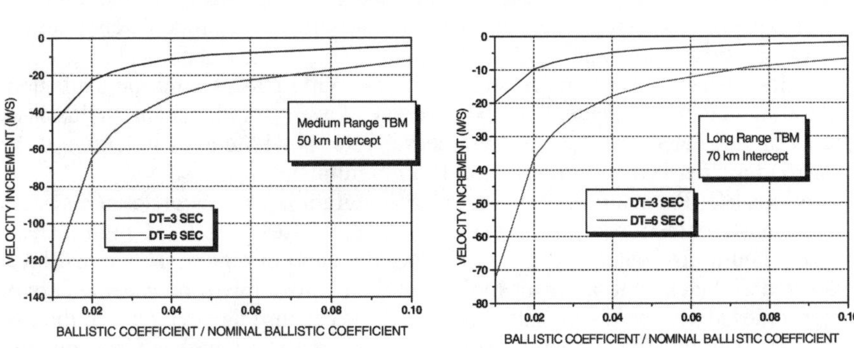

Non Separating TBM Separating TBM

Fig. 18 Change in velocity as a function of damage.

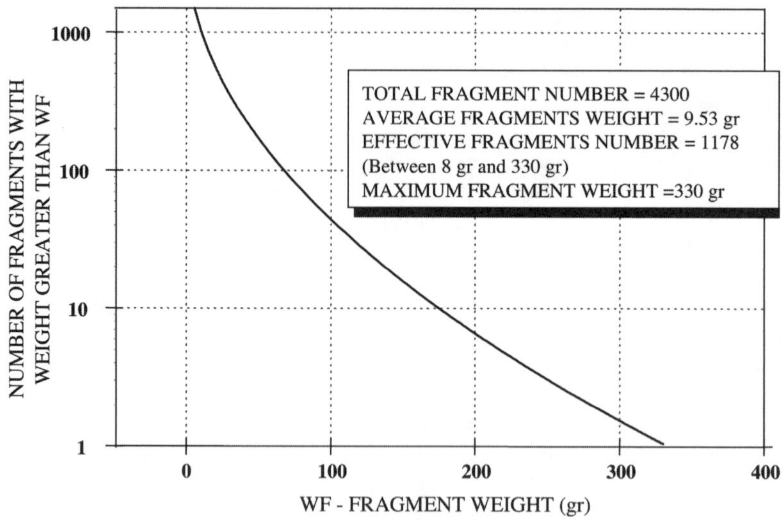

Fig. 19 High explosive debris distribution.

be undistinguishable of each other. In various geometries, a discriminator based on the derivative of the Doppler velocity processed through a Kalman filter will identify the change in trajectory much more quickly than assessing the trajectory out of position measurements. This can enable discriminating and assessing a kill at much higher altitude.

The residuals of the RV envelope can also increase the probability of correct assessment of a killed warhead. Those fragments have an average RCS between thousands and tens of thousands of a square meter and relative velocity of thousands of meters/second. Figure 19 presents the distribution of fragment sizes that are generated in a representative explosion calculated using the Mott equation.

Though these quickly disperse to a density that is not detectable, early after the explosion the fragment cloud will be clearly distinguishable by the radar in a range/Doppler map. A schematic representation of the range/Doppler gate map of a radar for the no-kill and kill cases is shown in Fig. 20. Assuming that the fragment cloud expands as a sphere, there are two possible situations. Immediately after the explosion, the entire fragment cloud is within a single radar beam and is detected as a wide distribution of ranges and velocities. Within 1–2 s after the explosion, the fragment cloud is greater than the coverage of a single radar beam. In this case, the radar will detect two sets of "symmetric" returns within a given region of the range/Doppler coverage (ignoring range ambiguities).

Various EO/IR sensors are candidates for integration in a theater defense system for the early detection of postboost and reentry phases of a TBM flight. These sensors could also detect explosions in the interception region. The signal level expected at the entry to a sensor looking at the explosion will be many orders of magnitudes above the RV signature level. This is because the area ratio of the two is above 30 dB and the temperature of the explosion is much higher. Consequently a detection range of many hundreds of kilometers is possible, limited only by attainment of line of sight and atmospheric phenomena. Admittedly, because the fire ball lasts less than few tenths of a millisecond, a scanning IR sensor is very

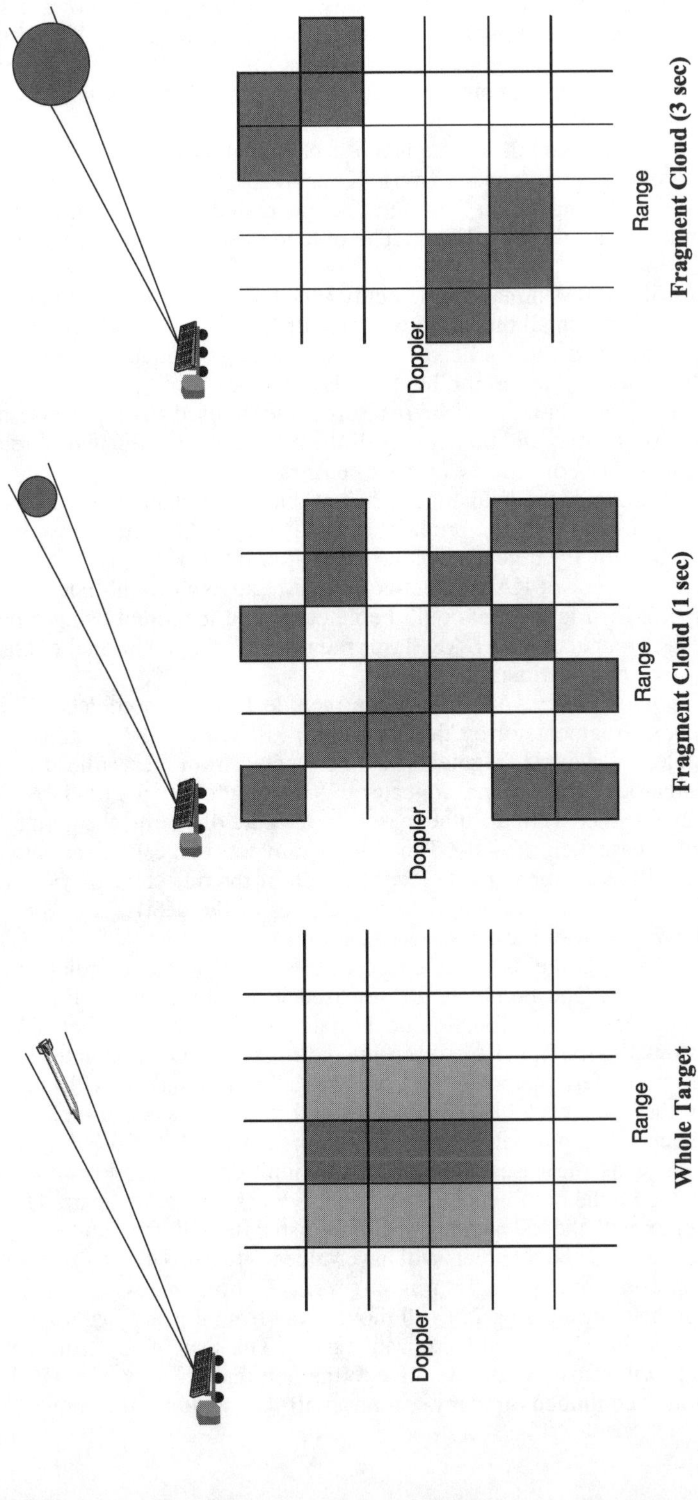

Fig. 20 High explosive kill range/Doppler map.

inefficient because of a very low probability (almost zero in fact) of the sensor beam being active and looking at the explosion's spatial location at the right time. Nevertheless, there is a very good chance of assessing an explosion from an EO/IR sensor having a clear line of sight to that location, provided the sensor was cued by the fire control radar.

Chemical bulk: The kill mechanism of a chemical bulk threat is based on the pyrolization of the agent (usually by HTK) or the explosion of the warhead and the dispersion of the agent via the ram effect generated by the penetration of the lethal fragments into the liquid bulk. The outcome of the kill can be one of the following:

1) Most of the TBM remains essentially intact while the warhead has a large opening through which all the liquid was expelled.

2) An explosion of the warhead resulting in a large amount of debris and a payload cloud (somewhat resembling the HE outcome).

The main parameters that can be measured and be used for a kill assessment are 1) relative velocities and trajectories of the fragments (debris) and 2) released payload signature (IR or millimeter wave sensors).

The modification of the ballistic coefficient due to the change in the mass and the drag coefficient as well as a probability that the threat becomes nonstable may modify substantially the trajectory of the TBM after it has been killed. As with the HE warhead, this type of KA is effective only at relatively low altitudes.

The dispersed warfare agent could be detected and identified using a passive long-wave IR or an active LADAR (laser radar) providing additional confidence in the kill assessment estimation.

Cluster submunitions: A warhead can include 100–200 bomblets. When hit by high-energy fragments or by the interceptor kill vehicle (KV), damaged and intact bomblets as well as fragments will be ejected from the warhead and will be dispersed around the nominal trajectory. With a high-energy kill, TBM debris also will be generated as in the other cases. In the case of chemical submunitions, some might release their payload. The main parameters that can be measured and used for the kill assessment are 1) identification of the trajectory of the released submunitions, 2) relative velocity and trajectories of the debris, and 3) released payload signature (IR or millimeter wave sensors).

Figure 21 presents the path and shape of the bomblet "cloud" relative to the nominal trajectory. The bomblets are released in all directions, with a certain velocity component in the direction of the interceptor relative to the TBM. The relatively slow dispersion velocity presents returns in few Doppler gates for most fire control radar (few meters/second of Doppler resolution). It will take many seconds for the bomblets to disperse into several range gates because of the small relative velocity. The non-kill reference case is shown in Fig. 20 (whole target). Figure 22 presents the case of a cluster submunitions (CSM) kill after a few seconds. After 1 s the bomblets will be dispersed less than 50 m apart. They will appear together with the RV nucleus within the usual (no kill) few range gates. The velocities of the detected bomblets will have values between 0 to $\approx$100 m/s relative to the RV, presenting doppler returns in several Doppler gates. A few seconds later the bomblet cluster (Fig. 22) will move away from the nominal trajectory in range and populate a large number of range gates. The span of velocities between the bomblets will remain biased relative to the nominal velocity of a TBM. This phenomenon, if continued for many seconds, will "concentrate" the bomblet cloud

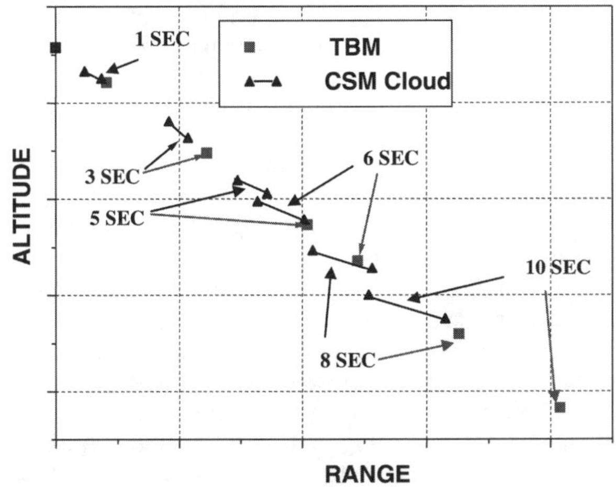

Fig. 21 Bomblet cloud after kill.

return in a few Doppler velocities in each range gate, while spreading the cloud over several range gates.

The main useful effect for kill assessment is the unique spread of velocities that could provide a quick assessment if enough resolution is available. As with the other warheads, for purposes of KA, the trajectories of the debris have limited usefulness at high altitudes. Signature identification of the payload could be a better solution.

D. Debriefing

The ATBM systems are sophisticated, state-of-the-art weapon systems designed according to the best available information, at any given time, about the threats. Qualification and validation capability of ATBM systems is limited because of the

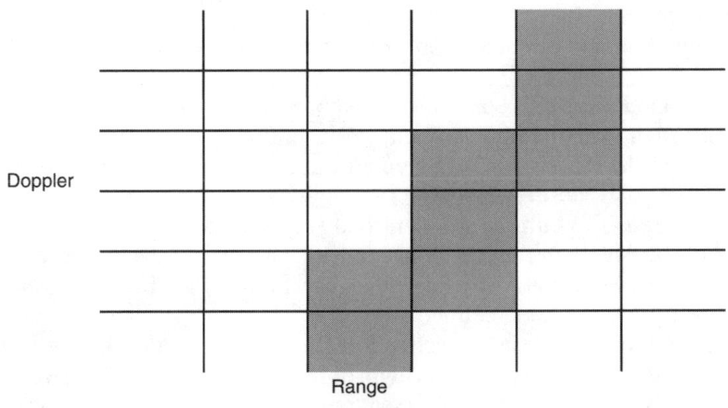

Fig. 22 Bomblet kill range/doppler map.

following: 1) There is very limited actual experience with relevant threats. 2) It is very expensive and complex to test the system. In particular there are difficulties in testing against the actual threat or against simulations with all predicted behaviors and parameters. 3) The threats are continuously developing, including the addition of new capabilities.

As a result, an important phase of the defense process is the postattack debriefing. This phase must include assessment of the success/failure of the mission against each threat and identification of failure causes and "almost" failures where elements of the system functioned incorrectly.

The debriefing process has three main phases, including data collection from all defense system elements, data reduction, and analysis.

Analysis can be performed two times. *Immediate debriefing* is performed to identify failure causes that can be immediately dealt with, using the existing systems and their capabilities. *Long-range debriefing* is performed to provide the required modifications of the existing system or generate requirements to be implemented in new systems. Long-range debriefing can use statistical data from a large number of interceptions to reach conclusions. The best debriefing would provide the failure cause in all cases and recommended solutions in both the long and short term.

The debriefing system is the tool or set of tools that enables the system users (operators, commanders, analysts, and engineers) to identify the causes of system failure and the appropriate responses. Near-real-time debriefing is relevant during a war. It has to identify, as quickly as possible, the success or failure in the handling of each TBM (performing an interception), the reason for the failure, and analysis of the behavior of each subsystem. The system should recommend the quick fixes that will improve the performance of the system, within the capabilities of the system. These will include in most cases changing operating modes or improving the data with which the immediate operational decisions were made. For example, changing the interception altitude in response to new information about the adversary's TBMs or interceptor characteristics.

The amount of relevant data in the case of the ATBM system is very large. The issues are complex and it is not always clear what questions need to be asked to reach the correct conclusions as to the failure cause or recommended action. A semiautomatic analysis tool could provide an important contribution to the debriefing process.

The main elements of such a tool are presented in Fig. 23. These include the following.

1) Failure database: This consists of a list of possible failures and the method of identifying each. The methods are analysis routines to be performed on the data collected from the defense system elements and the required results that indicate the occurrence of a failure.

2) Failure tree: The failures are identified according to more and more in-depth analyses of the events in the intercept process. The structure is a tree where each node is a possible failure. At each stage, the failure identification routine (the required analysis routine) is defined.

3) Analysis tools: Because for each failure the method of identification is defined, a set of data reduction and simulation algorithms is required to perform the analysis.

4) Tree tools: Routines that enable scanning the failure tree, as well as updating the system as more information is collected, are required.

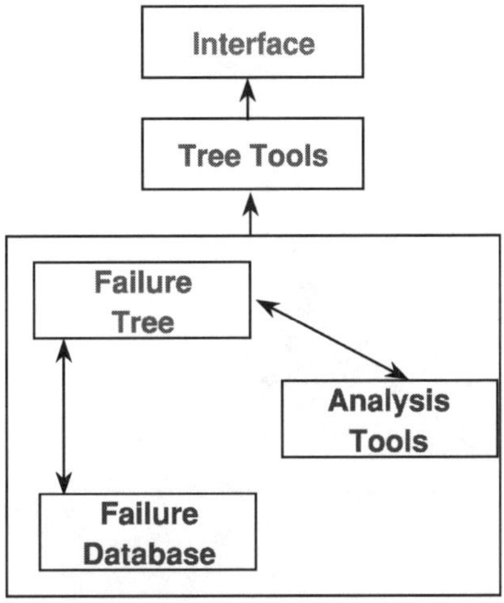

Fig. 23 Debrief system main elements.

The debriefing system includes both human analysts and computerized tools. The division of tasks between human and machine is determined by the capabilities of each. The task of the computerized tools is to serve as memory and processor to store and collate all relevant data, to provide the analysis tools in a form that is simple to operate and gives understandable results, and to perform automatically a set of predefined analyses that focus the area of the problem. The task of the analyst is to identify and analyze new and unknown situations. The systems under discussion are complex and multidisciplinary, making it impossible to predefine or even know all possible relevant phenomena. The analyst's job is to think beyond the understood system parameters and to reach new, imaginative solutions.

Figure 24 presents an operating logic for such a near-real-time-debriefing system. All relevant data about a mission from the sensors, BMC and interceptor (via downlink), together with the results on the ground, enter the automatic system. The automatic system performs a set of analyses that may or may not lead to a conclusion as to the reason why a specific TBM caused damage on the ground. If there is a conclusion, it will be verified by the human operator. An incorrect conclusion or a result of "don't know" requires analysis by the expert human operator. This includes performing additional analyses using the existing tools and data, as well as using tools and data from external sources. If the additional analyses use the existing tools and data, it is possible to "teach" the automatic system the analysis procedure and the conclusion (failure cause), thus increasing the knowledge base for the next interceptor. An inconclusive analysis will result in the data being stored and analyzed at a later time by specific experts using more complex tools.

In the near term, as long as the combat environment is unknown, the knowledge base is very limited. The types of failures that will be identified automatically at the first stage are obvious technical failures (the failure of a specific component in the interceptor or radar) or conflicts between sets of data: the database in the BMC that was used for planning and the actual data (targets, interceptor performance) collected during the actual interception. In addition, the automatic analysis will be

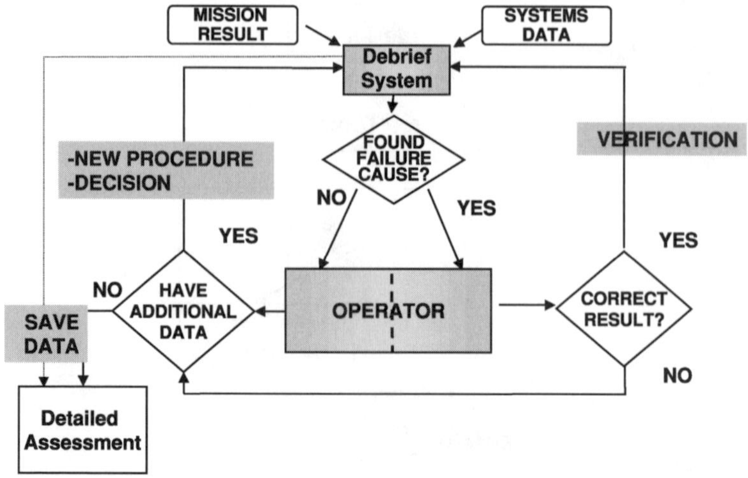

Fig. 24 Debrief system operating logic.

able to identify at what stage the failure occurred, thereby streamlining the work of the human analysts.

With learning capability, it is possible to continuously expand the knowledge base, where the human operator will identify additional failure causes and predefined analysis routines that the automatic system can learn. This process occurs not only during an actual conflict but can also be based on the results of simulations and tests. In this way the system could be more and more useful with time.

V. Defense Process Measures of Performance

The previous sections of this chapter have discussed each phase of the defense process, including the main relevant parameters that need to be considered to perform each phase and the overall interception successfully. To determine the optimal configuration of the defense system, or to assess its contribution within an architecture, it is necessary to define clear measures of performance that summarize the overall performance of all the elements in all the phases.

Single TBM measures of performance include *battlespace*, which is the volume in space in which an interception can be performed successfully, and *footprint*, which is the impact area (of the TBM) on the ground that is defended by the defense system. The main additional measure that is used when assessing a TBM salvo is the defense system *capacity*. This is the number of simultaneous TBM that can be successfully intercepted by the defense system.

A. Battlespace

The battlespace of the defense system is a measure of the performance of a defense system in the intercept volume. It is provided as the probability of kill (P_k) of a single interceptor at each location in space relative to the defense system, where the P_k is the estimated value of the probability of successfully neutralizing the TBM (in particular destroying the warhead). The P_k is the successful culmination of the entire defense process and includes the following probabilities:

$$P_k = P_D \times P_I \times P_P \times P_k \text{ (ROE)}$$

where the subscripts denote the following: D = correct detection, I = correct identification given detection, and P = Planning given identification; additionally, P_k ROE = probability of kill of the executed ROE.

The main parameters that affect each of the probabilities have been discussed before. For a given threat P_D is dependent on sensor deployment and performance parameters. The emphasis in *correct* detection is that it occurs sufficiently early to enable correct defense performance. P_I is the probability to correctly identify the target out of all accompanying closely spaced objects. Sensors (ground and onboard) and analysis capability, as well as available intelligence data, determine the likelihood of success. The time of correct assessment of the attack scenario is also an important parameter that must be matched to interceptor capabilities. P_P is the probability to generate a defense plan in time. This includes both initial planning as well as updates resulting from improved track and discrimination data. P_kROE was described previously as the probability of kill of a given ROE and is a function of SSP_k and kill assessment. This includes the correct functioning of the ground-based sensors and fire control system, as well as the capabilities of the interceptor compared to the capabilities of the TBM. This is also dependent on the kill method of the interceptor and the TBM warhead's payload and structure.

For most defense systems, it is most simple to present the battlespace as the capability in a defined plane (TBM approach, defense system deployment direction). It is important to remember that most systems function differently when the interception occurs outside of the defined plane.

General battlespace maps that identify the boundaries of the defense system's performance and limitations can be generated using simple simulations of all system elements. In this case, the requirements of each element (accuracy, timelines) must be assessed separately. This level of appraisal is useful for architecture evaluation.

Detailed battlespace maps that include sensitivity to various threat performance parameters and defense system distributions can be generated using detailed simulations (six degrees of freedom) of all elements. This is time consuming and highly sensitive to performance assumptions but is usually necessary for a detailed understanding of defense system engineering issues.

B. Footprint

The footprint of the defense system is the ground area that can be defended using the defense system. Each point in a footprint is a specific TBM trajectory. The footprint calculation takes into account the time line of the defense process and the capabilities of all the defense system elements and provides a final result of what can be defended. The footprint summarizes the battlespace relative to the defended assets.

The footprint provides the simplest display of defense system capabilities. It is used both for deployment planning in the initial phases of the defense system life cycle and for defense planning during a battle, where it is used to choose the appropriate defense system to perform an interception. Figure 25 shows an example of a simple coverage footprint.

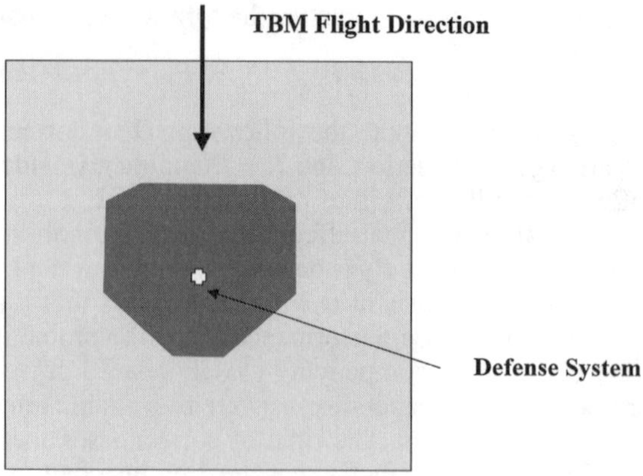

Fig. 25 Simple footprint.

The basic footprint calculation is the time line of the interception process. If detection and accuracy limitations are ignored, the contour of the footprint is the maximum effective coverage provided by the interceptor. Addition of radar detection capability, tracking accuracy, and planning requirements enable the calculation of the coverage provided the entire defense system. Parameters that can be included are radar search patterns, BMC processing time, launch preparation time, and coverage limitations. Interceptor limitations can be included either as P_k (battlespace) in which case the resulting footprint is the maximum P_k achievable per TBM trajectory and/or as specific interception limitations such as sensor coverage requirements, interception angles and velocities or maneuvering capability.

The footprint presentation method can be used to demonstrate system capability in various cross sections. These include the coverage at a given altitude, the coverage of a given ROE (shoot-shoot, shoot-look-shoot), a summary such as maximum intercept altitude for each trajectory or maximum P_k for each trajectory. Figure 26 shows an example of a two-layer footprint.

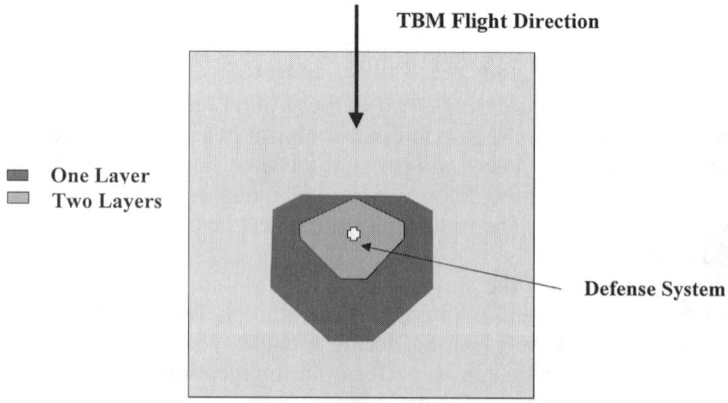

Fig. 26 Two-layer footprint.

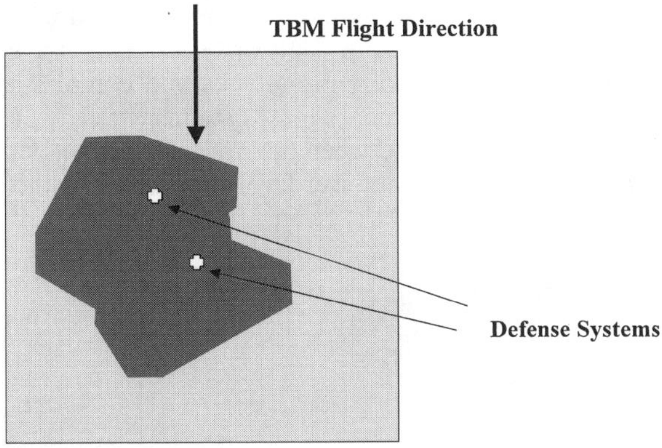

Fig. 27 Architecture footprint.

C. Capacity

Analysis of the performance against a simultaneous attack by a large number of TBMs includes, in addition to the previous measures per each single TBM, the capacity of the defense system. This is the number of TBMs that can be handled successfully in a salvo. Successfully in this case means that each TBM is handled at the required defense level. The parameters that affect this measure include the search and tracking capability of the sensors, the data-handling capability of the BMC, simultaneous interception limitations, and the uniformity of the battlespace that provides flexibility in the location of the interception point.

Capacity assessment provides both the limits of the defense system (number of simultaneous interceptions, number of simultaneous targets) as well as the performance degradation of the process as the number of targets increases. Such a measure is necessary to quantify the impact of resource management capabilities.

D. Expansion of the Measures

We have described the previous measures as they relate to a single deployment of a single defense system. Both footprint and capacity are also used to describe the performance of an entire defense architecture. Figure 27 presents the footprint of an architecture that includes two deployment sites of a defense system. The calculations in this case have to take into account the impact of the interaction between the systems as well as the performance characteristics per system. These include coordination issues such as the time required for coordination, the effect of coordination on BMC capacity, the impact of coordination errors on system capacity, and the effect of the ROE chosen and limitations placed on each defense system (for example limiting a specific system's area of responsibility).

VI. Summary

The purpose of this chapter has been to provide an overview of the TBM defense process, to identify those specific issues that need special consideration, and to present proposed solutions.

The TBM threat is highly energetic and hard to kill. This results in the need for a long-range, high accuracy sensor system and fast, accurate interceptors. The likelihood of massive saturation attacks and complex evolving threats requires intelligent battle management center systems with advanced data processing capabilities. The interaction between the defense system elements is what finally will determine the available defense level provided and the effectiveness of a given system.

III. Interoperability, Battle Management, and Strategic Considerations

Chapter 8

Interoperability Between Defense Systems

Dror Cohen* and Eitan Yariv†
WALES Ltd., Ramat-Gan, Israel

I. Introduction

THE *Dictionary of Military Terms* defines interoperability as "the ability of systems, units or forces to provide services to and accept services from other systems, units or forces and to use the services so exchanged to enable them to operate effectively together".[1] This ability is fundamental to theater missile defense (TMD) systems in particular. The reason for this is twofold.

First, future wars (as already evidenced in current world affairs) are likely to be fought in coalition settings. This means that the forces of two or more nations are likely to participate in countering a common aggressor. A number of nations are developing defense systems and sensors for countering the tactical ballistic missile (TBM) threat, thus the opportunity for interoperability among systems belonging to different coalition partners clearly presents itself.

Second, TBMs are difficult weapons to counter. Systems and sensors currently in operation or under development have partial, often complementary, abilities in countering them. The TBM travels large distances in a relatively short time, and in each phase of its flight presents defense systems with different problems and intercept conditions. A single system cannot hope to cope with the entire range of these conditions, whereas joint operation of a number of systems with different capabilities offers the possibility of improving overall effectiveness.

Being able to operate different systems and sensors jointly, in a smooth manner, is therefore one of the major considerations guiding defense systems planners. Indeed, the U.S. Ballistic Missile Defense Organization (BMDO) has coined the term "family of systems" to describe its commitment to develop systems that will be able to complement each other and work together as a seamless whole. In this chapter, we will take the view of the planner of defense architecture rather than that of the builder of a weapon system. From this point of view, we shall attempt to define and quantify the possible advantages to be gained by interoperation of defense systems and sensors, as well as the pitfalls that should be avoided. We

Copyright © 2000 by the American Institute of Aeronautics and Astronautics, Inc. All rights reserved.

*President. Member AIAA.
†Team Leader, Interoperability, External Cueing, and Concept of Operations. Member AIAA.

shall attempt to link between the level of complexity of the chosen implementation of interoperability and the extent of advantages gained. We will also try to highlight some of the problems that may be encountered in implementing various interoperability features in weapon systems, without stating specific solutions or preferences. As a general guideline, we chose to treat this chapter as a survey of the tradeoffs between the complexity of the adopted implementation, the advantages to be gained, and the potential problems. The reader may than choose an adequate working point, using the guidelines and thought processes outlined in the following sections, bearing in mind the qualities specific to the systems comprising a particular architecture and the anticipated threat.

Finally, because interoperability may be implemented between task forces of different nations, in a coalition setup, a few remarks regarding the operational implementation will be provided. These remarks are intended to highlight the problems involved in the operational application of interoperability and not to offer specific schemes or doctrines. Clearly, the writers' position in a small country, which may become the "host" of interoperating parties in an attempt to defend its own territory (as happened in the 1991 Persian Gulf War), influences our views in this respect, and the reader should take this into consideration and make the necessary adjustments to other possible situations. We chose to limit ourselves in discussing the operational issues relevant to ballistic missile defense (BMD) units and avoid dealing with the more general problem of the integration of BMD units in the overall war effort. Such a discussion would entail treatment of the connection between BMD units and air traffic control, passive defense assets, forward deployed fighting units, etc., which is out of the scope of the present volume.

II. Benefits and Drawbacks of Interoperability

In this section, we will try to define in general terms the major benefits and drawbacks associated with interoperability. Some of these benefits and drawbacks lend themselves easily to quantification and will form the backbone of the discussion throughout the rest of this chapter. Others are more qualitative in nature and are mentioned here for the sake of completeness. Theater- and situation-specific considerations should be applied, in order to properly take these factors in account.

Let us begin with the definition of benefits that may be expected from the application of interoperability. These are as follows (in random order).

Sizing: The most obvious benefit, and probably the easiest to make use of, lies simply in the added firepower that additional weapon systems offer the theater defense planner. However, as will be discussed at length later on, simplistic application of the added firepower may be insufficient for the requirements of the combined defense architecture, and may even lead to the emergence of problematic situations.

Footprint: This is a related benefit to that of added firepower. The addition of defense assets to an existing architecture may either be applied to thicken the defense at a given sector or to widen the borders of the defended region.

Better probability of kill (P_k): The existence of varying interception solutions vs a given TBM allows the selection of an optimal plan, optimizing the defense against the specific threat.

Robustness and mutual backup: Having overlapping assets defending a given region allows better robustness in case of system failure resulting from malfunction, resource overload, or enemy counter measures. This quality is intensified if the interoperating systems have different features (e.g., different radar operating frequencies or different interception altitudes allowing multitiered defense), making it much harder for the enemy to neutralize the combined architecture.

Early warning and external cueing: These benefits result from interoperability with longer range sensors than those of the original defense architecture. They are the subject of a separate chapter, and therefore will not be analyzed at length here.

Dealing with a broader range of threats: Added defense systems may incorporate qualities allowing the combined architecture to deal effectively with threats that could not otherwise be countered.

Support in defense processes: Data from additional sources may assist in the application of defense system algorithmic processes such as discrimination (for example between TBM warhead and separated motor), kill assessment, etc.

Cost effectiveness: Ultimately, the aforementioned advantages of interoperability may be utilized to achieve a more cost-effective defense in a specific theater than would have been achieved through a "monochromatic" architecture, based on only one type of defense system.

The benefits of interoperability do not, however, come without an associated cost. The main pitfalls to be considered are the following.

Complexity: Various applications of interoperability require connecting defense systems through elaborate communication protocols and also defining algorithms and interfaces. All of these factors complicate the structure and operation of the combined architecture as well as that of each of the participating systems.

Errors: This problem is related to complexity. Interoperability processes may induce errors that could otherwise be avoided. Examples include wrong correlation of tracks and wrong interception solutions. The effect of such errors, as well as their causes, will be analyzed in depth in the following sections of this chapter.

Load: Interoperability processes generate large amounts of data to be processed in the participating systems. If the added data are not treated wisely, the data may overflow critical components at certain points in time. An easy example is overflowing defense system radar with external cues because of the inability to correctly correlate tracks from several independent sensors. Another, less obvious example, is when a high-tier interception by one system clutters the sky-picture of a lower tier system with a large amount of debris, at the critical point in time when defense planning (possibly for a different threat) is taking place.

Dependency: Relying on systems that are not under immediate control of the ATBM defense planner to achieve a specific goal is risky because it may be that at the crucial moment these systems will not be made available to perform their assigned role. This may stem from political reasons, in cases where more than one nation is involved, but also from practical considerations regarding theater-specific situations. Examples include dual-use defense systems (e.g., air defense and missile defense, or ballistic missile and cruise missile defense) that may be diverted from their ballistic missile defense role according to the overall war situation.

Cost: Obviously, implementing interoperability between defense systems requires a certain amount of investment, which grows with the complexity of the chosen application. This added cost should be weighed against the expected benefits in overall cost-effectiveness assessments.

III. Levels of Interoperability

Interoperability between defense systems may be described as a continuum of possible connections, on one side of which lies the case of no connection. Each system operates on its own without regard to the existence of the other. On the other side is the case of full integration, where defense planning is done jointly, and each system is capable of using the resources of the others. To effectively analyze this spectrum within reasonable time and space, it is necessary to select a number of representative points along it and analyze each point in more detail. The points we selected are intended to highlight the growing capabilities of the resulting architecture. In each point (termed "level of interoperability") the BMD architecture gains the ability to perform an additional part of the defense process in a joint manner. Obviously, the level of complexity of the implementation increases as well.

The levels of interoperability are defined as follows: *level I*—no computerized connection (coordination may be attempted via voice channels); *level II*—single integrated air-picture achieved via computerized connections, external cueing mechanisms, and threat information sharing algorithms; *level III*—defense plan sharing by computerized means; *level IV*—defense planning/execution by one weapon system using data supplied by the other weapon system; and *level V*—full integration (centralized decision making, control, and guidance of the other system's interceptors).

This broad categorization leaves, of course, some options that do not exactly match any single category. An example is receiving external cueing without attempting to also integrate the sky-picture between the systems. In the sections to follow, we will address each level as containing the breadth of possibilities up to it. In the rest of this chapter, the various levels of interoperability will be analyzed through their influence on the defense process occurring in the combined architecture. The defense process is described in detail in a special chapter. A simplified definition is given below to form the background for the described analysis.

IV. Architecture Defense Process

The defense process starts offline, with the setting of defense goals (e.g., the assets to be defended, allowable leakage threshold), selection of deployment sites for the various elements, and coordination of search sectors and areas of responsibility between the systems comprising the architecture.

The online defense process may be described, using a rough approximation, as consisting of four major stages:

1) The air situation picture (ASP) describes the detection of objects and the classification, association, and maintenance of tracks.

2) Defense planning entails arriving at a suitable interception plan for each TBM deemed threatening to the architecture's area of responsibility. This stage includes coordination of the interception between different systems, if such coordination is required.

3) Interception is the execution of the defense plans arrived at in stage 2.

4) Debriefing concerns analyzing the results of past engagements and drawing conclusions for improving future conduct.

We will now proceed to discuss the effectiveness and implementation techniques of interoperability, in each one of the previously defined levels, at each of these stages.

V. Planning and Deployment

Planning and deployment are the first steps in any BMD operation. The deployment of defense assets is based on consideration of the assets to be defended, the allowable leakage rates, the characteristics of the expected threat, etc. The final outcome of this process is a set of decisions regarding the deployment of each system and sensor, primary target lines (PTLs) of the various sensors, and rules of engagement (ROE).

Interoperability with other systems not originally belonging to the architecture should also be considered in the planning process. The architecture's defense goals, deployment parameters and ROE may be changed according to considerations stemming from the possibility to operate in conjunction with other systems. The impact of interoperability depends on the type of connection (interoperability level) and the characteristics of the systems involved.

Some characteristic considerations may include the addition of a sensor to the architecture, whether as an external cueing source or as a sensor for a particular weapon system, which may influence the deployment of all other sensors in the architecture. A particularly easy-to-implement effect is a change in other sensors' PTLs to affect an optimal use of all sensor resources available.

Another characteristic is that defense goals may be changed because of added firepower (e.g., allowing the defense of otherwise nondefended assets).

If the implementation of the interoperability level selected calls for offline division of engagements (for example, the added system is to be given a separate defense sector), this may affect the deployment of other systems as well.

The level of expertise of the units that will be required to perform the real-time coordination and deconfliction tasks should be taken into consideration, and may cause a change in some units' deployment.

Because these considerations are mostly operational, rather than technical, and depend heavily on the specifics of the theater of operations and the particular defense architecture, they will not be developed here in greater detail. We turn our attention to more general considerations governing the real time operation of the architecture and the implementation of interoperability.

VI. Air Situation Picture

The first stage in the creation of an ASP is detection of objects. The contribution of peer systems to this process, through external cueing, is dealt with in a separate chapter. We shall, therefore, limit ourselves here to the discussion of the stages following detection, namely, classification and association. A special case, presenting more problems to the defense architecture, is that in which a TBM does not appear as a single entity, but is accompanied by related objects (a separating motor, decoys, debris from an earlier interception attempt, etc.). In this case, discrimination of the true target among the variety of objects in the air is also required.

Let us start our discussion in the case where all the objects in the air are legitimate targets for the BMD architecture (i.e. TBMs). The first problem facing the architecture is how to form a single integrated air picture (SIAP) in which each defense system is aware of all the tracks, or at least all the tracks relevant to it, and each system associates a common identifier to each track.

To analyze this issue in more depth, let us define two generic defense systems. The first, designated "system A" is an area defense (higher tier) system. It has a

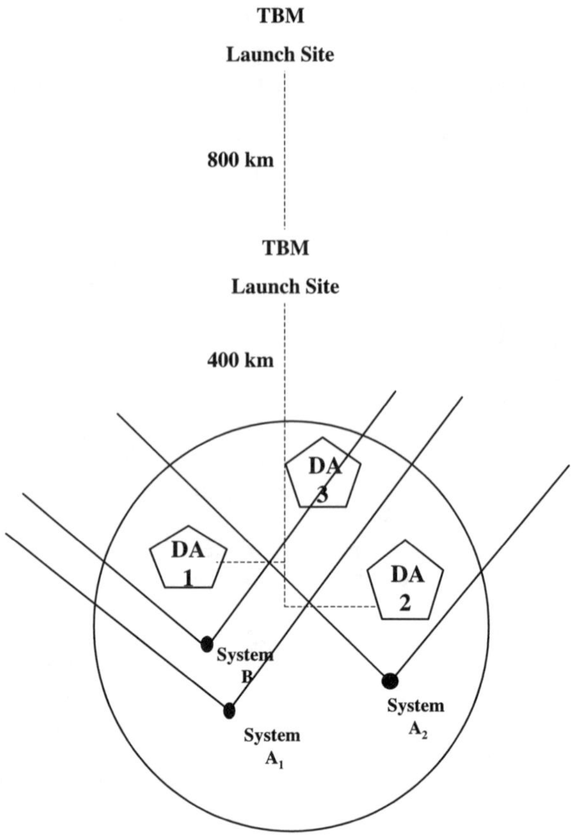

Fig. 1 Defense architecture layout.

radar that is capable of detection of TBMs at 700-km range (for simplicity, we assume a constant detection range). The second system, "system B," is a point defense (lower tier) system, with a detection range of 350 km. Both systems have a detection sector of ±45 deg in azimuth, and 0–85 deg in elevation (for the purpose of SIAP analysis, we need not bother with the definition of the matching interceptors). Our defense architecture is composed of two systems of type A and one system of type B, deployed to defend three defended assets (DAs), as depicted in Fig. 1.

One TBM launch site is located 800 km from the center of DA3. Let us assume a salvo of 30 TBMs, 10 aimed at each DA, according to the time line depicted in Table 1. TBM launches start at the designated time and a 2-s interval is assumed between consecutive launches. A second TBM launch site, capable of firing shorter range TBMs, is located 400 km from the center of DA3. This site will remain dormant in the present example.

Let us now look at the emerging ASP, when no attempt is made to correlate it between the participating defense systems. Figure 2 shows the number of tracks in each system as a function of time. Figure 3 shows the same data, for DA1 only. Looking at these graphs the problem of correct association presents itself clearly.

Table 1 Attack scenario

Time, s	TBM launch
0	Six at DA3 Three at DA2 One at DA1
60	One at DA3 Three at DA2 Six at DA1
120	Three at DA3 Four at DA2 Three at DA1

Each one of the defense systems is "seeing" a different sky-picture. In the case presented, we did not clutter the picture with interceptors, debris, and other objects. However, in real life the picture will be cluttered, and in particular when it comes to the picture observed by system B.

The first task of systems wishing to operate together is to unify the sky-picture. This could be attempted via voice channels (level I interoperability), but this would require extremely adept and well-trained personnel in both systems, and will be limited to relatively sparse attack scenarios.

The other alternative is to create an algorithm dedicated to associating tracks reported through interoperability. This process is called threat information sharing (TIS). A few remarks as to the implications of this process are in order, even before we turn to a discussion of the algorithm itself and its effectiveness.

First, each one of the defense systems involved in the process is routinely performing association tests to compare new tracks (initiated by its own sensors) to

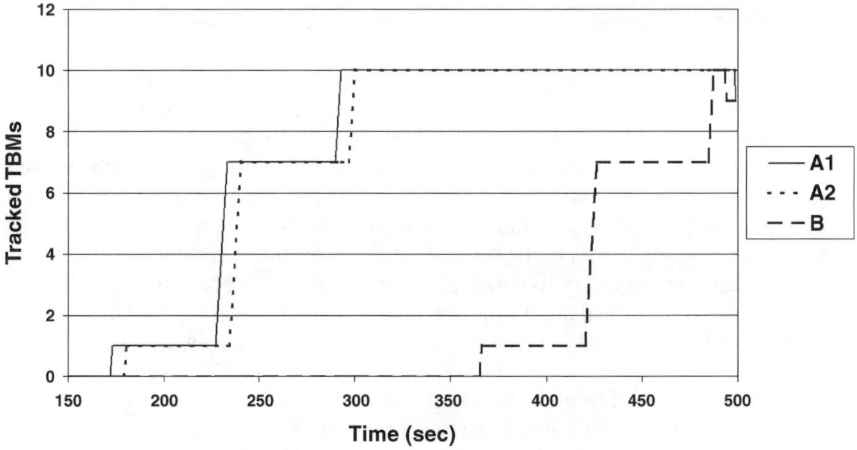

Fig. 2 Number of tracked TBMs vs Time: DA 1, 2, 3.

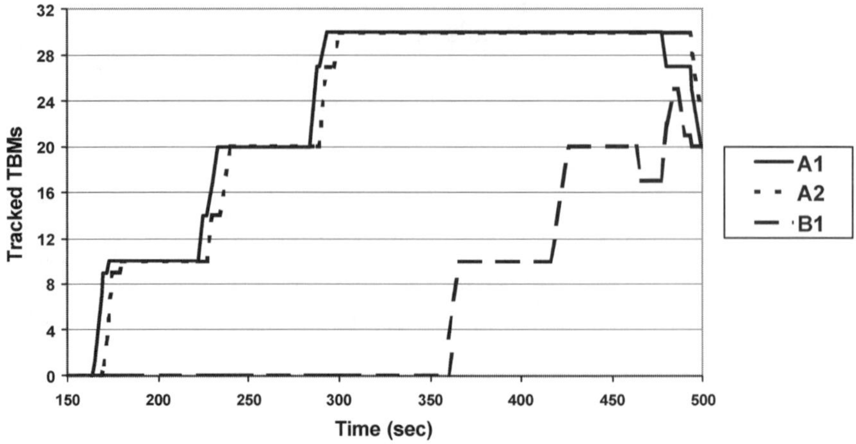

Fig. 3 Number of tracked TBMs vs Time: DA 1.

known system tracks. Problems may arise if the test used in a "joint" TIS process is different from that employed by the system in its regular operation (two tracks may be associated by one of the tests and not associated by the other).

On the other hand, because in the general case one cannot assume that the two systems in question employ identical association techniques (e.g., because they were produced by different countries), a common method—either one of the methods employed by the systems or a third algorithm—should be agreed on. Alternatively, the issue of how to deal with errors stemming from the use of different tests and algorithms, should be dealt with by the joint process.

A third point that should be taken into account is that data supplied by one system will not necessarily be in the same format used by the other. Not all of the data items required may be supplied, update frequencies may vary, and the accuracy of the data may not be known. All of these issues should be dealt with by the TIS algorithm, or regulated through the data link and communication protocol used.

TIS processes have already been defined, developed, and implemented among a number of different systems. The U.S.–developed communication protocols include provision for all the types of data that may be required by such processes. However, we are not aware at the time of this publication of cases where these algorithms were tested under actual battle conditions, against a large number of TBMs and other objects simultaneously in the air. Any such algorithm has the potential for causing errors in the process. It is important to know in advance what sets of conditions are likely to cause these errors and to prepare means by which they may be avoided. We shall now formulate the general processes involved in the TIS algorithm and analyze the causes of errors in the process through a specific example.

The first step in the TIS algorithm is dealing with a new track message provided from the peer system. This step is shown in Fig. 4. The process we are outlining assumes that all of the data relevant for the creation of a track file in the receiving system has been supplied. The receiving system first uses an extrapolation algorithm for each of its own tracks to bring it to a common time with the peer system

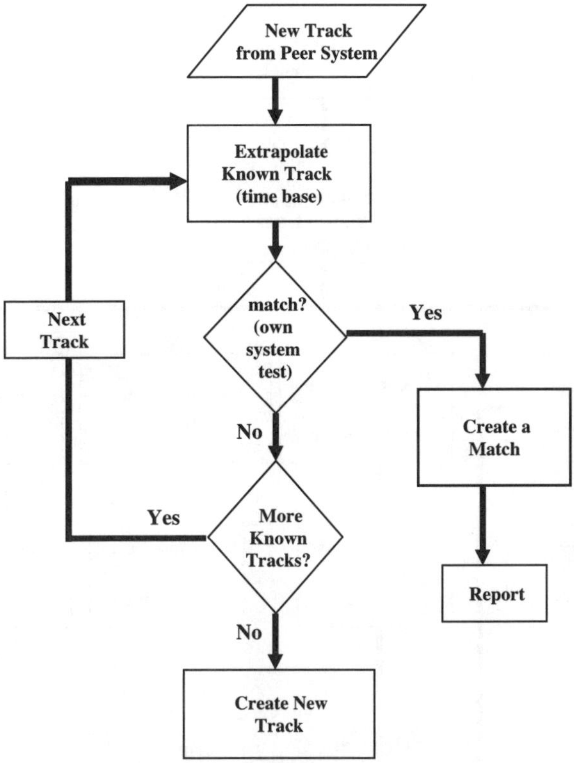

Fig. 4 TIS: dealing with a new track.

report, and then uses its own association test to find whether or not the two tracks are matched. If no match is found, the system creates a new track file.

If the track is, indeed, new, the receiving system may now take a number of steps to acquire it. This process is described in a separate chapter, dealing with external cueing. Therefore, we need not elaborate it at this point in time.

If a match is formed, the system links together the two tracks and issues a report to the sending system. As mentioned earlier, the possibility of a mistaken association should never be neglected. The way to deal with that possibility is to identify any out-of-place matches (in this case, a "new track" that turns out to match an existing track) and resolve the match by reporting and rechecking.

Let us return to the case of a truly new track. The peer system updates the report of the track at regular intervals. At some point in time, the receiving system also picks up the track and a match is achieved. Now, two possibilities exist as to how to treat the data about this track. Each system may choose to use a combination of the tracks and thus attempt to improve the track quality, to rely on the higher quality track, or to choose its own track regardless of the quality of the track provided by the peer system. The implications and possible benefits of these approaches are discussed at length in the chapter on external cueing. One important observation, though, is that to avoid further complication of an already complex procedure, both systems should agree on the same procedure for choosing the data to be used.

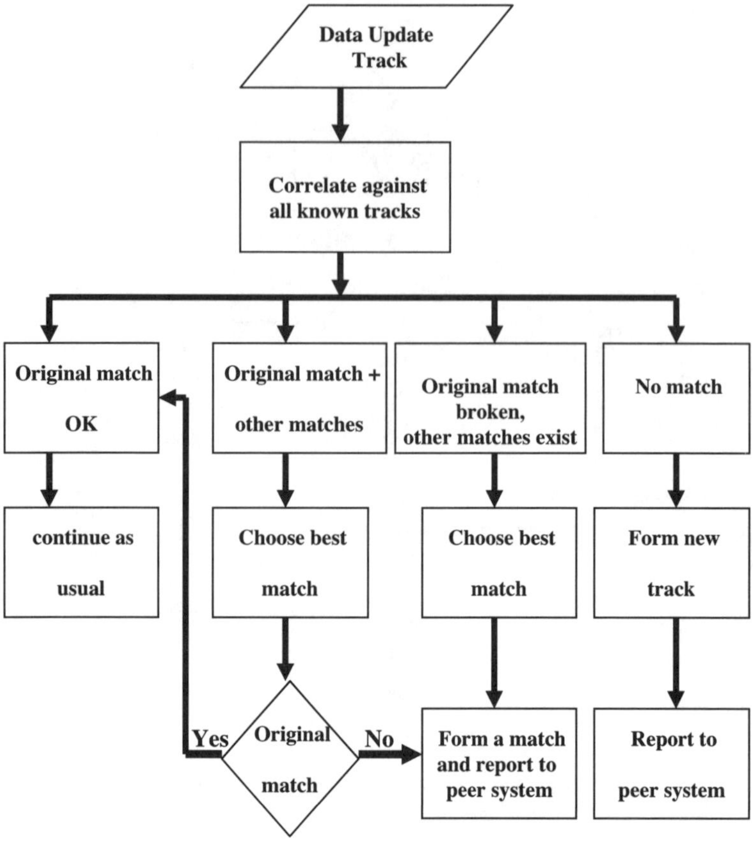

Fig. 5 TIS: update message.

Upon receiving an update to an existing track, no matter if it is provided by the peer system or by own system sensors, a correlation check should be performed to determine if the original match was broken or if another one is formed. Several outcomes are possible from this process, as depicted in Fig. 5: 1) the original match is kept, 2) the original match is kept but another track also matches the updated data, 3) the original match is broken and no existing track matches the updated data, and 4) the original match is broken and one or more new matches are formed. All of these cases except the first, represent anomalies that should be treated in coordination with the other system. In any such case, appropriate precautions should be taken to avoid a process of constantly breaking and reestablishing matches (e.g., not declaring a break of a match before several consecutive updates indicate it, and setting appropriate thresholds for association tests).

Two further comments need to be made about the nature of the TIS process, before we turn to analyzing its effectiveness. First, the process of resolving conflicts between the ASP observed by the interoperating systems has to include a method for taking preference in case an agreed upon match is not achieved. Such a mechanism may choose to prefer the system that first reported the TBM, the one reporting higher track accuracy, the one in whose area of responsibility the TBM is supposed to hit ground, etc.

Second, an important aspect of the TIS algorithm is to unify the track identifier presented to the human operator in both systems. This requirement has several reasons, the most important of which is that interception coordination (see also in the next section) is a process that will either be conducted by human operators, or at least monitored and approved by them. Human-in-the-loop experiments conducted in the Israeli test bed simulation facility showed that the existence or lack of a unified sky-picture is the single most important factor affecting the quality of coordination between weapon systems. When dealing with unifying the sky-picture as seen by the human operator, one should keep in mind that changes in the displayed track number influence negatively the performance of the operator. It is, therefore, recommended to separate the internal track number (which may change as a result of association problems) from the displayed track number, which should remain constant. Conflicts occurring in the TIS process should also be presented to the operator.

The effectiveness of the TIS process is highly affected by the performance of the association test employed by each system, and by the inherent qualities of the sensors used. To see this, let us return to the example presented in Fig. 1. We will now look more closely at a small part of the attack scenario—two consecutive TBMs launched at DA3. We will concern ourselves only with the two area defense systems, A1 and A2. Because these are identical systems, we assume that they use the same association test. Our aim is to show what type of conditions cause such an association test to fail, creating a situation where two different TBM tracks may be processed as one, or vice versa.

The association test we chose to implement for this example is the χ^2 test. The χ^2 statistic is applied to the difference between the two state vectors in position and velocity. If we designate ΔX as the difference along the X axis between the two vectors, ΔV_X as the difference in the velocity along the X axis, and likewise σX as the standard deviation in X, etc., then χ^2 is calculated by

$$\chi^2 = \frac{(\Delta X)^2}{(\sigma_x)^2} + \frac{(\Delta Y)^2}{(\sigma_Y)^2} + \cdots + \frac{(\Delta V_x)^2}{(\sigma V_x)^2} + \cdots + \frac{\Delta X \Delta V_x}{\sigma (X V_x)^2} + \cdots \tag{1}$$

The χ^2 statistic is applied on the Cartesian state vectors (x,y,z,v_x,v_y,v_z) containing each radar's measurements. A value of $\chi^2 > 12.6$ indicates a 95% confidence that the two objects tracked are different.[2]

Let us look now at two TBMs as already described, launched at exactly the same time, and let us assume they are separated by a certain distance X (one case) or 5.5 X (second case) along the X axis. Figure 6 shows the χ^2 in both cases. As can be seen from the graphs, the test achieves clear discrimination when the two TBMs are widely spaced, but fails to separate them when the distance between the launch points is only X meters. Figure 7 shows the same analysis for two TBMs launched from exactly the same location, but with a time difference. The graph shows that the test fails only in cases of a very small separation $\mathrm{d}t$.

These two generic examples point to the fact that closely spaced objects in time and/or space may mislead the TIS algorithm. The actual conditions under which a separation test is misled will depend on the nature of the test itself and the qualities, in particular in terms of the signal to noise ratio S/N, of the participating radars. Analysis of the type shown in Figs. 6 and 7 should be conducted in advance so

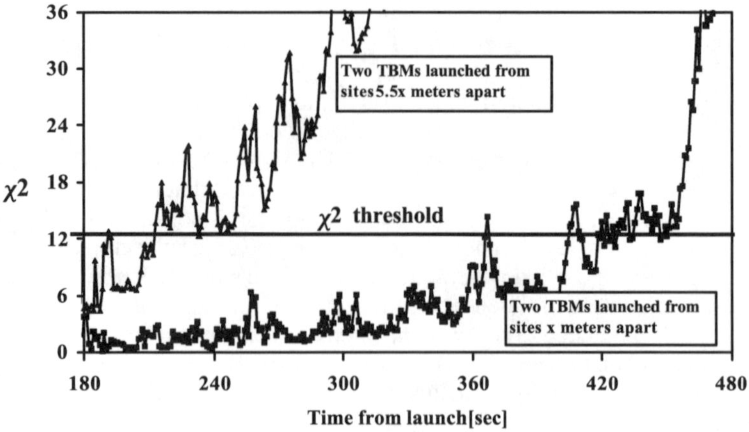

Fig. 6 **χ^2 Analysis launch location difference.**

that the limitations of the particular implementation chosen are well understood. Before leaving the χ^2 example, let us explore one more point, which was only briefly mentioned earlier. The issue is that of not knowing exactly what is the quality of the track provided by the peer system. In particular, the biases involved in the tracking of the other system may not be known. A quasi-linear model was used to simulate biases. The model is summarized by the following formula[3]:

$$\delta R = c_R \tag{2}$$

$$\delta A = c_1 \tan(E)\sin(A - c_2) + c_3 \tan(E) + \frac{c_4}{\cos(E)} + c_5 \sin(A - c_6) + c_7 \tag{3}$$

$$\delta E = c_1 \cos(A - c_2) + c_8 \cos(E) + c_9 \sin(E - c_{10}) + c_{11} \tag{4}$$

where A and E are the azimuth and elevation as measured by the radar; δR, δA, δE

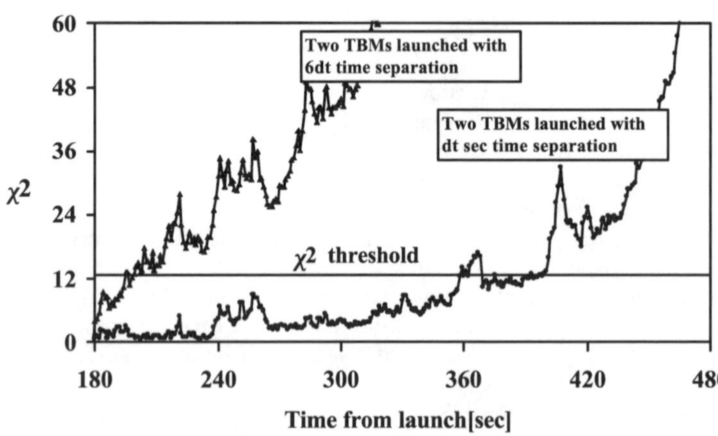

Fig. 7 **χ^2 Analysis: launch time difference.**

Table 2 Bias model coefficients

Notation	Error
c_1	Leveling error amplitude
c_2	Leveling error phase
c_3	Orthogonality error
c_4	Colimation error
c_5	Azimuth eccentricity error amplitude
c_6	Azimuth eccentricity error phase
c_7	Azimuth offset
c_8	Droop
c_9	Elevation eccentricity error amplitude
c_{10}	Elevation eccentricity error phase
c_{11}	Elevation offset
c_R	Range measurement error

are the biases in range, azimuth, and elevation; and the coefficients represent different errors according to Table 2.

Figure 8 presents a case where a single TBM is viewed by the radar of systems $A1$ and $A2$. $A1$ has no bias, but $A2$ reports are corrupted by severe biases. The result is that up to 240 s before impact, the TBM is regarded as two separate objects. This phenomenon has severe implications, which may include waste of resources (cueing A1's radar, for example), and may even lead to unnecessary launch of interceptors. To solve this problem, we use the fact that the development of the difference between the vectors in time is much less sensitive to biased measurements (because they are nullified by the subtraction) than the original state vectors.

We turn, therefore, to test the time derivative of $\chi^2 - \mathrm{d}\chi^2/\mathrm{d}t$. In Fig. 9 the results of $\mathrm{d}\chi^2/\mathrm{d}t$ are shown for the same measurements that were used for Fig. 8. The result is a clear indication that there is only one object in the sky.

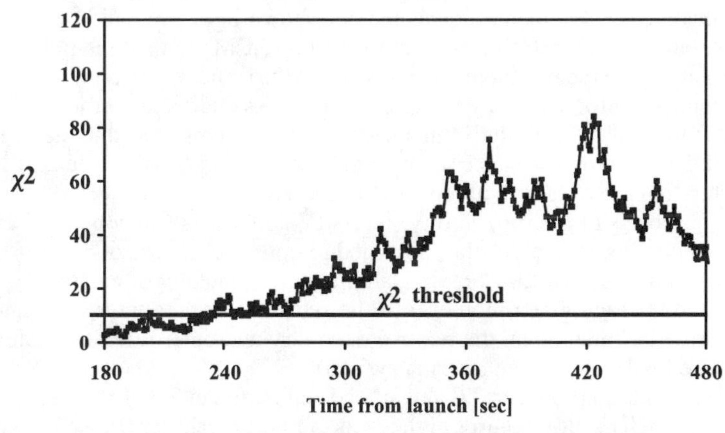

Fig. 8 χ^2 Analysis: one TBM in presence of severe bias.

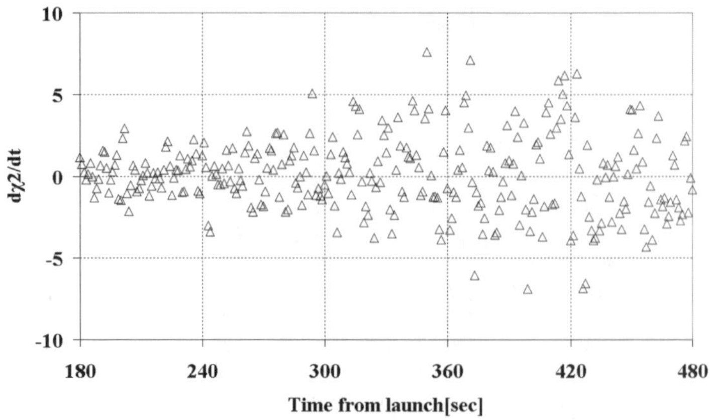

Fig. 9 Time derivative of χ^2: severe bias.

Because the nature of the peer system with which interoperability will be practiced, and the conditions under which it will have to function, are not known in advance, the planners of TIS algorithms should apply considerations akin to those outlined previously to arrive at association tests that are as robust as possible to biases, and to other system errors (e.g., false alarms).

Up to now, we explored the need for SIAP via automatic TIS algorithms, as a cornerstone for interoperability of level II and above. However, it should also be noted that SIAP contains, by itself, several possible advantages, even when it is not considered as part of the coordination of interceptions. The possible uses and advantages of these procedures include the following.

1) External cueing. A separate chapter in this book is dedicated to cueing and its implications.

2) Robustness. Correlating and integrating the sky-picture between two or more systems carries the advantage of being less sensitive to problems in any one of the sensors involved. Phenomena such as the one shown in Fig. 8 could be attributed to biases, but also to electronic counter measures (ECM) against the radar of A2. If, for example, the radar systems do not work at the same wavelength, it becomes almost impossible for an enemy to block both at the same sector at the same time. The SIAP formed by TIS algorithms serves both systems, and thus negates the effects of degraded performance in any single sensor and adds redundancy to the architecture in case of failure of any one of the sensors.

3) Higher levels of interoperability (levels IV and V). TIS may be used as part of a more complex joint algorithm designed to optimize the use of radar or other sensors resources across the complete architecture. Tracking of each object may be entrusted (at each given moment) to the sensor(s) best equipped to handle it at that particular time, given the relative geometry and other relevant parameters (such as the load experienced by each system).

4) Discrimination (between TBM warhead and motor, or TBM and decoys) and kill assessment. This use requires high levels of interoperability (IV or V) because of the strict accuracy and time line requirements involved in these processes.

VII. Interception Coordination

Following the creation and understanding of the sky-picture, the next stage in the defense process is defense planning. In this stage a specific plan of interception, for each TBM threatening the designated defended assets (DAs) is to be reached. The defense plan (DP) consists of a combination of tracking and firing entities (radar and fire units) and their activation time. If more than one planning entity (e.g. battle management center) is included in the architecture, then deconfliction, or coordination, of the interception has to take place. This is also the case where interoperability with systems outside the architecture is concerned.

Let us return now to the attack scenario example defined in Table 1. Assuming that no effort was made to coordinate the interceptions between the defense systems, and that each system launches one interceptor vs any TBM threatening a DA in its footprint, this 30 TBM scenario would result in a launch of 50 (assuming system B does not defend DA3) to 60 (in case it does) interceptors. This, when in theory 30 interceptors would suffice to provide an adequate level of defense (assuming that one interceptor per TBM is enough to provide the required level of defense). This high ratio of interceptors/TBMs is clearly unacceptable. At the very least, it is unacceptable not to be able to influence it when the need arises. Obviously, in almost any situation involving the deployment of several weapon systems, coordination of the interception tasks will offer considerable benefits.

Coordination of interceptions can take place at any of the previously-defined levels of interoperability. It can take the form of drawing a clear dividing line between the areas of responsibility of any two systems and then act according to that division at each system (level I interoperability), or of actively performing coordination of each TBM answering to specific characteristics either by voice (level II interoperability) or via computerized algorithms (level III). It may even take the form of a dual-system defense plan in which a lower tier system serves as a second layer to an upper tier one (levels III–IV). The most extreme version may take the form of central planning of interceptions, drawing upon a "bank" of available resources from the involved systems (level V). We will discuss each of these options in turn, focusing most of the analysis on verbal and computerized coordination, as these are, from our point of view, the more probable versions to be actually implemented in the field.

A. Offline Coordination

The simplest way to perform interception coordination is, obviously, to do it offline, in advance. The defense systems may divide the responsibility among them according to defended assets or TBM launch sites/countries. Another option is to allow, as a rule, the first system that has a DP to engage the target and halt the engagement process in the other system (this procedure is frequently described as a "shoot and shout" policy). These solutions have the benefit of not requiring real-time coordination and the complex processes involved in it. However, they entail several major drawbacks:

1) Sometimes, as in the case of system A1 and system B in our example, it is simply impossible. This situation, in which a point defense (lower tier) system will be deployed inside the area of responsibility of an area defense (higher tier) system, is a very probable one in real deployment.

2) Defense systems vary in their capabilities. System B for example, which is a less capable, smaller footprint system than system A, may not be able to defend against longer range, faster TBMs, although it may perform as well as, or even better than, system A against shorter range TBMs. Dividing responsibility according to simplistic area division may thus lead to a situation in which the provided defense is not adequate.

3) Also, one should keep in mind that the information about a track is different in different systems. Some factors, such as the nature of the (suspected) TBM warhead, or even the type of TBM, may be calculated (or derived from intelligence information) by one system and not known in the other. These factors, although they may be important for differentiating between the two systems' ability to intercept a specific threat, cannot be used for a priori differentiation, but only in real time, during an actual engagement.

4) Finally, this type of "offline coordination" fails to provide a lot of the benefits already described, which an architecture planner would like to achieve through interoperability. Having two systems capable of defending a common region allows for mutual backup, alleviating load problems from any single system and optimizing the defense on a track to track basis or for a whole TBM salvo. All of these benefits cannot be achieved using offline, strict division of labor.

For the reasons just outlined, we consider coordination by offline decisions as an inferior option to real-time coordination.

B. Real-Time Coordination

Real-time coordination may be achieved at various levels of interoperability. It may be applied by voice channels (level II), or by automatic defense plan sharing (DPS) algorithms (levels III and above). In the following discussion, we will attempt to identify the major issues affecting defense coordination, and also demonstrate its effectiveness in various situations. Finally, we will discuss the causes and effects of coordination errors, and possible ways to avoid them.

C. Time Line for Coordination

The first issue to be considered regarding defense plan coordination at all levels is that of the available time. To understand this problem more clearly, and to get a hint of its magnitude, let us return to our ongoing example from Fig. 1.

Because we are now dealing with the interception of TBMs, we have to introduce into the example the qualities of the defense planning process. As we are only interested in this chapter in the effects of the coordination between the systems, we will allow ourselves to use a very simplistic model for these qualities.

In our model the interceptors of both systems are flying a straight line to a chosen interception point, at a constant velocity. The boundaries of the available battlespace for each system are fixed in range and altitude. For the moment, we will not bother with the interceptor's P_k. The only defense planning parameter that we introduce is a requirement that the TBM be tracked for a certain period of time before a defense plan can be produced. The parameters of the two types of defense systems are presented in Table 3. These numbers do not represent any known defense system. However, they are representative numbers that may be used to draw initial conclusions, relevant to the actual situations an architecture planner might encounter.

Table 3 Defense systems characteristics (example)

System type	Interceptor velocity, m/s	Interception altitude, km Min	Interception altitude, km Max	Interception range, km Min	Interception range, km Max	Required tracking time, s
A	1500	20	100	5	300	45
B	1200	5	30	5	50	15

Let us now define what we mean by "the time for coordination." To do this, let us look at Fig. 10. In this figure, a TBM is launched at time t_0, and is supposed to hit ground at the attacked target at time t_{end}. The first system to detect the TBM, system 1, detects it at t_1; this system takes n_1 s to plan a DP, which is ready at time t_3. The DP of system 1 has to be executed at t_{11}. Meanwhile, a second system (system 2) detects the TBM at time t_2. This system now takes n_2 s to plan a DP of its own, at time t_4. The time available for coordination between the two systems is the time between t_4 (system 2 knows whether it can intercept this TBM and with what parameters) and t_{11} (system 1 has to activate its DP). In other words,

$$t_{\mathrm{co}} = t_{11} - t_4 \tag{5}$$

where t_{co} is the time for coordination.

Clearly, the more time given for coordination, the better. As can easily be seen from Eq. (5), the only way that the systems involved in the process can influence the time available (other than using external cueing to achieve earlier detection), is by changing t_{11} (t_2 is determined by the radar qualities and the TBM trajectory,

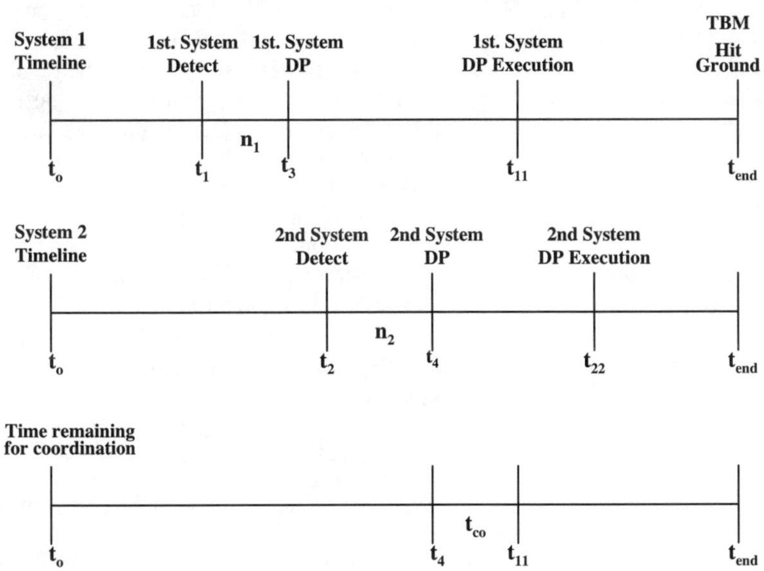

Fig. 10 Time for coordination.

Table 4 Time for coordination: "A" intercepts at highest altitude

TBM range, km	Time for coordination, s B-A1	B-A2	A1-A2
400	87	72	155
800	16	−1	155

and n_2 is a system parameter). Time t_{11} is affected, of course, by t_1 and n_2, which cannot be changed. However, it is also affected by the choice of interception point. In our simple example, t_{11} is directly proportional to the altitude of interception because if the interception is to take place at altitude $\boldsymbol{a}$ and range $\boldsymbol{r}$ (from the launcher), then

$$t_{11} = \frac{\sqrt{\boldsymbol{a}^2 + \boldsymbol{r}^2}}{V_{\text{interceptor}}} \tag{6}$$

where $\boldsymbol{a}$ and $\boldsymbol{r}$ are related through the TBM trajectory. This relation between the interceptor launch time and the chosen interception altitude may be used to maximize the available time for coordination, by choosing the lowest possible interception altitude.

Let us look at the concrete example of our three systems: A1, A2, and B. Clearly, since A1 and A2 are identical systems, they detect the TBMs at nearly the same time, and the time to coordinate is almost identical to the time from end of defense planning to interceptor launch in any one of the systems. The situation is drastically different between any one of the A-type systems and system B, because of the large differences in detection and interception envelope. For this example, a 800 km TBM and a 400 km TBM were launched to DA1, and the time available for coordination was calculated for each pair of defense systems. The results are presented in Tables 4 and 5. In Table 4, the A systems plan to provide defense at the highest possible altitude. In Table 5, A systems plan for the lowest altitude (20 km) to allow the maximum time for coordination. System B detects TBMs at the 350-km range, and then plans a DP based on the parameters in Table 3.

Looking at these tables, a few observations can be made:

1) Although the time available for coordination between the area defense systems is adequate, the time for coordination between point defense (lower tier) and area defense (higher tier) systems may be expected to be extremely short. This effect

Table 5 Time for coordination: "A" intercepts at lowest altitude

TBM range, km	Time for coordination, s B-A1	B-A2	A1-A2
400	179	156	230
800	88	66	221

grows in magnitude for longer range, fast TBMs. In some deployments, there may be negative time for coordination (one system has to launch an interceptor before the other picked up the target).

2) The relative deployment geometry between the coordinating systems and the attacked asset affects the interception solution (DP) adopted by each system, and thus the resulting time for coordination. In our example, we chose a relatively small deployment area. However, in real life the deployment area may be much larger. An example is the case where one of the systems is a naval system, which has to deploy at a safe distance from the shore.

3) Lowering the interception altitude increases the time available for coordination. However, one must keep in mind that this practice is detrimental from the point of view of defense quality. For most systems, going to lower altitude means a loss of P_k, and the ability to perform shoot-look-shoot processes is sometimes lost, as well as the ability to compensate for any unexpected problems during the interception process.

The question of how to conduct the coordination of interceptions—by voice or by computerized process—now becomes a question of the nature of the defense systems performing the coordination, the chosen deployment, and the expected threat. For humans to conduct verbal coordination, tens of seconds are required. This means that if only voice coordination is available, the defense planner must use a mix of predefined rules of engagement, and various means to increase the available time such as lowering interception altitude, cueing the lower tier system, or attempting to predict its ability to intercept a given TBM before it has actually detected it. One should also keep in mind that verbal coordination entails other problems, mostly concerning the operation of the human-operator in the coordination loop. Problems relating to language barriers, different conceptions of defense plan quality, different command structure, and even the simple fact that the two systems do not display the same set of data items to their operators, have to be discussed and resolved before such a solution can be considered.

D. Methods for Interception Coordination

Whether the coordination of interceptions is to be conducted verbally by the defense systems operators, or via a computerized algorithm, the most important issue to be resolved in defining the coordination procedure is to select the most important parameters of the defense plan and the defense system status to be compared during the coordination. Obviously, verbal coordination allows fewer parameters to be compared, whereas computerized algorithms are almost limitless in the number of parameters available. However, even when a computerized algorithm is considered, it pays to keep the number of compared parameters to the minimum required for effective coordination. There are a number of reasons for wanting to impose such a constraint:

First, the higher the number of compared parameters, the more complex is the resulting algorithm. Although this allows for more control over the resulting defense plan, thus enhancing its optimality, it also creates very complex comparison mechanisms and more opportunities for errors in the process. (A more thorough discussion of coordination errors is provided later on in this chapter.)

Second, current communication protocols allow for automatic transfer of only a few of the parameters associated with a defense plan. It is possible to design and implement special links and protocols, but the outcome has to be weighed in terms of improvement over what can be achieved using a smaller number of parameters.

Third, in planning coordination algorithms to be implemented in any defense system, one should keep in mind that the partner system for interoperability is not necessarily decided on in advance. This is especially true for systems that are planned to be deployed for defense of forward-deployed troops or as part of a coalition in different theaters. Not all of the defense systems with which interoperability may be enacted use the same parameters for building and evaluating defense plans. Thus, using many parameters as part of the coordination algorithm may increase its theoretical effectiveness, while at the same time harming its real world usefulness.

In this section we will try to quantify the contribution of various methods of coordination to the results achieved by the antitactical ballistic missile architecture. We will focus the discussion on coordination using three parameters, which we consider to be the most important for defense planning.

1) *Probability of kill* (P_k): This parameter (together with the number of interceptors to be used) indicates the quality of the defense plan as a singe entity (without taking into account cumulative effects of any kind). Other parameters could also be taken as representing DP quality (e.g., interception altitude, maneuverability ratio) but we believe this is the most representative.

2) *Inventory:* The number of remaining interceptors at the time of planning is reflected here. This number gives no indication of DP quality, but is indicative of the possibility of future problems the defense system may face through interceptor shortage.

3) *Load on defense system assets (mainly the radar):* This number gives an indication of possible problems that the defense plan may face when the time to execute it arrives. The more loaded the system, the more chances that the interceptor launch will be delayed, or even cancelled, because of the need to perform higher priority tasks (e.g., interception of TBMs aimed at higher priority DAs). In this chapter we will be using the immediate load at planning time as an indicator. It is possible to perform a prediction of expected load at the time designated for interceptor launch, either using the data available in the system itself, or using external cue data, information regarding future events. It remains to be seen whether these more complex considerations are justified in the context of coordination between weapon systems. (For more information on these topics, the reader is referred to Chapter 9.)

As can be seen from these definitions, the parameters to be compared describe different aspects of defense system operation. Because of that, they are seen as complementary, allowing for maximal added value of each one to the overall defense effectiveness.

To quantify the contribution of each of these parameters to the effectiveness of the coordination function, we return now to the example presented in Fig. 1. We will deal in the following examples only with coordination between the two area defense systems, A1 and A2. Notice that for A1 and A2, the defended space may be divided into three subareas 1) S_1, which includes DA1, where only A1 can provide defense (disregard, for this example, system B), 2) S_2, which includes DA2, where only A2, can provide defense, and 3) S_{12}, which includes DA3, where both systems can provide defense. This quality will have an important role in our example. (The fact that such a division is possible is trivial. The fact that each subarea contains

Table 6 Reference P_k table (example)

Defense system	DA	TBM range 400 km	800 km
A1	1	0.86	0.84
	2	0	0
	3	0.83	0.78
A2	1	0	0
	2	0.86	0.84
	3	0.85	0.8

exactly one defended asset, which is separated from the other DAs, is a simplifying assumption). Furthermore, we will make another simplifying assumption: TBMs are only fired at the designated assets. That is to say, no TBM is fired at a point that lies between the designated DAs, and no TBM misses its intended target (through statistical dispersions and CEP). We will now introduce P_k values for our two defense systems, to be used while coordinating the defense. Table 6 presents P_k for each system against TBMs of the two types presented earlier, in defense of each of the three DAs. Notice that while the two systems are identical, P_k for each asset is different. Also notice that we assign to each system zero P_k in the domain of responsibility of the other. The P_k given by the table is the single shot probability of kill (SSP_k).

The scenario consisted of 30 TBMs of 400 km range, and 30 TBMs of 800 km range. Out of these 60 TBMs, 40 were aimed at DA3 (the asset over which coordination is performed) and the other 20 were evenly divided between DA1 and DA2. Let us look now at the effect of various methods of coordination on the results achieved by the combined architecture vs this attack scenario.

Figure 11 shows the number of leakers suffered by the architecture as a function of the initial interceptor inventory in each system (the number of interceptors is identical in both systems). Two graphs are shown. In the first graph, no coordination was conducted. Each system fired at each TBM, provided it had a nonzero P_k, until no more interceptors remained. In the second graph, coordination by P_k was

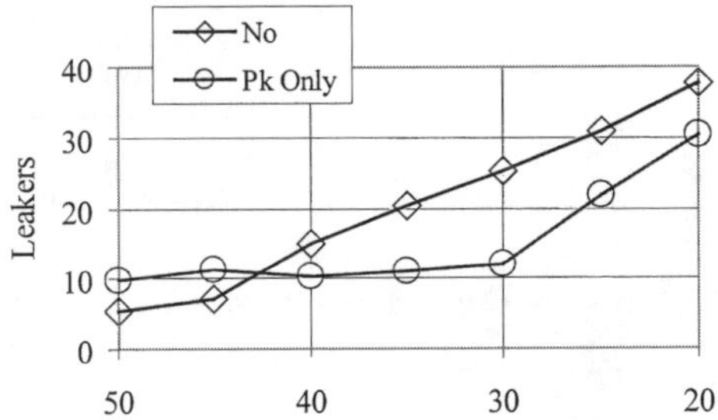

Fig. 11 Coordination by P_k vs "no coordination."

conducted on the TBMs aimed at DA3. The system with higher P_k was chosen, unless it was out of interceptors.

When the architecture has a large number of interceptors (on the left side of the chart) we can see that the results (expressed by the number of leakers) are better if no coordination at all is performed. This is simply because the P_k for each interception over DA3 is improved (two interceptors instead of one). However, this is achieved at a price of launching 100 interceptors (both systems fire at the 40 TBMs aimed at S_{12}, and 20 TBMs are intercepted by one system only) instead of 60 in the case that coordination is performed.

As we move to the right of this figure the results of the "no coordination" case deteriorate quickly, because the interceptors are depleted before the end of the attack. The coordination by P_k scheme, on the other hand, achieves almost constant results until the point where there are fewer interceptors than TBMs, and only then its performance is degraded. These results show clearly the benefits that the architecture may derive from even the crudest form of coordination. The resulting architecture performs in a much more robust fashion, enabling the defended nation to counter different attack plans and scenarios. However, there is also another way of looking at this graph. If we subtract one line from the other we can immediately get the maximal benefit of interoperability, expressed in terms of consumed interceptors. There is a tradeoff between acquiring more interceptors and conducting interoperability, and there is a limit to the investment that should be made in interoperability. Sometimes, the "rich man's solution" of simply adding more firepower, can turn out to be less costly. Our simple example is, of course, too crude to be used as a "meter" for studying the cost-effectiveness of various forms of interoperability. Cost-effectiveness considerations should be applied on the basis of intimate knowledge of the two systems to be connected, as well as a detailed description (as much as possible) of the foreseen threat.

Let us now add to our example another form of coordination. This time the systems coordinate according to the immediate inventory; i.e., the system with more available interceptors is the one to fire. The results of this form of coordination appear in Fig. 12, in addition to the "no coordination" and "coordination by P_k" cases. Looking at this graph, a few observations can be made:

First, the major gain from interoperability between the systems is achieved by the mere fact that coordination is enacted. The actual parameter by which coordination is conducted is less important. Second, the "obvious" parameter for judging the

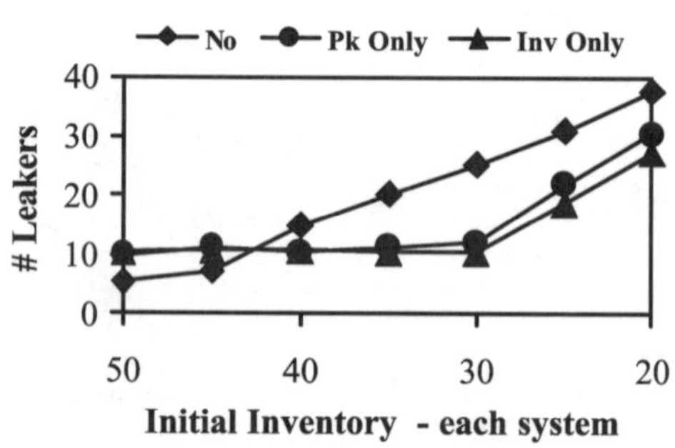

Fig. 12 Coordination by inventory.

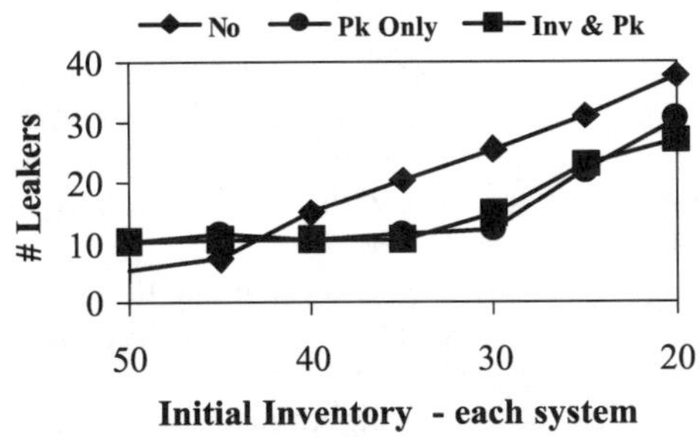

Fig. 13 Coordination by P_k and inventory.

quality of defense plans is not always the best. In this example, where the system's P_k values are close one to the other, coordination by inventory manages to achieve the same level of performance as coordination by P_k, and it is even slightly more robust toward the right side of the chart, where inventory levels are low. This occurs because coordination by P_k only may cause situations in which one system becomes short of interceptors, whereas the other still has a sufficient number. If TBMs are launched to the area where only the first system can engage, the result will be a large number of leakers.

To gain the best of both worlds, a combined coordination rule is introduced and plotted in Fig. 13 alongside the "no coordination" and "coordination by P_k" graphs. In this mode or coordination, the system with more interceptors launches, unless its P_k is lower than a predefined threshold value (in our example -0.79). The results indicate, again, achievement of equivalent level of performance to that of coordination by P_k only, but in a more robust manner.

There are, of course, many other parameters that may be considered as candidates for supplying a basis for coordination between defense systems. The most important one, in our view, is the load experienced by each system. The load on the system could be taken as the instantaneous load at the time of defense planning, or, using external cue data, predicted load at the time designated for interceptor launch. (For further discussion of this topic see Chapter 9.) Load may be factored into the coordination procedure using a threshold mechanism similar in nature to the one already introduced for inventory and P_k coordination.

E. Coordination Errors

Although coordination between defense systems offers many advantages, as was already shown, it also entails a few problems. An obvious problem is that of the cost of implementation and the added complexity of operation, as well as the timing problems already mentioned. Another problem associated with coordination, which we would like now to highlight, is that of coordination errors.

Conducting real-time coordination of interceptions between two or more weapon systems inevitably leads to a certain number of errors. We shall first discuss some of the reasons that errors occur in the coordination process, and then we will proceed to classify them into separate groups and evaluate the impact of various error types on the performance of the combined architecture. Errors in the coordination process stem from several different sources.

1) The actual sky-picture. As discussed earlier, closely spaced objects may induce mistakes in TIS processes, which form the backbone of any computerized coordination algorithm. Obviously, the same closely spaced objects also may confuse the human operators engaged in verbal coordination. Other forms of problems associated with the actual sky-picture, such as decoys, remnants, or ECM, will have a similar effect.

2) The computerized models involved also contain the potential for errors. None of the algorithms employed by any of the systems is immune to problems. Nevertheless, the main problem is associated with different systems employing slightly different measures, parameters, and weighing functions. The interpretation of the various parameters exchanged may be different, and some parameters needed by one system in defense planning may not be considered at all by the other. Errors will generally increase with the complexity of the chosen algorithms.

3) Human operators in the two systems are not necessarily thinking in the same terms. In the general case, they may not even be speaking the same language. The goals of the defense architecture, as well as its ROE and CSOP (combined standing operating procedures), may not be fully agreed upon in advance, especially in cases where defense is conducted by a multinational architecture.

4) Last, but not least, is the time line issue, which we discussed earlier in this chapter. Interoperability errors are one of the manifestations of this problem. In this respect, it is also important to remember the physical links and communication protocols involved, which also contribute to the timing problems and also introduce errors in the data transmitted.

Let us now turn to the classification of coordination errors and assessment of their impact on architecture performance. We find that the most convenient (albeit, not the only) way to classify coordination errors is by their result in terms of a specific interception. According to this approach, coordination errors may be divided into three groups.

1) No interception: Situations where each defense system assumed that the responsibility to intercept a specific TBM rests with the other system. The result is that none of them engages the TBM, which leaks through.

2) Double interception: A case where both systems assume they are responsible for intercepting the TBM, and both fire at it. The result is a waste of interceptors, while at the same time also increasing the P_k for that specific intercept.

3) Wrong interception: A case where a correct interpretation of prevailing concept of operations (CONOPS) and ROE would mean that one system should engage, but the coordination process assigns the interception to the other system. This is the most elusive type of error. The result in terms of architecture performance depends on the set of parameters by which coordination is conducted, as well as on the specific systems used.

We shall now turn to a simple demonstration of the way in which coordination errors affect architecture performance, and use again our previous example, of the coordination between systems A1 and A2. We keep the same attack scenario, and, for the sake of simplicity, conduct coordination by P_k only. Figure 14 shows the original graphs for "no coordination" and coordination by P_k, together with three graphs representing various levels of "no interception" errors.

Looking at this graph, the following observations can be made: First, errors obviously diminish the cost-effectiveness margin of coordination. At some point (which may be even at low error values), they may even lead to a case where it is not worthwhile to conduct coordination between the systems at all. Second, the general effect of "no interception" errors is to "lift" the coordination graph while retaining its

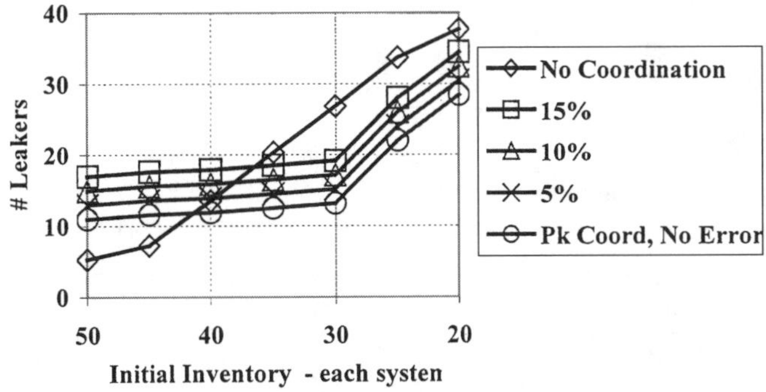

Fig. 14 "No interception" errors.

shape. This is because this type of error results in a direct increase in the number of leakers. Third, this type of error is severe from the point of view of the architecture planner, since low levels of errors result in significant performance degradation.

Figure 15 shows the same graphs for different values of "double interception" errors. Again, some observations are in order. First, at high levels of interceptor stock (the left side of the graph), this type of error actually improves the architecture performance, because it improves the P_k for specific intercepts. Second, as the number of interceptors available decreases relative to the attack size, double interceptions are punished by early depletion of interceptors and, as a result, more leakers. Thus, a rapid decrease in architecture performance is observed. Third, the sensitivity to this type of error (the percent of errors that cause significant decrease in performance) depends on the ratio between the available inventory and the (expected) attack size. Generally, it may be stated that this type of error is less severe from the architecture point of view than the "no coordination" errors.

Finally, Fig. 16 illustrates the effect of "wrong interception" errors. This effect is marginal in our example, because of the small difference in the P_k of the two systems. However, this type of coordination error should not be neglected in decision-making processes. It should be evaluated according to the actual parameters of the defense systems involved, the exact coordination scheme contemplated, and the envisioned threat.

Coordination errors will be a part of any process, be it verbal or automated. However, their presence may be controlled and contained by careful consideration at the definition phase, and constant training of the relevant personnel. (The issue

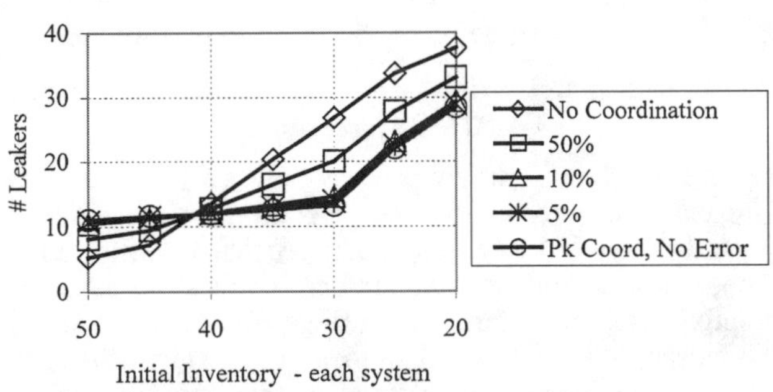

Fig. 15 "Double interception" errors.

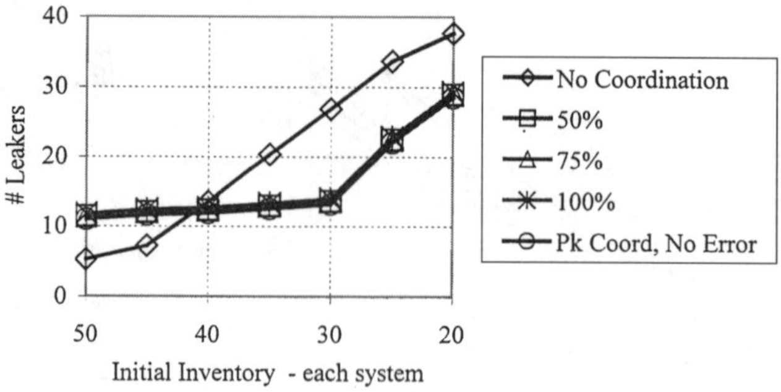

Fig. 16 "Wrong interception" errors.

of training for interoperability will be developed further toward the end of this chapter.) Computerized processes, such as TIS algorithms, may be tuned so that a specific type of error will occur with a lower probability. (An easy case is "preferring" double interception to no interception errors by controlling the threshold distance under which two tracks are considered as one object.) Architecture planners and defense system designers should be aware of this issue and develop the necessary tools to deal with it effectively.

F. Real-Time Interception Coordination—Summary

Real-time coordination of interceptions offers significant benefits to the missile defense architecture. We have shown that many of these benefits may be achieved by relatively simple procedures. The resulting architecture will be both more effective and more robust in terms of being able to counter deviations from the planned-for threat. Mutual backup possibilities are an added benefit, as is the enhanced ability to defend against threats to the defense architecture itself.

However, these benefits do not come without an associated cost. The cost of coordination is multifaced. It consists of the actual cost of linking the systems, the added complexity in the algorithms, and the inherent possibility of errors in the process. Defense architecture designers should consider carefully the cost-effectiveness of each proposed implementation, and strive to adopt the simplest possible approach for the specific architecture at hand. To effectively conduct this analysis, good knowledge of both defense systems concerned is required, as well as a thorough consideration and assessment of the expected threat. Some of the considerations and techniques discussed here, as well as in other chapters of this book, may be of value in deciding on the best way to perform this task.

VIII. Interception

The next phase in the interception process, following defense planning, is the actual carrying out of the interception. Interoperating systems may take part in this process also, and in any kill assessment activity that follows it in a shoot-look-shoot situation. Let us follow the interception process stage by stage, discuss the benefits that interoperability offers at each stage, and determine the requirements that may be imposed to take advantage of them. Following the successful creation of a defense plan, a tracking regime is defined, with the goal of reaching a sufficient accuracy at the time required for interceptor launch. This regime is to be carried out by the radar of the system that is about to engage the TBM. However, the initial plans may be disturbed by a large number of occurrences, from jamming, to attack on the radar, or simply to excessive load caused by the need to perform other tasks (e.g., engagement of higher priority targets).

If the defense system is working on its own, these occurrences may result in a change of the defense plan (e.g., lowering interception altitude to gain more time) and, in the worst case, even in aborting a specific interception. Interoperating systems may provide a "safety net," by taking over the tracking of the target at a specific point and returning it to the system chosen to engage with improved accuracy. Such a process would require intimate knowledge of the details of the tracking regime and its goals by the interoperating system. Therefore, it would require interoperability of level IV or V. Implementing such a high level of interoperability, particularly among systems belonging to different nations' task forces, entails very complex changes in both systems. The cost-effectiveness of such solutions should be weighed, based on the attributes of the actual systems involved.

Another possible use of interoperability at this stage, as well as in the actual launch and interception stages, is to have the peer system prepare a defense plan of its own to be used as a backup in case the first system fails in any stage of the process. This can be done relatively easily, using only level II or III interoperability (not level I, because some information on the target, and possibly the current plan, has to be shared). However, this is a wasteful process, doubling (or almost doubling) the resources devoted to a single interception over the entire architecture.

The next stage in the engagement process is the actual launch of the interceptor and supplying it with information until some predefined point in its flight via uplink. (For more information on these topics, the reader is referred to Chapter 7.) Again, interoperating systems may be used to assist in this process. Several options, at various levels of complexity, exist.

1) The peer system may actually guide the first system's interceptor (level V interoperability). This is the most complicated approach, bringing to the fore problems of compatibility of wavelengths, uplink/downlink messages, etc. If the two systems will not be jointly planned to include this capability, implementation at a later stage would entail very large investments and considerable development risks.

2) The peer system may supply information to the original system, which would use it to update the interceptor (level IV interoperability). This could be done throughout the interceptor flight, requiring very good knowledge on the part of the peer system of the data type and accuracy required by the interceptor. Alternatively, it may be done up to a predefined point where the engaging system has to acquire the target on its own, simplifying the process and the data requirements involved.

3) An alternative defense plan may be placed on hold in the peer system, as a backup in case the interception fails at any point in the process (level III interoperability and up).

This last option brings us to the last stage of the interception process. The assessment of the engagement result and the possible launch of a second tier interceptor.

IX. Shoot-Look-Shoot Applications

A defense system applying shoot-look-shoot involving a kill assessment mechanism may use information supplied by a peer system to enhance the effectiveness of the process. (For more information on kill assessment processes, see Chapter 7.) Obviously, this requires that the receiving system be aware of exactly what type of information is being supplied, from which location (since relative geometry is very important), etc. It is questionable, however, how beneficial is this approach, especially in cases were the constant presence of the peer system cannot be relied on (as is the case in most situations involving coalition warfare). Shoot-look-shoot can also be conducted as a combined defense plan, where one system provides the first layer and the other provides the second layer. Indeed, this appears to be a very natural procedure when one of the interoperating systems is an area defense system and the other is a point defense system.

The application of combined defense plans brings about two issues that have to be resolved: 1) How is kill assessment to be conducted? 2) What is the effect of the time intervals involved on the effectiveness of the process?

The first question is not an easy one to resolve. Combined kill assessment (KA) brings about even more complex problems than those already discussed for assistance by one system in KA performance by the other. If only one system is to perform the kill assessment, the question is which one will it be. On the one hand, the system that performed the interception has the most knowledge about the way its interceptor behaved during the interception (including the most up-to-date downlink data prior to interception), and is also the most aware of the type of sky-pictures resulting from its interception. It is therefore the best equipped to decide on the kill result. On the other hand, if the system that has to perform the second layer fails to identify the target, the result of the kill assessment process is meaningless. If KA is performed by both systems, whose judgment should be preferred in case the results do not match? There is no clear-cut answer to these questions, nor is there at the moment sufficient experience in kill assessment and kill pictures to support such an answer.

The second question just posed brings us back to the issue of the time for coordination, which was already discussed earlier in this chapter. In its current incarnation, the problem takes the form of assessing the effect of the time taken by the kill assessment process on the defended footprint of the lower tier system.

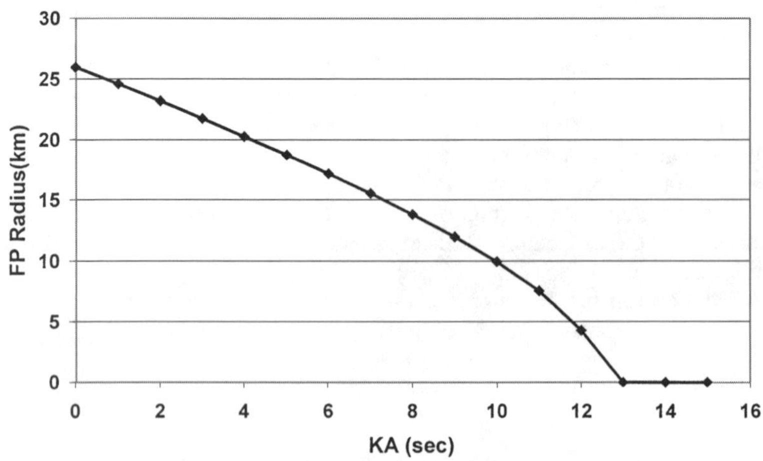

Fig. 17 Footprint radius as function of kill assessment time.

One should bear in mind that the time involved includes the KA time, the communication time, and the reaction time of the activated system.

To get a feeling for the effect of this type of time line problem on defense system performance, we return to our familiar example from Fig. 1. We will now focus on an 800-km TBM, attacking DA 1. System A, the area defense system, attempts to intercept it at 60-km altitude. If it fails, system B, the point defense system, is to perform a second layer interception at 20-km altitude. Figure 17 shows the size (radius) of the defended footprint by the lower tier system, as a function of the time taken for kill assessment and related activities. As can be seen from the graph, the problem is by no means negligible, and should be considered whenever such joint procedures are contemplated.

X. Debriefing in an Interoperability Environment

Debriefing is an integral part of any military operation, and debriefing capabilities should form a part of every defense system. In the field of TMD, the debriefing capabilities are especially important, and should be as extensive as possible, because of the relatively small amount of data currently available and the rarity of actual data (the difficulty in actively training for TMD). The situation is even worse where interoperability is concerned, for a number of reasons:

1) Training and actual operation, in any particular interoperability setting, will be extremely rare. This means that any such occurrence should be used to gather as much data as possible.

2) The data relevant for analysis of the combined operation of interoperating systems are much harder to accumulate than the data relevant for analysis of a single system operation.

3) The ability to implement the lessons learned from debriefing (especially in the short time allowed to respond within the same war), is also constrained by the fact that two nations' task forces may be involved.

Let us take a minute to elaborate on the second issue (the first will be discussed later on). Analyzing interoperability operations requires gathering information on activities (e.g., coordination processes) conducted between the systems, rather than at each system individually. As an example, let us look at the data required to analyze the results of a single interception, which was coordinated between two defense systems. We assume that an automatic TIS algorithm handled track correlation, and the interception coordination was done verbally.

First, we need to establish that the systems were indeed talking about the same target. For this, we need to know the following: 1) What was the information at each system at the time of track correlation and what data were transmitted across the communication network. 2) What was the interpretation given to the data at each system (as we can not assume that both systems perform the same association tests). 3) What data were actually displayed to the human operators performing interception coordination at the time the coordination occurred (which may be different from the final results of discrimination algorithms stored in the system's files). 4) Was the TBM correlated really the one talked about by the operators (they may have talked about one TBM but conducted operations on a different target).

Following this analysis, we should turn to analyzing the coordination process and its results. For this, we need to know the following: 1) What were the prevailing rules of engagement at the time of coordination (because ROE may change dynamically during the war). Specifically, what were the rules set by higher command concerning the priority assigned to each defense system vs the specific threat? 2) What were the defense plan options available to the operators in both systems. We need to know what options were available inside each system, which of them were actually discussed in the coordination process, what was the basis for the decision-making process (which parameters were discussed), and which was the selected defense plan? 3) What was the timing involved in the process, when was the process started, how long did it take, and what was the time allowed for coordination?

The next step in the process is the debriefing of the actual interception. To properly analyze this phase, we need to know what each operator in each defense system did (e.g., activate DP, place DP on hold, change specific parameters), at what time line, and what was reported to the peer system. Finally, a similar process should occur for the kill assessment and launch of the lower tier interceptor, if this were a part of the defense plan executed.

Looking at this one example, it is easy to see some major problems that are involved in debriefing operations involving interoperability: First, for the debriefing to be effective, the data files of both systems should be analyzed together. This will inevitably cause a problem in the general case, where the systems do not come from the same nation's task force. Second, coordination is, by nature, an act of decision making. Even if we can reconstruct the database and time line that was available at the time the decision was made, several interpretations of the data are probably legitimate. A "schoolbook solution" doesn't exist in most situations. Third, coordination is a decision-making process that takes place at more than one point in space (i.e., it occurs *between* the two systems using, ultimately, human conversation across a verbal communication net). This means that complex analysis of verbal communication protocols is required.

The question of how to conduct efficient debriefing in an interoperability setup has to be resolved on a case-by-case basis. It is important that this issue not be overlooked whenever interoperability between defense systems, particularly systems belonging to different nations, is being discussed.

Before we leave the subject of interoperability, we feel that a short discussion of human-in-the-loop issues is in order. These issues are not particular to the case of TMD systems, but some aspects are singular, due to the special nature of the TMD war.

XI. Human-in-the-Loop Considerations

As has been continually stressed throughout this chapter, the major differences between interoperability in TMD and interoperability in any other military operation, are the short time intervals under which decisions have to be made and carried out and the uncertainty as to the actual battle picture, stemming both from its complex nature and from the small amount of data available and real combat experience. These two characteristics lead to two important requirements for TMD systems wishing to operate together. These are 1) the need for constant training/exercising and 2) the need for operator assistance tools.

We will discuss each of these requirements briefly, not attempting to provide general solutions, but rather to provide some useful observations and guidelines.

A. Training for Interoperability

The complex nature of the processes involved in interoperability, together with the lack of real-time operational experience and the timing problems involved, create a need for constant training, both at the single system as well as the multi-system (or nation) level. However, these same factors also impose difficulties on joint training and exercises. The problem is somewhat alleviated when several nations use equipment manufactured by a common source, but even then problems of compatibility between various versions of the same system, not to mention problems arising from different doctrines and modes of operation, and even national culture, will doubtless arise.

Thus, there is a need for constant training and exercising to reach proficiency in operating a joint architecture, but the opportunity to conduct such joint exercises is rare. Exercises involving live firing are even rarer, yet some aspects of interoperability can only be tested and exercised in them.

A partial solution to the problem lies in the use of simulations and simulators. Simulations can be used with relative ease. Using today's distributive interactive simulation (DIS) protocols, exercises can be performed in remote locations. Yet, even so the performance of such exercises is a costly and complex undertaking. Moreover, these exercises are good for testing issues such as combined standing operating procedures (CSOP), language problem, time line, etc., but they are not adequate for testing, for example, the physical link between the systems. (More information on the use of simulations in interoperability exercises may be found in this book, in Chapter 14.)

There is a need, therefore, for establishing a training regime for any two systems wishing to interoperate. This regime should include periodic exercise in different forms, and it should touch on all of the aspects of interoperability. Specifically, one may define the following aspects as describing the elements that should be trained and exercised.

1) Engagement coordination: The ability to perform efficient coordination of engagement, either automatically or through voice channels.

2) CONOPS/CSOP: The existence of commonly accepted rules and organizational structures able to support the required level of joint operation.

3) ASP correlation: The ability of the joint architecture to create (either automatically or by voice) a common "sky-picture."

4) Equipment connectivity: The ability of the two systems to physically connect one to the other and send and receive all the data required for performance at the agreed upon level. This includes both automated and vocal procedures.

5) Time line/response time: The available time for the aforementioned activities, in a real engagement.

6) Mutual debrief: The ability to jointly reach conclusions, within a reasonable time, as to the effectiveness of the joint operation, and ways to rectify the problems identified.

7) Other joint procedures: The ability to jointly conduct activities such as discrimination, kill assessment, etc.

8) Logistics: Readiness of the joint architecture in terms of being able to support actual deployment of forces and supplying their material needs, and the required infrastructure for connecting the systems.

Several types of exercises are available to train the combined architecture. They are 1) simulations (including human-in-the-loop models), 2) war games, 3) joint

Table 7 Interoperability exercises

	Exercise type					
Attribute	Simulation	War game	Plan meeting	CPX	Deployment	Live firing
Logistics		+	+	+ (+)	++	+
Equipment connectivity			+	+	+ (+)	++
CONOPS/CSOP	+ (+)	+	+	++	++	++
ASP correlation	++	+			++	+ (+)
Engagement coordination	++	+			++	+ (+)
Other procedures	+ (+)	+			+ (+)	++
Mutual debrief	+ (+)	+	+	+ (+)	++	++
Time line	++				+ (+)	++

planning meetings, 4) command post exercise (CPX), 5) unit deployment, and 6) live firing.

Obviously these methods may be combined. For example large-scale exercises may involve several units actually deployed in the field whereas other units are participating via simulations. Such an exercise may even culminate with one or two units conducting live firing of interceptors. To fully train and test the combined architecture, a carefully defined mix of the previously defined exercise types is required. To see why this is so, one needs to look at a table of each of the elements of interoperability, such as Table 7, which shows the level of testing achieved in each type of exercise. In the table, one plus sign (+) means that the attribute in question is partly tested by the specific exercise type, a plus followed by a plus in parentheses (+(+)) means that an attribute is almost fully tested, and two plus signs (++) mean that it is fully tested.

A few notes regarding Table 7 are in order. First, as can be clearly seen, only live testing, including firing, can accomplish true testing of all the attributes of interoperability. However, it is possible to test a lot of the attributes to a large degree by simpler means. Second, we assume that even in large-scale exercises live firings will be conducted against single targets and not salvos (this seems to be a natural assumption, at least in the general case). This is why, for example, live firings do not fully test the engagement coordination capability. And third, the contents of the table reflects the authors' experience and beliefs and is, of course, debatable. However, no matter what other views are held by the reader, the main message of the table will remain this: No single type of exercise fully tests the ability of two systems/units to conduct interoperability at any specific level.

We strongly believe that the level of training and testing by the involved units/systems will play a major role in the success of TMD interoperability operations. A training regime should be set, based on the specifics of each case, to include a combination of the different exercise types. Simulations and war games probably will play an important role in any such training regime, but we must not delude ourselves into thinking that they can, by themselves, fully test the combined architecture.

B. Operator Support Tools

Interoperability between defense systems probably will be conducted by a combination of computerized algorithms and communication between human operators. The grave nature of the decisions being made (affecting directly the probability of assets being hit by TBMs) lends itself naturally to human decision making, or at least human monitoring and approval of computerized decisions. On the other hand, the short time available for decision making puts extreme pressure on the human operator and may even, at times, make human intervention impossible. The immediate conclusion from these observations is that designers of TMD systems who wish to operate jointly, should invest a lot of effort in supplying their human operators with adequate support tools to carry out this complex mission.

The goal of support tools should be twofold: To allow the operator to "see" the picture viewed by his peers in the other system, as accurately as possible (situation awareness tools), and to alleviate the timing problems by providing as much advanced information as possible. (Decision support tools).

We conclude this brief discussion with some comments regarding specific operator assistance tools and their utility.

1) TIS algorithms are almost a must when it comes to coordination between weapon systems. The time required for verbal correlation of the sky-picture is prohibitive from the point of view of effective battle management. Care should be exercised in careful design of the algorithms so that changes in the sky-picture representation at the system level are not automatically repeated at the operator level. (The system may take a number of "trial and error" steps to correctly discriminate, for example, a warhead from its associated decoys. Displaying all of the interim stages of this process to the user may overload him or her.)

2) Early knowledge of any event in the sky is important. Displaying external cue information to the operator allows for early correlation and coordination procedures, and lets the operator prepare for the tasks to follow. On the other hand, too much advanced information, or too early a presentation of the data, will clutter the display and make it more difficult for the operator to understand the immediate sky-picture. The best mix of data to be displayed is particular to each system, and is affected by the display capabilities and the role the operator is expected to play in the interception process.

3) For effective coordination of interceptions, or monitoring of a computerized coordination process, the operator needs to be made aware of most, if not all, of the parameters being exchanged and weighed. It is very important for the operator to be able to understand what is to be contemplated, and reach a decision based on known and clear rules.

4) Other, more advanced, methods for saving coordination time may be suggested, based on the specifics of the systems being connected. An example is that an upper tier system may attempt to predict the capability of a lower tier system to intercept a given track, by an algorithm representing the qualities of the lower tier system. Alternatively, a lower tier system might be fitted with the capability to conduct its defense planning process based on external cueing data, without self-detection of the target. Both methods allow longer time for coordination, and each entails its own benefits and drawbacks. (For example, planning according to cue data allows for a full coordination process by the system that is actually going to carry it out. On the other hand, it takes resources off other tasks, and may wind up allocating resources to a target that will not be detected or intercepted.)

The human operator involvement in interoperability processes, both offline and online, is an issue that requires more analysis and thought. It is the view of the authors that this will turn out to be one of the core issues for interoperability studies in the near future.

XII. Summary

Although interoperability has been, in recent years, the subject of many studies and analyses, as well as actual progress in working out the details for connecting specific systems, it is the authors' view that we are still just scratching the surface of this issue. Many of the important questions and parameters discussed in this chapter were completely unknown a few short years ago. Many more, we feel, are still lying in uncharted regions of this vast field.

We have, however, learned a lot in recent years. Treatment of interoperability has advanced from neglect, to fervent study and analysis, and to actual implementation of some algorithms, links and protocols, designed to accomplish at least a part of the tasks discussed in this chapter. As implementation continues to mature, and is tested and trained in various drills and exercises, the knowledge base will continue to grow, and our understanding of the fundamental issues governing interoperability will be heightened.

Just as in many other areas in TMD, we are still trudging the road toward a full understanding of interoperability. We hope the present chapter helps, if not actually to navigate us onward, at least to chart the course we have already covered.

Acknowledgments

The authors would like to acknowledge the work of Karel Pick and Yuval Karakookly in preparing material for this chapter.

References

[1]*Dictionary of Military Terms*, U.S. Dept. of Defense, Greenhill Books, London, 1995.

[2]Spiegel, M.R., *Theory and Practice of Statistics*, Schaum's Outline Series in Mathematics, McGraw–Hill, New York, 1961, App. IV.

[3]Blackman, S.S., and Banh, N.D., Hughes Co., "Track Association Using Correction for Bias and Missing Data," *Signal and Data Processing of Small Targets*, Paper 2235-34, Vol. 2235, edited by Oliver E. Drummond, Society of Photo-Optical Instrumentation Engineers, 1994.

Chapter 9

External Cueing

Dror Cohen,* Eitan Yariv,† and Ayala Gur ‡
WALES Ltd., Ramat-Gan, Israel

I. Introduction

THE process of external cueing, i.e., supplying/receiving target-related data from sources external to the defense architecture, is a special form of interoperability. Interoperability between defense systems is discussed in some detail in Chapter 8. However, we feel that external cueing, because of its relative ease of implementation (compared with other forms of interoperability) and its many uses, merits a chapter in its own right. The basic process of external cueing is depicted graphically in Fig. 1.

The external cue source detects the target before it is detected by the defense system radar. It transmits the target data to the defense system, enabling earlier detection and allowing more time for the defense system to react to the threat. This can either increase effective radar coverage by providing detection at greater ranges and angles than the radar can effectively scan or increase effective radar capacity by freeing radar resources (both in search and track). The main commodity exchanged in this process is time. On the one hand, time is "gained" in terms of earlier detection. On the other hand time is "lost" in terms of the requirement for the defense system to invest extra resources (long-range cued beams) and to track the incoming tactical ballistic missile (TBM) for a longer time. The balance between the time lost and the time gained provides the benefits of external cueing. These benefits are a function of the threat, properties of the cue source, the intended use of the cue data, and the defense system capabilities. The purpose of this chapter is to map the relationships between these elements and their impact on the effectiveness and utility of the cue.

The cue source is any sensor that is not under the control of the defense system. It may be a sensor dedicated for this purpose, such as a surveillance satellite, or a sensor performing external cueing as a secondary activity, such as a forward-deployed radar of another weapon system. It may even be an "opportunity-based

Copyright © 2000 by the American Institute of Aeronautics and Astronautics, Inc. All rights reserved.

*President. Member AIAA.
†Team Leader, Interoperability, External Cueing, and Concept of Operations. Member AIAA.
‡Senior Systems Analyst. Member AIAA.

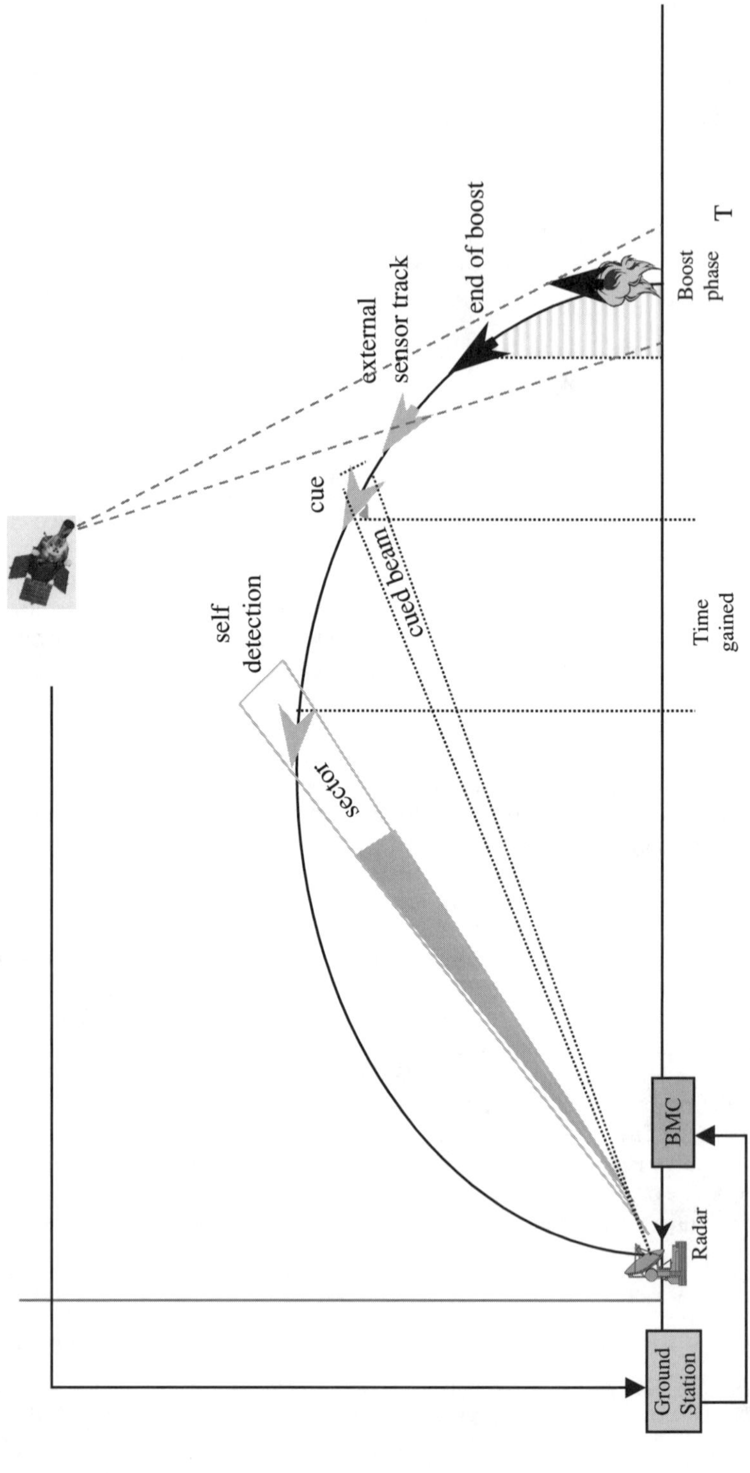

Fig. 1 External cueing process.

cue" supplied by aircraft that happen to observe a TBM launch. Cue data, likewise, may vary from general early warning and up to a very accurate state vector. Cueing may be provided once or continuously as long as the remote sensor is tracking the TBM. Delay in providing the cue may be anything from a few seconds up to minutes. The effective use of the cue data depends on correct implementation based on the cue charateristics.

There are a number of possible ways to map the connections between the elements mentioned above. In this chapter, we chose to start with defining the possible uses of cue, from the point of view of the defense system. We will then analyze each possible use and identify the merits that may be gained, the pitfalls that should be avoided, and the requirements posed by each specific use on the participating systems. For the sake of convenience, we shall limit our discussion to the relatively simple case of a single radar/single cue source throughout most of this chapter. The case of multiradar/multicue sources will be discussed only briefly, in a separate section. Finally, we shall construct a table summarizing the connections between cue source qualities, cueing system qualities, and cue use.

II. Possible Uses of External Cueing

The possible uses of external cue data are listed, arranged by order of complexity.

1) *Early warning:* Using the early data provided by the cue source to warn the population at the predicted impact point of the TBM. In this use, there is no benefit to the active defense system, but the importance of a few minutes of early warning to the passive defense layer need hardly be stressed.

2) *Early calculation of TBM launch point:* A companion use to early warning. External cue data are used to activate and guide forward deployed forces, as counter force. Since this book deals only with defensive aspects of the ballistic missile war, this will not be dealt with in great detail.

3) *Early detection:* The "classic" use of cue data. There are a number of variants here, but we shall deal mainly with two of them: First, cue as a companion to search, where the defense system radar continues its normal search functions while devoting some resources to cued acquisition at longer ranges or extreme angles. Second, cue instead of search, where the defense system radar does not perform autonomous search, but relies entirely on cue data for target acquisition and performs solely in fire control mode. Obviously, there are numerous options between these two extremes, but they can be treated as a continuum involving different "doses" of the two extreme solutions.

4) *Defense planning based on cue data:* Delaying own radar acquisition of the TBM to the last possible moment before launching an interceptor, while relying on the data supplied by the cue source for all defense planning functions. There is a range of options between assistance in acquisition through full defense planning.

5) *Interceptor launch using cue data:* In this application, cue data is used to launch, and possibly even guide, the interceptor toward its intended target.

The aforementioned definitions of possible uses, though somewhat crude, provide a good background for continuing the analysis. It is, of course, possible to refine the division presented, but we feel that for our present goals, this level of refinement will suffice. The remainder of this chapter will consist of analysis of each of the possible uses of cue as defined. The main emphasis will be placed on uses 3 and 4, because we believe they are the ones most cue users are likely to pick as providing the highest gains, in terms of cost-benefit, to their systems.

III. Early Warning

The first use of cue data to be discussed is early warning. The goal is to provide an accurate warning earlier than is possible by the defense system's own radar. This is a relatively simple case, involving two main parameters: time and accuracy. The time gained is proportional to the range of the TBM from its impact point when the early warning is provided. Figure 2 shows three representative TBM trajectories. The X axis presents the range to the TBM impact point, and the Y axis presents the time to impact. From this graph it is easy to deduce the amount of time gained from early warning per TBM type, relative to own radar capabilities. It can be seen, for example, that if a TBM is detected at a range of 1000-km, the early warning time is between 6 and 7 min. If the same TBM is detected at a range of 800 km the early warning time is approximately 5 min. Again, if detection occurs at the 300-km range, the early warning time is reduced to less than 3 min. One may draw the following conclusions. An external sensor's contribution to early warning is significant for those TBMs of longer range than the defense system (or other detection assets) radar detection range. Additionally, the gain in time for each kilometer of detection is greater for shorter range TBMs (this is seen from the gradient of the graphs).

A point regarding accuracy should be made here. The accuracy of impact point prediction by the defense system (or by the cue source itself) depends on the accuracy of the cue supplied. Although it is not necessary to pin-point the impact point for early warning, the uncertainty ellipse should be small enough to support warning the population in specific areas. For this reason, although the gain in time for earlier detection is greatest during the TBM's boost phase, data before the TBM end of boost is of limited use.

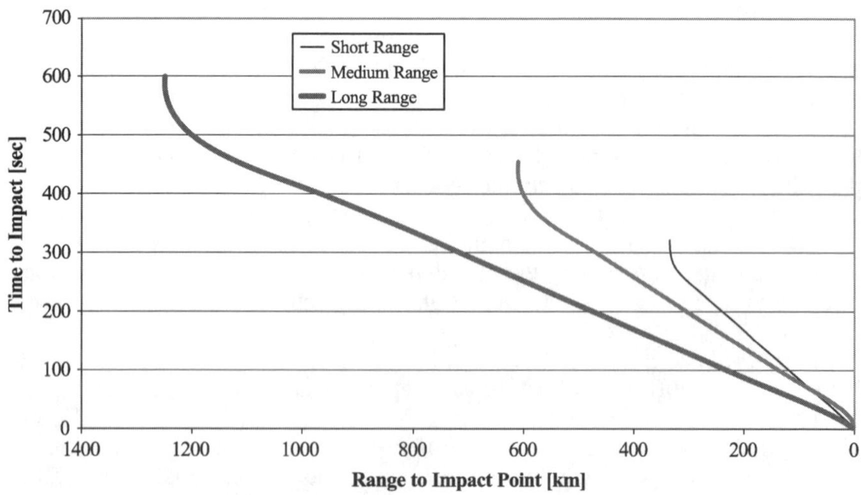

Fig. 2 TBM range vs flight time.

IV. Calculation of TBM Launch Point

Another possible use of external cue data is the early calculation of the TBM launch point. This can be done either before the TBM is acquired by the defense system itself (relying on cue data only) or after self acquisition (combining the data from external cueing and the system's own sensors). Because, obviously, it is important to estimate the TBM launch point as early as possible, the first option should be given high priority. The applicability of launch point calculation based on cue data alone depends on three parameters.

1) Arrival time of the cue. The cue should arrive before the system acquires the TBM by itself. (A more elaborate discussion of this issue will be given in the next section.)

2) Cue data. The cue data should include either the state vector of the TBM as close to launch as possible or the launch point itself. In this case waiting for end of boost is unnecessary.

3) Cue accuracy. The level of accuracy should be sufficient for the defined task.

This last point requires some elaboration. Obviously, the accuracy of the resulting launch point prediction (i.e., the size of the uncertainty ellipse) depends on the algorithms used. However, in all estimation algorithms the results will be directly related to the errors in the cue data. Figure 3 presents the length of the major axis in the uncertainty ellipse as a function of the (average) error in the cue data. In preparing the graph, we used a simple model for track calculation (assuming a Keplerian track). Looking at such a graph, based on the algorithms used in a particular system, and knowing the accuracy required for the launch point location, the reader may deduce the required accuracy of the cue source, to enable it to be used for launch point (LP) estimation.

Combining the data from two or more sensors can, of course, provide a higher accuracy than is obtained by each sensor on its own. However, achieving this higher accuracy requires implementing data fusion algorithms, and the results may not always justify the effort. To see this, we may look at Fig. 4. This graph shows the accuracy of the LP calculated by a combination of data from two sensors, as a function of the accuracy of each sensor data by itself. We have assumed a common time base, i.e., that all track reports are correctly synchronized in absolute terms. The fusion algorithm used was a simple best estimate trajectory (BET) algorithm. The BET algorithm calculates a weighted average of corresponding

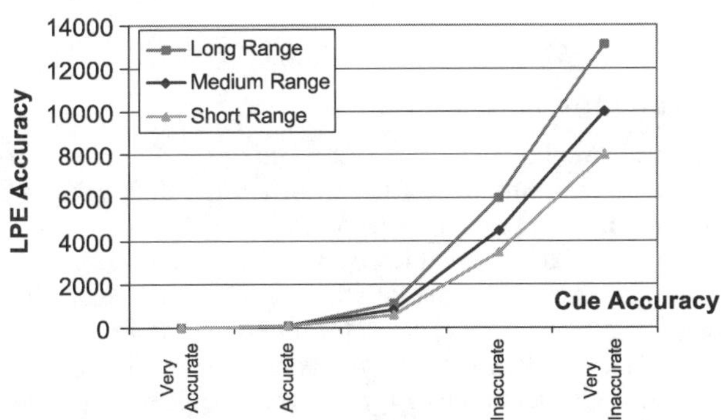

Fig. 3 Uncertainty in launch point estimation as a function of cue accuracy.

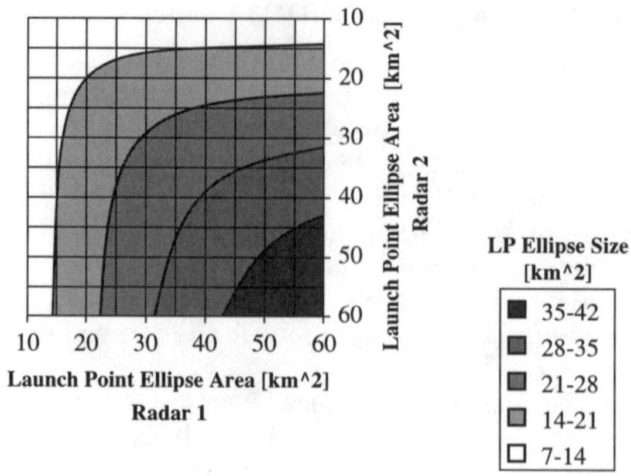

Fig. 4 Combined launch point estimation accuracy using best estimate trajectory.

track components, i.e.,

$$\bar{X} = \left[\frac{1}{\sigma_1^2}\bar{X}_1 + \frac{1}{\sigma_2^2}\bar{X}_2\right] \Big/ \left[\frac{1}{\sigma_1^2} + \frac{1}{\sigma_2^2}\right] \tag{1}$$

where $\bar{X}_1$, $\bar{X}_2$ are the measurements of each sensor and $\sigma 1$, $\sigma 2$ are the corresponding covariances. The maximum contribution is expected when the two sensors have similar accuracies.

Combining this graph with the graph in Fig. 3, one may deduce the contribution of external sensors relative to own system characteristics, the cue sources available, and the data fusion method considered. However, it is important to note here that data fusion should also be considered for other uses of cue data.

A word of warning should be inserted here. The results in Fig. 4 are obtained knowing the accuracy of the data from each of the sensors. In reality, the accuracy of each track may not be known. The actual measurement errors come into play here, and so does the sensor's bias, sometimes resulting in an inability to accurately define the accuracy of the combined track. If the LP itself is provided, the method of calculation must be known in order to know the size of the uncertainty ellipse.

V. Cued Acquisition of TBMs

A. Acquisition Improvements

The most "natural" method of using external cueing is for increasing acquisition coverage (range and azimuth) vs self detection by the defending system's radar. Obviously, this use requires specific capabilities in the radar itself, namely the capability to generate cued acquisition beams designed to search a limited area at a longer range or extreme angle relative to the usual search coverage. The characteristics of this beam should be determined as a function of the radar and threat qualities and its coupling with the weapon system being used. Let us assume for example, that for a specific TBM type, given acquisition, the defense system takes t_1 s to prepare a defense plan and that the time of flight of the interceptor in its longest possible trajectory is t_2 s. Then it is clear that $t_{max} = t_1 + t_2$ is the longest

Table 1 Acquisition range gain using external cue

TBM range	Characteristics (approximate)	Cued acquisition range	Acquisition range gain
Short	$R_{TBM} < R_{MSD}$	$R_{[EOB+T_D]}$	$R_{[EOB+T_D]} - R_{SDS} <= 0$
Medium	$R_{MSD} < R_{TBM} < R_{max}$	$R_{[EOB+T_D]}$	$R_{[EOB+T_D]} - R_{SDS} > 0$
Long	$R_{TBM} > R_{max}$	R_{max}	$R_{max} - R_{SDL} > 0$

time the system needs for intercepting any TBM. Detecting a TBM at $t > t_{max}$ before impact (TTG = time to go) is therefore useless from the point of view of the defense system. Because the basic equations determining TBM trajectory are well known, t_{max} may be used in conjunction with the TBM data to determine the desired cued acquisition beam range.

The actual cued acquisition beam range will generally be smaller than the maximum already defined. The actual range is a result of an optimization process based on available radar resources, the dependency of t_1 on acquisition range, the resulting energy requirements, and radar technical characteristics. For example, let us take a defense system with a given radar and cue supplied based on TBM end-of-boost data. Define R_{MSD} as the maximum self detection range of the radar search regime, and R_{max} as the maximum radar acquisition range (the range of the cued beam). In addition, R_{TBM} = range of TBM, T_D = time of detection process (radar and cue source) as well as data transfer delay, $R_{[t]}$ = range between the TBM and the radar at time t, and R_{SDX} = range of self acquisition (per TBM of type X). One may now define the maximum potential gain in acquisition range by utilizing external cueing based on end of boost (EOB) detection, as shown in Table 1.

B. Acquisition Resources

The gain in acquisition time does not come without a cost. Let us assume that a specific TBM is acquired in normal operation by a single beam with a specified probability of detection (Pd), at a given range R_1 from the radar. Assume now that using external cueing a beam is planned for acquisition at range R_2, with the same Pd. The situation is depicted in Fig. 5. Because the required energy of the beam is proportional to the range raised to the fourth power, we can state that

$$\frac{E_1}{E_2} \cong \left(\frac{R_1}{R_2}\right)^4 \tag{2}$$

where Ei is the energy needed for acquisition at Ri.

Equation (2) may be used to define the cost, in terms of radar resources, required to generate a cued acquisition beam for a certain range R. However, here too, the cue accuracy comes into play. If we assume (for simplicity) a pencil beam, then the area covered by a single beam at range R may be approximated as a circle (in two-dimensional space, where the third dimension is taken in the direction of the radar) whose radius is directly related to the radar bandwidth (BW) and the range

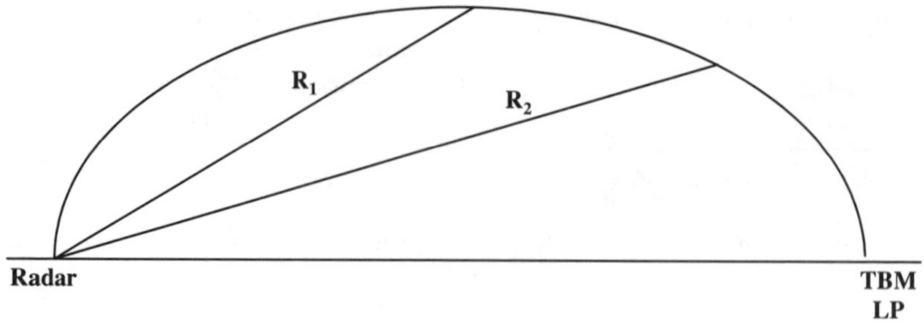

Fig. 5 Cued acquisition.

itself:

$$r = \frac{\mathrm{BW(rad)}}{2} \cdot R \tag{3}$$

The number of beams required to cover a certain area may be calculated as the number of circles required to cover that area, as seen in Fig. 6. If the cue accuracy is (σ_x, σ_z) along the x and z axis (the y axis is taken in the direction of the radar and may therefore be neglected), to guarantee that the TBM is detected, we need to search an area of $6\sigma_x \times 6\sigma_z$ in size. The number of beams required is given by

$$N = \frac{6\sigma_x \cdot 6\sigma_z}{(2 \cdot r \cdot N\_0)^2} \tag{4}$$

where N_0 is the nonoverlap ratio between two circles, given by

$$N\_0 = \frac{k}{2r} \tag{5}$$

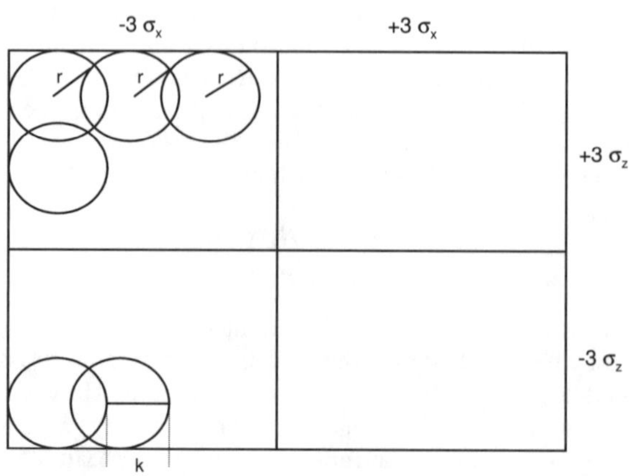

Fig. 6 Number of beams required for search.

C. Cue Contribution: Footprint

The time gained by early acquisition of the TBM may be used by the system in a number of ways. The most obvious use is to enable defense against TBMs that otherwise could not be intercepted. In other words, to increase the defense system's footprint.

Generally speaking, defense system footprint is directly related to detection range (and thus to detection time). Earlier detection of a TBM results in earlier preparation of defense plan, and therefore in the ability to launch the interceptor earlier, thus allowing the interceptor a longer time of flight (greater range) and increasing the footprint.

Quantifying the effect of earlier acquisition on the defended footprint is, however, a complex endeavor. The footprint is affected by radar coverage (both azimuth and range), interceptor trajectory (time of flight), and homing method. It requires an intimate knowledge of the weapon system and its relevant performance parameters. As a simple example, let us assume a defense system in which the interceptor flies a straight line, at constant speed, with no geometry limitations. Figure 7 shows the gain in forward footprint range as a function of the acquisition range.

In general, the following rules of thumb can be stated regarding footprint increase as a result of early detection.

1) The defense system has a maximum footprint size dependent on interceptor performance parameters.

2) If the capabilities of the radar and interceptor are well matched, the system reaches its maximal coverage without cueing

3) The contribution is expected to be larger for longer range TBMs, as long as they are within the interception abilities of the system.

4) Other benefits in interception volume may be expected, higher interception altitude, for example. These will be more significant the closer you come to the

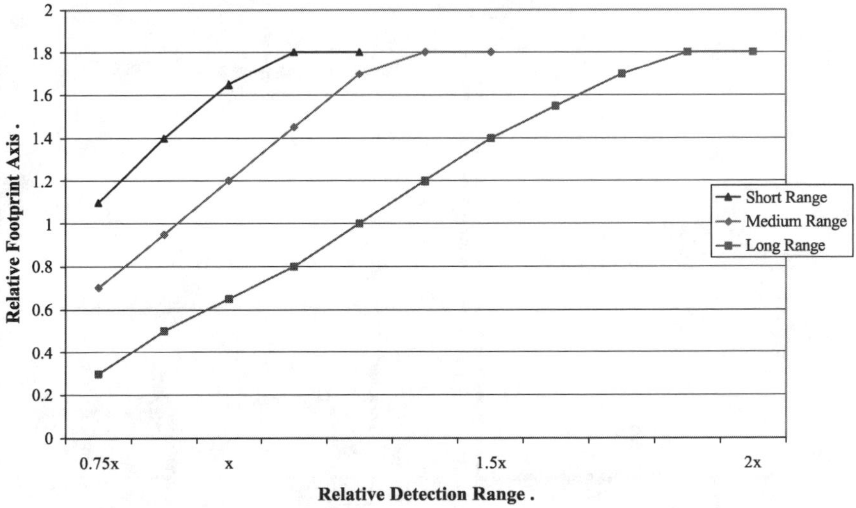

Fig. 7 Footprint gain as a function of acquisition time.

footprint boundaries, where there is more room for improvement relative to the normal operation of the system.

5) Contribution to the defense capabilities at the center of the system's battlespace is expected to be marginal.

D. Cue Contribution: Resources

The direct increase in footprint is not the only possible contribution of cueing in this mode. Early acquisition gives the defense system more time to react. Using this added time the system can now plan its use of resources more effectively, both for the specific TBM and for an entire TBM salvo (assuming cueing is available for all TBMs). To see the possible effect of using cueing to plan the tracking regime, let us look at a specific example.

Our example involves a single long-range TBM. If the system detects it by itself, there is a peak of resource allocation at the detection time. This peak is caused by the need to properly initiate a track for the TBM. This peak is avoided when external cueing is available, because the initiation of a track may be done based on the cue track. The average energy may be increased as a result of this use of long-range tracks or decreased resulting from the greater time available (lower track rate). If the cue is relatively accurate, it may be possible to delay the actual acquisition until some future point in time (delayed acquisition will be discussed later in more depth), thus both avoiding the resources peak at acquisition and investing fewer resources in the entire defense process. This basic situation is described qualitatively in Fig. 8. In this example, to enable interception using self-acquisition, a high track rate is required; however, if acquisition occurs at the long range provided by the cue, a low tracking rate is sufficient.

Other options of using the radar in the presence of cueing exist. If we assume that the cue source is constantly available and is sufficiently reliable (in terms

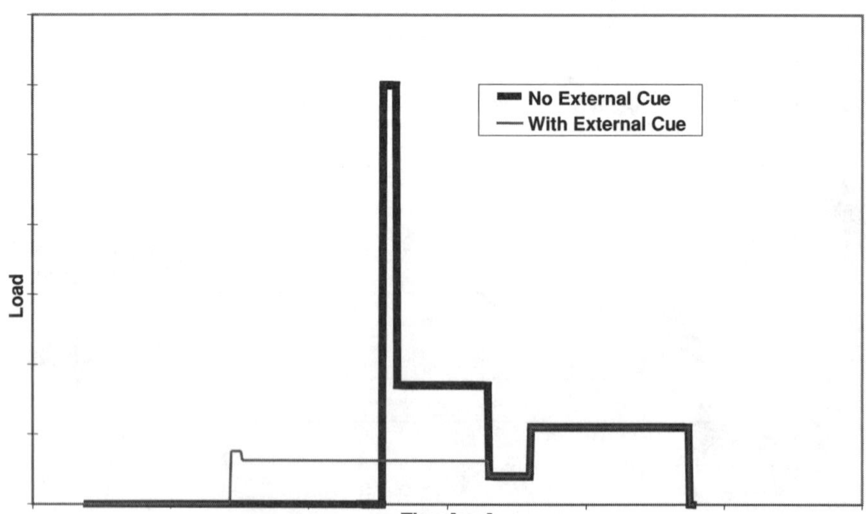

Fig. 8 Tracking load as a function of time.

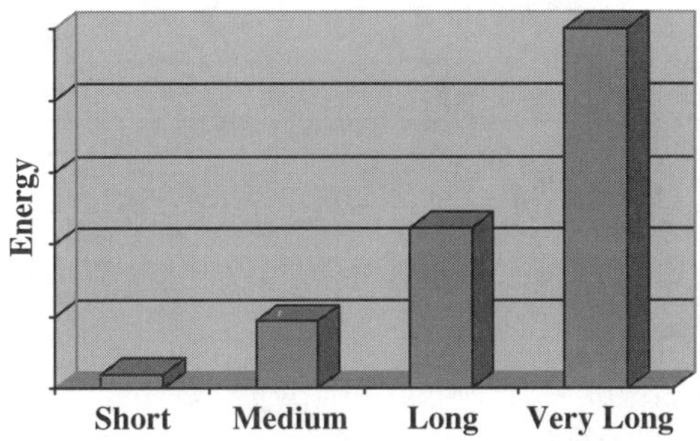

Fig. 9 Relative required energy (no cue).

of miss/false alarm rate), the defense planner may consider using cueing as a substitute, or at least a partial substitute, to search. Such practice would save radar resources, which can then be used to track and intercept more TBMs (in case the same radar is performing both search and fire control functions) or to increase the track accuracy per TBM.

Let us look at some simple examples. In the first example, a radar devotes a certain amount of energy to search. (For the current discussion, it does not matter if the radar devotes all of its energy to search or only a partial amount.) The radar searches constantly for TBMs at short, medium, long, and very long ranges. Regardless of the search mechanism used, the relative amount of energy devoted to search a given sector at each range will behave in the manner depicted in Fig. 9, i.e., in a form of an exponential function.

If a decision is made to stop searching at the very long range, and rely on cue data and cued acquisition, the resources devoted to search and acquisition are shown in Fig. 10. The resources devoted to search at very long ranges are significantly decreased, and the exponential function correlation is broken. Note, however, that the resources devoted to search at the very long range are still higher than those devoted to search at the short range. This is because of the large number of resources taken by each long-range cued beam.

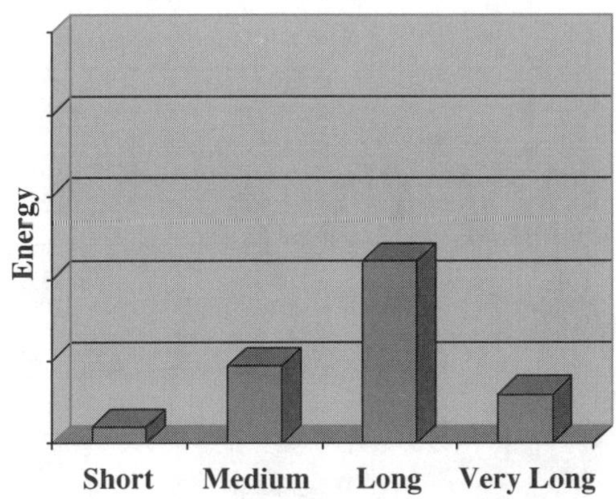

Fig. 10 Relative required energy (with cue).

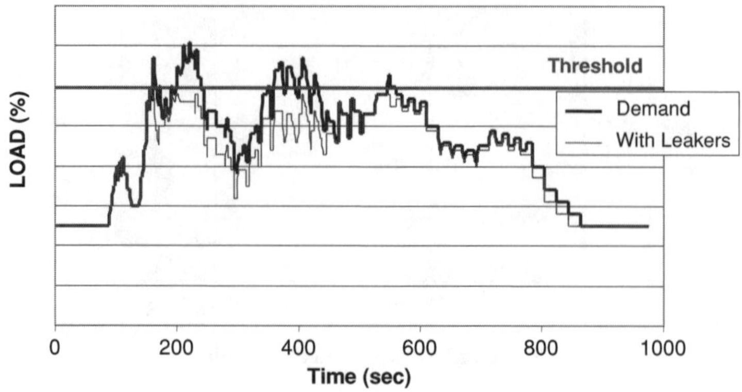

Fig. 11 Radar resources (no cue).

In a second example, a single radar has to deal with a heavy TBM attack in a short time period. In Fig. 11, the required radar load is depicted (the upper graph). Because this load exceeds the available resources, the actual results of the run indicate that a number of TBMs were not engaged and leaked because of lack of resources. The actual radar resource consumption is seen on the lower graph. Using the logic as described, of relying on external cueing for detection of very long range TBMs, the same scenario could be handled easily, without any leakers caused by resource problems (Fig. 12). Thus, wise use of external cue data may increase defense system capacity and robustness.

Having looked at this example, it is easy to construct a large number of possible search schemes, to be used in the presence of cueing, starting from not searching at all and relying on cue data for all acquisitions. Looking at the graphs presented in Figs. 9–12, it is obvious that the largest benefits are to be expected from avoiding long-range search. Partial schemes, such as diluting search as a function of radar load, not searching at a given sector, etc., may also be considered. When cueing is available, these can be performed while still providing the appropriate defense coverage.

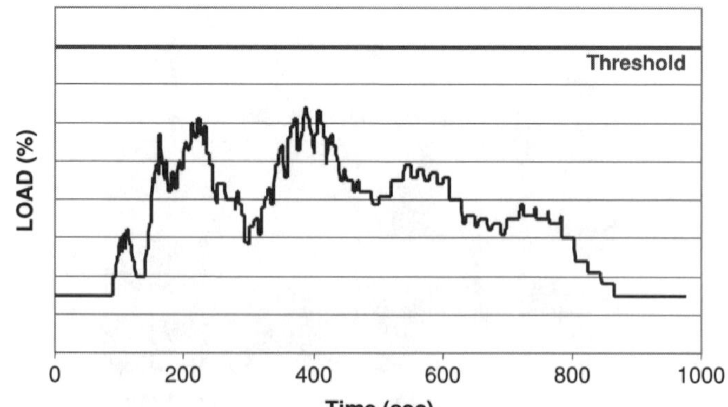

Fig. 12 Radar resources (with cue).

E. External Cueing for Acquisition: Summary

In calculating the cost vs benefit of cued acquisition per TBM type (or range), the accuracy of the cue is of the utmost importance. The cost in resources has already been discussed. While being the most natural method of using external cue data, cued acquisition entails defining special features in the defense system's radar, and also different forms of operational logic. Knowing the qualities of the cue source is important to achieve the highest benefit. We have seen, however, that with proper use the cue can provide significant benefits specifically in countering long-range TBMs (where the exact definition of "long range" depends on the qualities of the defense system studied) and radar load optimization.

These benefits become even more important when the system's performance is degraded, either because of jamming, antiradiation missile (ARM) attacks, or any other reason. Operation under degrading conditions will be discussed later in this chapter.

VI. Defense Planning Using External Cueing

A defense system establishes a defense plan against a specific target once the tracking data have reached sufficient accuracy to ensure that the target is threatening an area that the defense system is interested in defending and that the system has the capability to defend against the specific TBM (in terms of both battlespace and required resources).

Typically, the target will be tracked at a high rate up to this point, because knowing whether or not it should/could be intercepted is of utmost importance to the defender. After a defense plan has been initiated, a different tracking regime will be established for that particular TBM, which will bring the track to a required accuracy at the time of interceptor launch.

During the initial phase of the defense planning, the system has to devote a fairly large number of radar resources to reach the desired accuracy (e.g., time limitations, long range). It also has to reach decisions about the type of target being tracked, and in case the target is not alone in the sky-picture (i.e., it is accompanied by decoys, debris from other interceptions or from an earlier interception attempt by a higher tier system, a separated first stage, etc.), identification of the real target is required.

If external cueing data are available, and are accurate and detailed enough, they may be used to alleviate some of the load on the radar and also assist in the planning process.

Cue data may be used in several ways. First, availability of earlier data may be used to identify the true situation in the sky with which the system is faced. For example, if the defense system radar is tracking a cluster of objects, but cueing data were received only on one TBM along this track, it may be prudent to assume that the cluster contains only one real target, and the other objects being tracked are associated with it (motor, decoys, debris). If cueing is supplied continuously (for example, by an external radar), it may be that the history of cluster formation from the one real target is also known. All this added data could, of course, be very valuable in the defense planning process, but using it correctly requires special algorithms, and assumes a good knowledge of the cue source and its output. It also assumes that cueing is constantly available (at least in a specified sector), because the algorithm must make assumptions regarding the significance of certain objects not

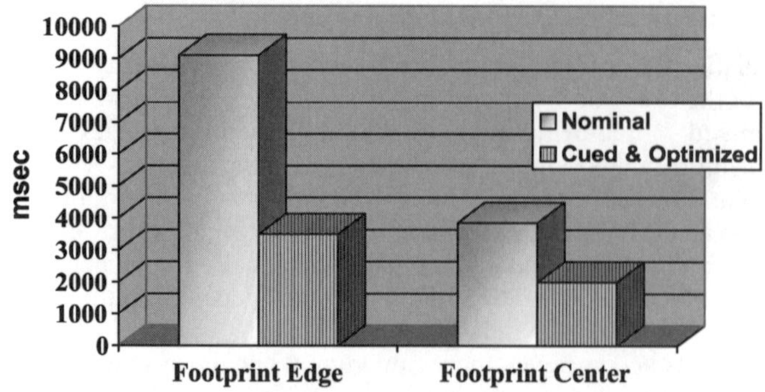

Fig. 13 Radar resources (delayed acquisition).

being reported (e.g., a cue report of one TBM, where the radar is now tracking several objects, would be interpreted as a case of breakup or decoys and not several TBMs).

If the data supplied by the cue source are accurate enough, an (initial) defense plan may be created without actually acquiring and tracking the TBM. This enables the defense system to plan a more economic tracking regime for the TBM, delaying its acquisition by the radar to the most convenient time. The most complex implementation of such a technique will be to attempt to optimize the use of radar resources over an entire salvo, based on the knowledge of future events supplied by the cue. However, such an algorithm is very complex to implement, and would almost inevitably have to make assumptions about cue availability and consistency that may adversely affect the performance in case the cue source, for some reason, does not function as required.

It is possible, however, to gain a lot of time and resources by simpler algorithms. An example can be seen in Fig. 13. In this graph the total amount of radar resources invested in tracking a single TBM aimed at different defended assets (located at the center of the system footprint or on its edge) throughout its flight are plotted. Two alternative tracking regimes are shown:

1) Detect and track by own radar without cueing.

2) Optimal detection based on cue data (minimum resources by either delaying acquisition to the latest possible time or tracking for a long time at a minimal tracking rate).

In both alternatives the same radar performs both search and fire control functions. The tracking regime in the cases plotted was designed to enable interception of the TBM at the same altitude (fixed defense capability). As can be seen clearly, it is possible to use cue data to save resources while maintaining the same defense level.

To illustrate the complexities involved in defense planning based on cue data, a simple algorithm is illustrated in Figs. 14 and 15. This algorithm implements a relatively simple use of cue data. It does not attempt to optimize the use of resources over an entire salvo but rather to delay self acquisition until a suitable time for tracking the target is found, based on defense system priorities and capabilities.

Figure 14 presents the main algorithm. The cue is handled by the defense system battle management center (BMC). It is only sent to the radar when the target (TBM)

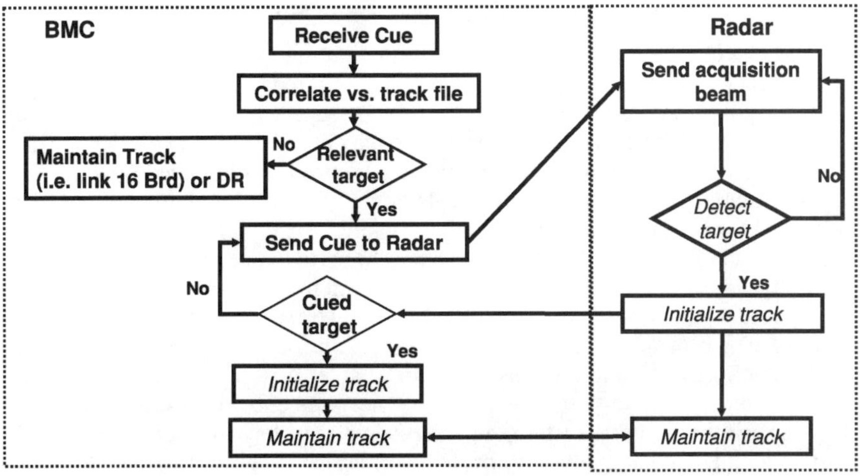

Fig. 14 External cue process flowchart.

is judged to be relevant for handling (acquisition and tracking by the radar). In Fig. 15 the process of deciding which target is relevant for acquisition is elaborated. The target is deemed "interesting" if it attacks an asset under the responsibility of the system. Targets are prioritized according to various preferences stated by the operational user (e.g., a target suspected of carrying weapons of mass destruction will have a higher priority) and according to timing considerations.

The processes in the flowcharts that are added or modified as a result of cue data are printed in boldface. It is important to note that even with this relatively simple algorithm, there are a large number of new functions that have to be developed. The exact cost-effectiveness of each cue handling policy ought to be determined by the weapon system designers based on detailed analysis of the benefits expected and the costs involved.

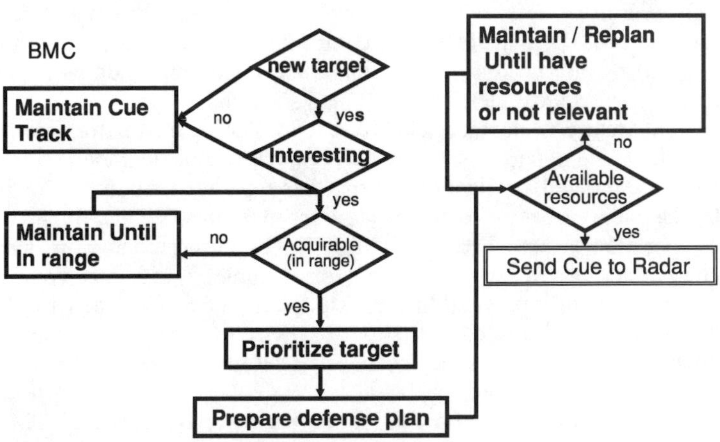

Fig. 15 Determining relevant target.

VII. Interceptor Launch Using Only Cue Data

The most complex use of cue data is for facilitating interceptor launch without acquisition by the defense system's own radar. This may be done as a first step in the engagement process, where the radar is expected to acquire the target during interceptor flight. Alternatively, the cue source may even be considered as providing the full interception solution, guiding the interceptor to its intended target.

This last realization falls, however, outside the realm of this chapter, because, as defined at the beginning of the chapter, we regard an external cue source to be any sensor not controlled by the defense system. In particular, its rate of tracking and reporting cannot be controlled by the defense system, and thus it may not be used for the actual guidance of an interceptor. In other words, we regard external cueing as a one-way transfer of data. Two-way interactions, including those required for guidance of an interceptor, are discussed in Chapter 8.

If the data supplied by the cue source are accurate enough to support a launch decision by the defense system, an interceptor may be launched without self-acquisition. The data received from the cue may be processed by the BMC and used to update the interceptor during flight. The interceptor itself, however, must be acquired and tracked by the defense system radar, if uplink capability is required.

This type of operation requires very good knowledge of the cueing system parameters, such as tracking and reporting rate, bias, etc. It also requires that the intercepting system has full confidence in the availability of cueing throughout the interception process. The defense system BMC and radar must include functions that provide the ability to operate in this mode.

The cost-effectiveness of this approach vs other uses of cueing depends heavily on the specific parameters of the defense system and cue source discussed, and will therefore be left to the consideration of each user regarding a particular system.

VIII. Radar Degraded Performance

The contribution of external cueing was analyzed so far with respect to a defense system operating in its nominal operational conditions. Contribution may be expected in a number of areas, as already described. However, it is safe to say that, in general, if the defense system is well balanced and the capabilities of the radar and interceptor are matched, the contribution of external cueing in normal operation will mainly be felt under subnominal conditions such as edge of the footprint effects, loaded attack scenarios, and so forth.

The whole picture is changed when one is looking at a situation in which the defense system, and in particular the radar, is experiencing degraded performance relative to the expected, or planned, levels. This type of situation may be brought about by the enemy's use of electronic counter measures (ECM), forced changes in radar operation in presence of ARM, or by any other change in one of the parameters affecting radar performance [for example, TBM radar cross section (RCS) is smaller than expected]. In these situations, a performance gap is created in which the system is limited by the performance of a specific element. External cueing is one of the possible means for restoring the original performance level.

Let us treat first the issue of ECM. When the radar is under an ECM attack, the general effect is an increase in the noise level, resulting in decreased *Pd* and thus in either reduced detection range or increased resources needed to maintain

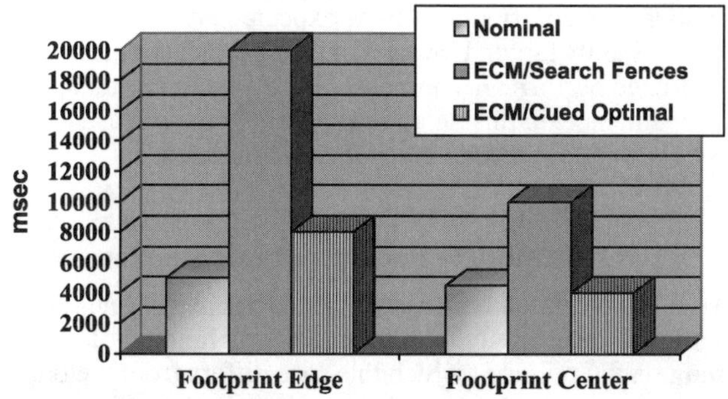

Fig. 16 Resources with and without cue under electronic counter measures.

the same detection range. External cueing data may be used instead of search at the longer ranges, according to the principles discussed in the section dealing with cued acquisition, to enable detection at longer ranges and thus restore system footprint.

Let us look at an example. Assume a defense system performance is degraded by ECM to 70% of its original value. Figure 16 shows the quantity of radar resources needed to intercept a long-range TBM at a fixed point 1) under nominal conditions; 2) under degraded performance, using the resources required to restore search performance (and thus neglecting some of the other radar tasks); and 3) under degraded performance, with optimal acquisition based on cue data.

In each case, the required tracking accuracy at any given time was the same; the radar detection range and track accuracy are a function of the case tested and the tracking rate was adjusted to achieve the required accuracy, at the correct time. Without cueing, there is a significant increase in required resources. With cueing there is an improvement.

It should be noted that to maintain the same level of performance, the case of cued acquisition under degraded performance is still costly in terms of required resources. This is because tracking under ECM requires many more resources than under nominal conditions. However, this process is much cheaper in resource consumption than attempting to restore performance using own search. In reality, given that the radar has a limited quantity of resources that should be divided among several tasks, this may spell the difference between succeeding in restoring the system to its original performance and having to accept a smaller footprint.

Another representative case of degraded performance is when the system has to shut down transmission of the radar in an intermittent or periodic fashion, for example because of the presence of an ARM threat. The system thus needs to compensate for being unable, periodically, to track a certain target or perform search functions, either in general or in a specific region. In this type of situation, defense planning and track maintenance using cue data, if sufficiently accurate cue is available, could allow the system to continue to provide defense. It is also possible to alternate between self track and cued track as the situation requires, while keeping watch of the combined track quality. This type of solution will naturally require suitable logic in the defense system BMC.

Situations of radar degraded performance cause a performance gap between the elements of the defense system, some of which may be closed by intelligent use of external cueing. The contributions to be expected are of the same type as under nominal conditions, only larger. However, it is important to note here that while the situation of degraded performance increases the utility of cue data, it also increases the system's dependence on this data. Thus parameters such as cueing availability and miss/false alarm rate, become much more significant.

IX. Multiple Radars and Cue Sources

Up to now we have limited our discussion to the case of one radar and one cue source. We will now deal briefly with the more general case of many sources and radars, touching on the points in which this case differs from the one-on-one case.

A. Single Radar/Multiple Cue Sources

Let us look first at the case of one radar receiving multiple cues. In principle, if all cue sources are reporting on the same net, using the same reporting protocol and rules (for example, Link-16), this situation may be avoided by use of internal network procedures. However, even in this case it is possible for two cue sources to report the same track because of mistaken association (i.e., tracks supplied by different sources are missmatched). Also, it is quite possible that one or more cue sources are not operating on the same network (for example, a forward deployed collection asset of the defended country may not be linked on the same net as a satellite cueing system).

When two or more cue sources are reporting objects in the same region in the sky, two problems arise: 1) How to associate the various reports to different tracks and 2) what data to use for each track.

The first question involves the use of threat information sharing methods designed to associate between tracks provided by different systems. It is dealt with elsewhere in this book, in the chapter dealing with interoperability. The second question deals with the decision as to what data to use for the cueing process. In all cases, an algorithm to select and/or combine the data has to be provided in the receiving system.

The two possible methods of using the multiple cue source data are either to choose one of the tracks or to combine them using a data fusion algorithm. The relative merits of these two approaches may be deduced from graphs such as the one depicted in Fig. 18. Two radar systems tracking the same TBM produced this graph. One radar is deployed closer to the TBM launch point and the other is located near its intended impact point. The two tracking histories are shown qualitatively in Fig. 17.

In Fig. 18, the accuracy (the major axis of the uncertainty sphere) of each radar track is depicted, together with the two options for track combination, the "choose best" method, and data fusion [using the same BET algorithm described in Eq. (1)]. An interesting feature to note is the abrupt "jump" at the point of transition between radar 1 and radar 2 in the "choose best" graph. In real applications of the "choose best" method, it may be that some smoothing function will have to be defined to deal with these situations.

The graph in Fig. 18 represents, obviously, a specific example. Comparison of the relative utility of the two approaches will have to be conducted according to the true situation (i.e., sensor parameters and deployment, expected number of sources, etc.).

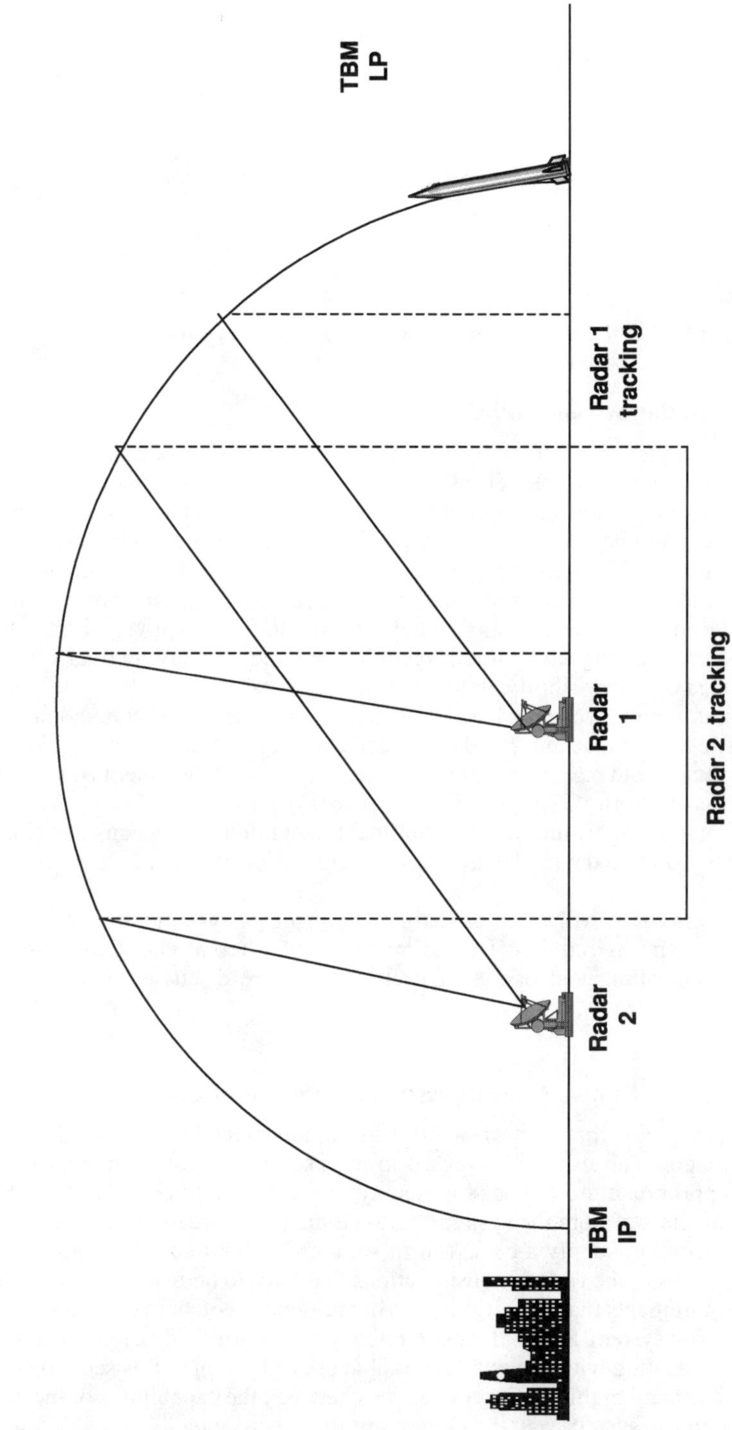

Fig. 17 Multiple cue sources.

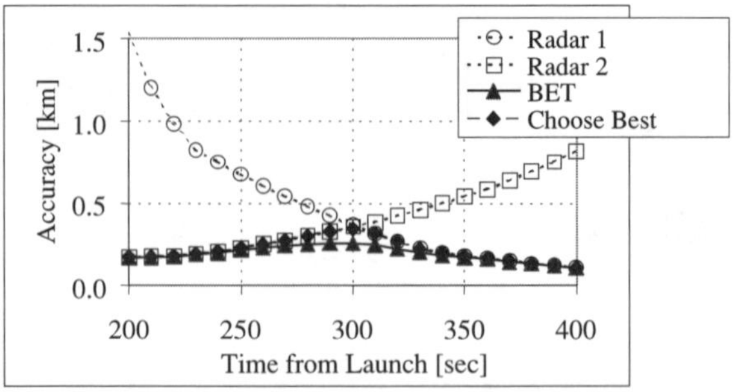

Fig. 18 Combined track accuracy ("choose best" vs data fusion).

B. Several Radar Sensors and Cue Sources

The most complex situation to be discussed with relation to external cueing is that of a number of cue sources serving a number of radar sensors, where the radar sensors are linked and form a single defense system. If the radar systems are not linked, the situation degenerates, to a duplication of the case already described. The main difference between this situation and the ones already discussed, is that a cue distribution mechanism is required. Cue data could be screened at a central unit that determines the radar responsible for each track. Alternatively, it may be distributed freely, having each radar screen the data and act only on tracks in its predefined area of responsibility, giving the same results.

The most complex process of deciding to which radar(s) the cue should be referred has to take into account 1) the attacked asset, 2) the radar coverage, 3) the load on the radar (both current and future projection), and 4) the other tasks of the radar (in terms of priority). Simpler processes can take into account less of the data resulting in simpler algorithms and less optimal functioning. These considerations will have to be combined with the timing and overall priority constraints described earlier.

The considerations involved in operating a multisensor system are much more elaborate than what is required for the treatment of external cue. Other issues involved in controlling and operating such systems are discussed at length in Chapter 8.

X. System Characteristics and the Use of Cues

The final part of this chapter deals with the most fundamental question to defense system developers and users with regard to the use of external cueing: How to choose the appropriate use of cues for their system, taking into account all of the relevant parameters of both the system itself and the cue source(s) available.

It is impossible to supply a closed-form solution to this issue. It is, however, possible to highlight the type of considerations that have to be made, and to point to certain requirements that the various uses of cues impose on both the cue source and the receiving system. Some of these requirements have already been discussed in the sections dealing with each of the possible uses. Our aim to this section is to complete the list and highlight the connections between the capabilities of the cue source, the defense system, and the chosen use for the cue data.

A. Cue Source Requirements

Let us look first at the requirements from the cue source. These requirements may be viewed from two points of view. If the cue source being discussed is a system that is under development, a potential user should influence its development to include qualities supporting their projected use. If, however, the cue source discussed already exists and is operational, analyzing its qualities (in relation to operational requirements) may lead potential users to a better understanding of the benefits and limitations of using that specific source in their system.

Requirements from the cue source are divided into the following categories.

1) *Availability:* The capability of the cue source to provide constant surveillance of specific areas. This attribute has both a technical side (time of deployment and operation, dependence on weather) and an operational/political side (the extent to which the cue operator is willing to commit the cue source for the needs of a specific cue user).

2) *Operational reliability:* The capability of the cue source to detect and supply up-to-date cue on all TBMs in its area of responsibility. This attribute is measured by two important parameters: false alarm rate and miss rate.

3) *Time delay:* The time gap between cue measurement and actual receipt of cue data. This factor includes both the calculation time in the cue source itself and the delays associated with dissemination of the data.

4) *Accuracy:* The errors in the cue data provided.

5) *Frequency:* The number of times that cue is provided and the time between consecutive reports.

6) *Type of data:* Data include position, full state vector, launch point estimation/impact point prediction, etc.

Table 2 connects between the possible uses of cues and the required attributes of the cue source. It is important to point out that the table includes the least severe requirement for each use. For example, in the case of "cue with search," the frequency requirement is one time. Obviously, a higher frequency will be useful, but it is not necessary as cued search can be conducted based on a one time report. Also, some of the requirements depend on the actual qualities of the systems discussed. In those cases, the methods of deducing these requirements were pointed out earlier in the appropriate sections.

B. Cue Receiving System Requirements

The requirements from the cue receiving system are stated in the form of required capabilities. These capabilities are mostly achieved through BMC algorithms and radar capabilities. Throughout this chapter, we have explained the need for these algorithms, and have hinted, to the best of our ability in the limited space of one chapter, to the principles governing their realization. Table 3 should be treated as a checklist where the specifics of each requirement depend heavily on the characteristics of the defense system(s) and the cue source. It is also important to note that the complexity of each required algorithm changes with the situation discussed. For example, a cue distribution mechanism that only has to deal with point defense systems, with no overlap in defense capabilities, will be much simpler than one developed to disseminate information between systems with large, overlapping footprints.

Table 2 Requirements from cue source

	Use					
Requirements	Early warning	Launch point prediction	Cue with search	Cue instead of search	Defense planning	Interceptor launch
Availability	Low	Low	Low	Very high	N/A	Very high
Reliability	High	High	High, to avoid wasting radar resources	Very high	N/A	N/A
Time delay	N/A	As soon as possible (to avoid launcher movement)	Depending on radar cued-search attributes	Like cue with search	Depending on defense plan algorithm requirements	Very small delay
Accuracy	Depending on size of population clusters	Depending on launch point prediction algorithm requirements	Depending on radar cued-search attributes	Like cue with search	Depending on defense plan algorithm requirements	Very good accuracy
Frequency	Once	Once	Once	Number of times/ continuous	Continuous	Continuous
Type of data	Alert	Track of launch point	State vector	State vector	State vector	State vector plot

Table 3 Requirements from the receiving system

	Use					
Requirements	Early warning	Launch point prediction	Cue with search	Cue instead of search	Defense plan	Interceptor launch
Cued search beam	N/A	N/A	√	√	N/A	N/A
Cue distribution mechanism	N/A	√	√	√	N/A	N/A
Defense plan logic based on cue	N/A	N/A	N/A	N/A	√	√
Radar load in presence of cue	N/A	N/A	√	√	√	√
Defense plan execution using cue	N/A	N/A	N/A	N/A	N/A	√
Multiple cue handling (data integration)	N/A	√	√	√	√	√

Tables 2 and 3, when treated on the basis of the analyses and observations provided in the other sections of this chapter, may be of assistance in selecting and implementing the proper use for external cueing in a given situation.

XI. Summary

External cueing is one of the mechanisms by which a defense system can be assisted by other forces or devices operating in its region. The basic commodity that external cueing has to supply is time. The time gained by receiving the cue may be used by the system in a number of ways, which have been defined and analyzed throughout this chapter.

The benefits that the system derives from external cueing may be expressed in terms of timing of critical processes, availability of resources at key moments, the ability to compensate for performance gaps caused by various counter measures, etc. We have shown a number of ways to quantify these benefits, which may be used for performing cost-effectiveness analyses of the various methods for using the cue.

These benefits, however, do not come without a cost. The cost of receiving external cues lies in having to implement the capability to treat them properly. This requirement, obviously, is more costly as the use of cueing becomes more complex.

The information provided in this chapter, along with the chapter dealing with interoperability, is intended to provide the reader with a mapping of the trade space involved in the complex problem of selecting and implementing appropriate mechanisms for connecting between defense systems. Exact solutions, however, should be defined by the reader based on specific situations.

Chapter 10

Battle Management

Haim Baruch*
WALES Ltd., Ramat-Gan, Israel

I. Introduction

THE emerging threat of the TBM is not new and neither is it a typical representative of 1990s warfare. Its roots go back to World War II. However, following a long pause, the 1991 Persian Gulf War tactical ballistic missiles (TBMs) emerged once again as a strategic threat in their "mighty splendor." On this occasion the TBM left an everlasting impression because of their overwhelming effect on the Middle East psyche. In a flicker of an eye it almost paralyzed the economy of a highly developed and modern country and terrorized one of the most advanced societies in this century—Israel.

The Persian Gulf War and its outcome were the main trigger for the acceleration of the development programs of new weapon systems, able to cope with the TBM threats—mainly the Israeli Arrow weapon system (AWS) and the American theater high-altitude area defense (THAAD). These events also piqued the interest of many of the industrialized countries in Europe. Concurrently with the development of the new weapon systems it became obvious that to properly use the new systems, revamped battle management concepts, better suited to the new environment, would have to be created.

In this chapter various aspects of battle management, along with the various BMC (battle management center) concepts are introduced and analyzed. Most of these are taken from the Israeli experience, accumulated during the AWS development program.

In what manner are the TBM threat characteristics different from those of the manned aircraft or helicopter threat, and what are the attributes that require BMC adaptation (as part of the weapon system) to the new environment? When we analyze the TBM threat we can point to several characteristics that differentiate it from fighter aircraft:

1) A TBM can be launched from almost any site once it is within the target's range. Thus the launch site can be very much unpredictable and imposes some difficulties on locating the antitactical ballistic missile (ATBM) systems.

Copyright © 2000 by the American Institute of Aeronautics and Astronautics, Inc. All rights reserved.

*Senior Expert.

2) The TBM trajectory, once detected, is very rigid, and its impact point can be predicted with high accuracy.

3) Reentry speed is very high, which reduces the engagement opportunities and therefore requires a consolidation of short battle management processes that will leave enough time for the interception itself.

4) It is quite likely that in the future we will face new TBM generations that will utilize decoys and other aids for penetration.

II. BMC Objectives and Tasks

A. BMC Objectives

Battle management comprises the accumulated activities of processing intelligence information, planning a mission, and managing it during its execution stage. Traditionally, when aerial offensive missions are discussed, battle management is considered to be a "force multiplier" tool. This is very much the case also during ATBM defensive operations. The ability to shift forces (launched interceptors) from one sector to another, on short notice, and the ability to change the main effort activity and possibly impose on the opponent (attacker) less-than-desirable directions of attack, are part of the yield of the defensive BMC activity. Although defense activities are by nature a response to the aggressor's moves, they can still contribute to the overall force multiplication effect.

Consumers of sensor resources can be divided into three groups. Those performing surveillance, those performing trajectory prediction, and those controlling the interceptions. And there are of course the interception weapons themselves, which by their nature are limited in numbers. It should be borne in mind that during saturation attacks it would be difficult to switch resources from task to task. In such a case the focus of the battle management contribution may change somewhat into another objective that can be summarized as "resource management." Thus the tasks of the BMC are as follows.

1. Create a Defense Plan

One of the battle management tasks is to generate defense plans against TBMs that are on a course toward defended areas. A defense plan is the answer of the battle management to an intruding TBM. This plan is a combination of decisions and resources that have been reserved to engage a target. It includes one or more interceptors allotted to intercept a particular TBM along with radar resources earmarked for the task.

2. Optimize Overall Defense

An effective ATBM layout may comprise several different weapon system types. Sometimes it even includes other nations' weapon systems participating in a collaborative ATBM effort (see Sec. II.A.3). The complete ATBM activity includes the planning of the total defense layout based on 1) a predetermined policy, 2) decisions concerning current intelligence information, 3) the importance of each one of the assets that one wishes to defend, and 4) the use of various weapon systems that are deployed in the area (AWS, Patriot, THAAD, etc.), in a manner that will provide more than one defense layer for each defended asset.

3. Utilize All Resources

Radar and interceptors, in particular, must be used optimally. Because TBM detection, tracking, and defense planning and execution are high resource-consuming procedures, there is a constant need to carefully measure the current resource consumption levels and compare them with the planned resource consumption to be able to provide radar and interceptor system requirements.

4. Control Systems According to Unified Concepts

As mentioned previously, several weapon system types can participate in the ATBM campaign. Each one of these systems is not necessarily confined to the same concepts and can perform its mission according to different sets of conditions, such as policy, sky-picture, and intelligence. Therefore, one of the main BMC tasks is to provide an integrated situation map to all of the participating weapon systems.

5. Improve Overall Defense Structure Efficiency

Each weapon system usually has its own efficiencies and deficiencies. This is a result of the subsystem's characteristics, such as sensor characteristics (detection range, engagement range, and resolution) and killing vehicle features (effective range, warhead, acceleration rate, and homing devices), etc. One of the BMC objectives is to augment the advantages of each one of the weapon systems and diminish the disadvantages by mutual interfacing, thus contributing to the overall defense layout efficiency. This efficiency is measured in terms of the number of killed TBMs out of the total number of approaching and intercepted TBMs—the leakage rate. The objective of the ATBM defense layout is to minimize the leakage rate.

6. Minimize Overkill Phenomenon

The overkill phenomenon is a situation where several weapon systems that are part of the same defense layout unnecessarily engage the same target. This is an obvious case where radar and interception resources are wasted. It is the responsibility of the BMC to avoid such occurrences and determine which is the best, optimized solution to engage a target, without also increasing the leakage rate.

B. BMC in the Era of Interoperability

One of the new phenomena that emerged as a result of the Persian Gulf War experience is that alliances are to be considered to fight the TBM threat. This cooperation brings up the problem that different weapon systems from different countries have to work in concert. This is termed "interoperability" and is reflected in many ATBM considerations, including BMC. Actually the BMC is the main link of integration between any two or more ATBM systems, coming from different countries, that have to operate in full harmony. Here we will discuss the command, control, communications, and intelligence aspects of interoperability.

The ability to use information that is received from external sources and to use it concurrently with (and integrate it into) one's own database is of a great advantage. The main contribution is in longer alert and cueing times. Such a contribution is appreciated especially when one bears in mind the long ranges that today's TBM are fired from and the deployment limitations (political and consequently geographical) that are imposed on the defender. Successfully implemented interoperability will enable one party, which is confined to deploying its defense weapons within its borders, to receive alerts and cueing from sensors that are deployed outside the country's boundaries, thus dramatically enlarging its defense layout's effective killing envelopes. Interoperability is one of the new issues that have been recognized and only lately addressed, and therefore is still not yet mastered. However, its potential, as revealed in studies and war scenarios, is enormous, and certainly calls for further exploration and implementation.

The BMC responsibility in this field is in the following areas.

1) Disseminating relevant information to other parties.

2) Collating the information that is received from other members of the same net and presenting to the operators a unified data map (sky-picture and other relevant information items).

3) Issuing external cues to local sensors (to acquire targets) through the data dissemination mechanism.

4) Coordinating between weapon systems originating in different countries that operating according to different doctrines but are confined to act according to the policy of the host country. This coordination includes all of the battlefield activities, including policy, rules of engagement (ROE), target allocations and engagements, and so on.

III. Battle Management Process

A. Main Battle Management Process

The main stages in the ATBM defense process are depicted in Fig. 1. The process comprises three main software blocks: sky-picture generation software block, resources management and defense planning software block, and battle management (execution) software block.

The sensor detects the target, or the target information is supplied from an external cue and then acquired by the local sensors. Once the target (or targets) is confirmed the BMC generates the sky-picture. According to the target attributes (such as classification, launch area, etc.), a defense plan is constructed and the required resources (radar resources as well as interceptors) are allotted. The BMC then waits for the launch time to issue a launch order.

The next step is for the BMC to monitor the interception courses of the target and the interceptor, to detect deviations from the optimal interception trajectories, and to intervene to issue midcourse corrections or interception termination command. The main process is subdivided into several events as described further.

B. Functions Along the Main Process

To accomplish an ATBM mission, the BMC has to perform several functions. The order of functions is according to the evolution of the threat. Actually the process starts long before the war, by collecting intelligence data about potential threats' attributes. In parallel a large number of battle scenarios are evaluated to learn the possible effects of each opponent's attack scheme and to give proper answers in terms of optimal deployment. This process is graphically described in Fig. 2.

Most of these functions are conducted sequentially with a successful completion of the former task usually being a precondition to start the next one.

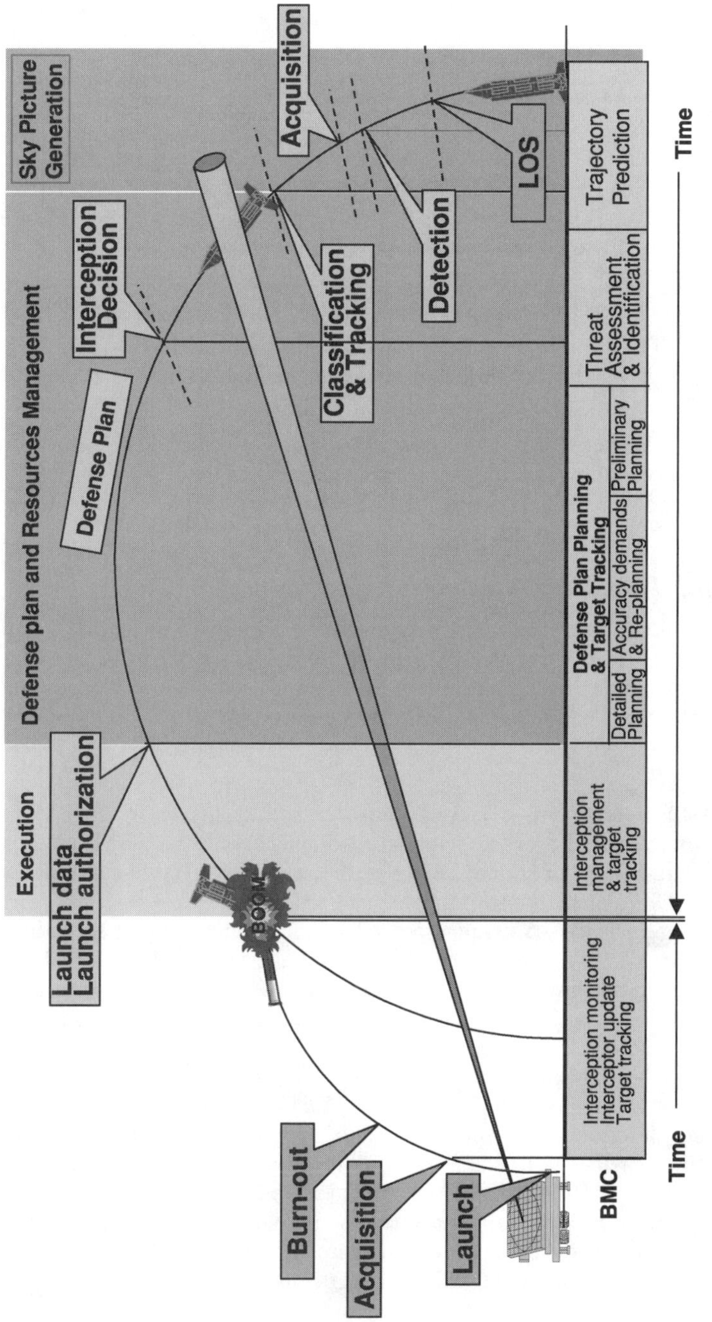

Fig. 1 Main battle management process.

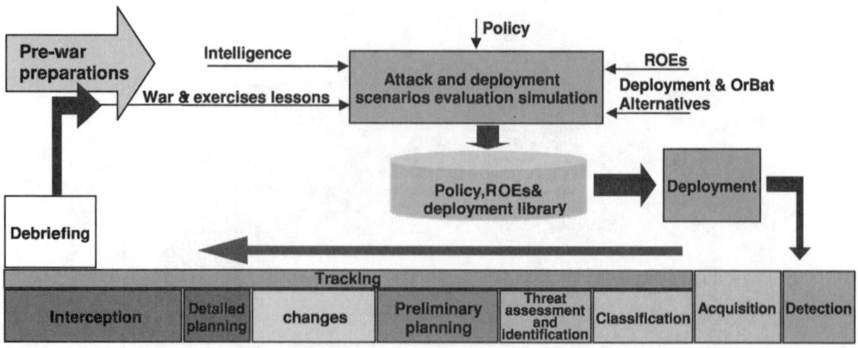

Fig. 2 Functions along the main process.

Obviously there are cases where new and updated information becomes available during the process. In such a case a new evaluation of the results gained so far is conducted and sometimes part of the tasks that have been completed have to be reevaluated or even repeated.

1. Defense Layout and Engagement Policy Planning

This task is conducted as an offline procedure, prior to a TBM attack and preferably before the war or the deployment of the defense systems. It includes high echelon decisions as to the placement of the radar sensors and weapon batteries and the policy that will be adopted at the beginning of the war.

2. Detection

Successful detection is a precondition for setting the entire ATBM defense system in motion. The problem with detection is that because TBMs are involved, a huge volume of space should be covered to enable a reliable surveillance, and this calls for special search techniques.

This being a phased-array radar, fence-surveillance or volume-surveillance are employed. In the first, one or more rows of radar beams create narrow-elevation "fences," which in azimuth extend the full width of the desired surveillance sector. Every ascending missile has to cross these fences and thus be detected. Unfortunately this technique is radar-energy intensive.

Volume-surveillance concentrates a sufficient number of radar beams to cover a much smaller volume of space, both in azimuth and elevation. While more frugal in resources, it requires prior intelligence to know where to look.

The choice of the particular technique to be used (or a blend of the two) is determined by the BMC, based on tactical as well as higher policy decisions. One of the BMC tasks is to arrange for the division of the surveillance volume among the array of sensors and yet to ensure sufficient overlapping to avoid any unwelcome leakage on the individual sensors' surveillance boundaries.

3. Prediction and Classification

Once a target is detected, it undergoes a number of evaluations. The first stage is to determine the trajectory of the target to find the answers to the following questions: 1) Is this a TBM? 2) What is the estimated launch point? 3) What is the predicted impact area? 4) What is the time to impact?

The answers to these questions are vital to the continuation of the entire process. The classification information serves as an initial filter in determining whether this particular TBM will impact within an area of interest. This information is important to the decision whether to intercept the TBM or let it go unengaged. It is also important to the civil defense authorities to alert the population at the impact point area. Impact time is among the parameters that are taken into consideration as part of the defense plan preparation. The knowledge of the launch point and its distance assists in the identification of the TBM, and it is vital to the counter-force planners.

4. *Identification*

Identification of the TBM type is a subset of the classification task. From the threat identification data one can learn about the type of the warhead and choose the proper ROE, the engaging weapon system, and the right interception parameters (number of interceptors, intercept altitudes, etc.).

Furthermore, if this is the opening move of a war, this information is of immense important to politicians, the military, and in essence to almost any government agency.

5. *Threat Evaluation*

Once all of the information is available, the threat evaluation task is performed. Actually, this task takes the information that has been achieved so far through the sensors and processed by the system's algorithms (prediction and classification) and compares it with the policy that has been embedded in the system. Once the findings match the policy demands, the system builds a defense plan. Obviously there are cases where the policy demands are not met by the system's capabilities or findings. In such a case the BMC will notify the operators about this situation and wait for further instructions.

6. *Preparation of a Defense Plan*

A defense plan is an implementation of a set of rules in the real-world picture as revealed through the eyes of the sensors. A defense plan is a sum-up of the following: 1) The level of threat as dictated by the policy and calculated by the system. A threat can be classified at several levels according to the importance of the area that is defended by the system or according to the missile/warhead type. 2) ROE. 3) Availability of resources (interceptors and sensors' energy). 4) Constraints, technical and doctrinal, such as a prohibition to launch all of the interceptors of the same defense-plan from a single site.

It should be emphasized that because of the short time intervals involved, the preparation of the defense plan is a highly automated (computer backed) process, and only in extraordinary cases would human intervention be required.

Once a defense-plan is prepared it waits for its execution time. As long as a defense plan has not been executed, it can be updated or replaced by a new defense plan, as a result of changes in the conditions and defense requirements. The need for changes can stem from various reasons such as new, arriving TBMs that have been detected or reported after the defense plan has been prepared and are of a higher engagement priority; sudden reduction in the availability of resources because of their sudden reallocation, battle damage, or technical reasons; and changes in operator decisions as a result of new policy or because of an individual's subjective judgment.

7. *Execution (Interception)*

Once the interceptor is launched, the last phase of the BMC task is initiated. At this stage this is mostly a monitoring task.

8. *Debriefing*

This is the last task that is performed by the BMC. The information is presented in a format that enables the operational analysis people to investigate the performance of both the system and the operators and to make the required changes in preparation for the next attack. It should be pointed out that in conventional air battles, let alone ground combat, debriefing may take place hours after the event without detracting from its usefulness. In the case of TBM warfare it is attempted to be done within minutes of the actual engagement to draw conclusions prior to the next salvo.

IV. BMC Types

A. Introduction

As part of the study of the BMC presented here, three BMC types were investigated. This study was conducted on a theoretical basis, though most of the inputs were taken from the AWS concepts. The three evaluated concepts addressed were delegated BMC, centralized BMC, and distributed BMC.

B. Delegated BMC Approach

The delegated BMC concept incorporates several operation centers (battery level BMCs) that are operating in conjunction, under a set of policies and ROEs that are delegated to them through a master BMC. (The reader is reminded that in addition to the interceptor launchers the battery has it own radar.) Each center is handed down a policy under which it performs its tasks within particular area of responsibility (AOR) boundaries. The AOR is dictated by the master BMC, based on previous know-how about the performances and capabilities of each one of the battery types and in accordance with the policy dictated by the higher echelon. The coordination level among the batteries and the cooperation requirements are also a part of the same policy that is delegated to the batteries. The master BMC is also linked to strategic information sources (satellite, intelligence, etc.). On the basis of this information and the current situation of each battery, the master BMC decides which of the subordinate batteries will be updated with this new information.

Once a battery has to make decisions that are not within its mandate, the local BMC has to address the master BMC and ask for permission to deviate from the original guidelines. The master BMC is the only element in the chain of command that is linked to a higher echelon. Through this link the current situation is reported and new policies are determined.

A delegated BMC is an evolutionary step of a system that is still undergoing a development process. This concept was included in the study because it is the initial and simplest one in the evolution from single battery layout to a complete ATBM architecture. A delegated structure is shown in Fig. 3.

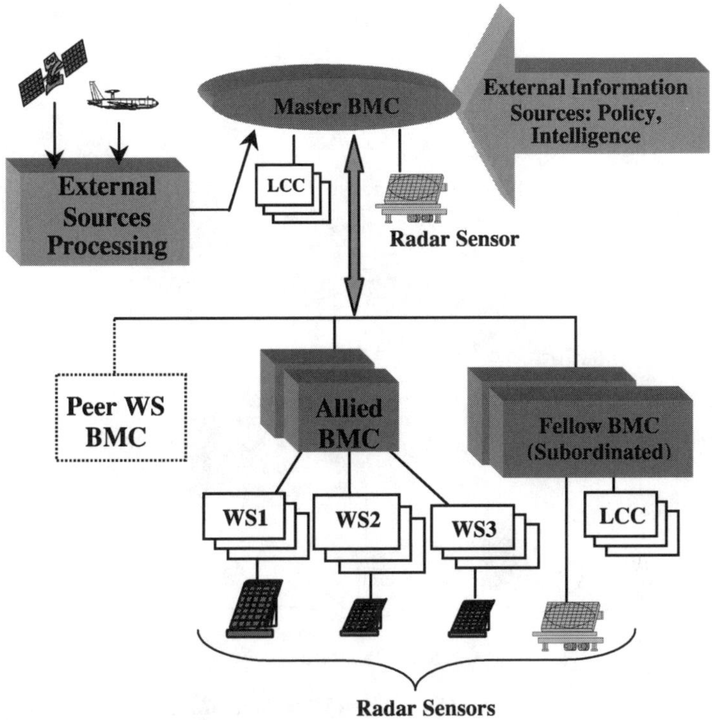

Fig. 3 Delegated BMC structure.

C. Centralized BMC Approach

The centralized BMC is a single operations center that integrates all of the information sources, and it generates a unified (fused) database. All of the sensors are linked directly to the central BMC and, based on their reports, a common sky-picture is generated. The central BMC is also responsible for the resource management of all of the batteries that are linked to it and for the optimization of the interception groups (radar and interceptor launch sites) that were created for engaging a target. In the cases where (because of the system's attributes) a direct link between the radar and the battery's own BMC is required to execute the interception (e.g., a Patriot battery), we assumed a three-staged process.

In the first-stage radar reports (plots, tracks, or any other combination, and including the batteries' own radar information) are sent to the main tracker in the central BMC. In the main tracker the data fusion process is performed and a common sky-picture is generated.

Based on the sky-picture that is generated in the central BMC, tactical decisions as to the engagement of the various targets are made. These also include decisions about the engagement priorities and the most suitable battery to carry it out.

In the last stage, the battery, by its own means, uses its radar to execute the mission.

The central BMC is connected to the higher echelon level where policy is determined. Apart from this, all other ATBM activities are under its total responsibility.

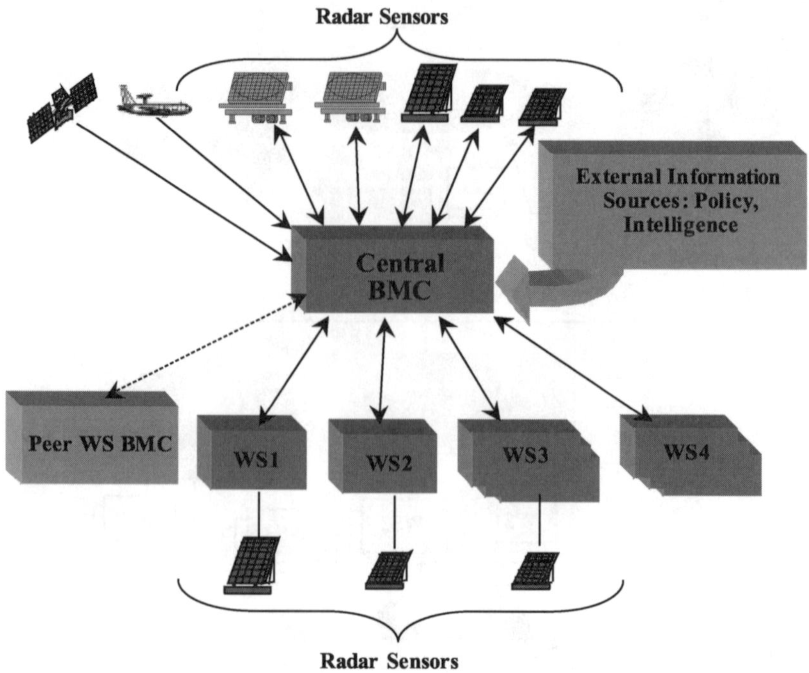

Fig. 4 Centralized BMC structure.

The central BMC consists of one command group (in contrast to multiple command groups, one per each battery in the delegated concept) that takes care of all of the required activities. The autonomy of the batteries is only for the execution level. All of the earlier tasks, such as trajectory prediction, target classification, and reparation of a defense plan, are under the complete responsibility of the central BMC. (The reader is reminded that in the delegated system, already discussed, all of these functions were carried out within the battery's BMC.) Once all of these tasks have been completed, the fire order is delegated to the battery that executes the interception and reports the results.

A centralized BMC structure is shown in Fig. 4.

D. Distributed BMC Approach

The distributed BMC approach accentuates the autonomy of the individual systems as opposed to the centralized approach. However, to enable a genuine level of cooperation between the individual weapon systems, a logic based on figure of merit (FOM) reports was established. According to this approach, every weapon system uses its own means to detect targets. Targets are acquired and reported through an L-16 (Link-16) bus to all other systems that are members in the net. Targets are reported with their track number, location coordinates, and the calculated local (at battery level) FOM that includes all of the engagement success probabilistic calculations of that target.

Other weapon systems that have not acquired the target by their own means will use this information as an external cue for acquisition. Once the target is acquired,

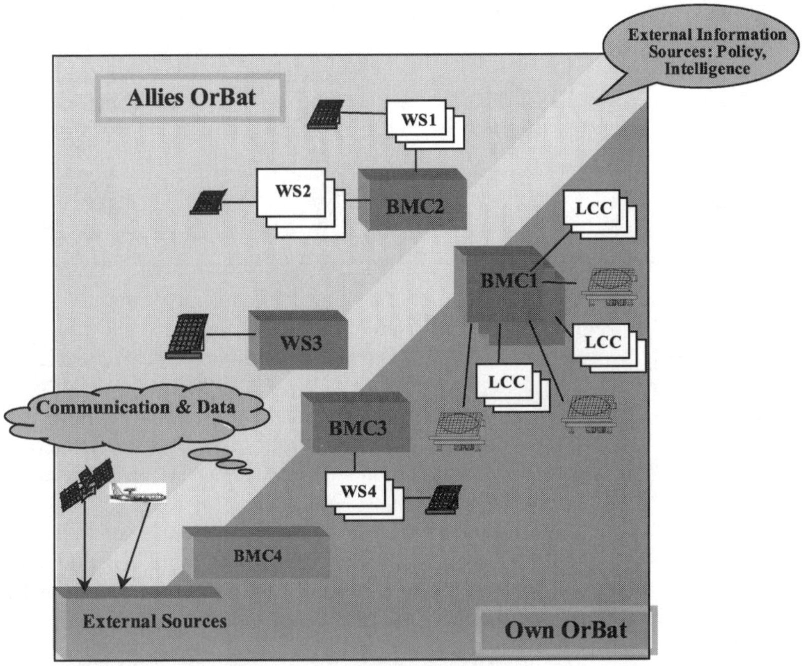

Fig. 5 Distributed BMC structure.

it is reported through the L-16 bus, with the new acquiring battery's calculated FOM. The system with the highest FOM engages the target, based on ROE that are predefined by higher echelons.

The sky-picture in this concept is part of the L-16 database that is disseminated among all the net members. There is no single place where a battery commander can see the entire picture, and only the higher echelon has a complete picture of the battle. A schematic picture, of a distributed BMC architecture is depicted in Fig. 5.

E. Evaluation Method

To measure the efficiency of each one of the three BMC types, a parametric model that measures the delay times caused by the different BMC processes was developed. This was done because the only measurable parameter in the BMC process, and the one that can be used as a common denominator for all BMCs, is *time*, or in other words, time delays caused by the BMC processes. The objective of the simulation runs was to evaluate the contribution of the different BMC concepts in terms of destroyed TBMs and consumed interceptors.

F. Conclusion

The results of this simulation are presented in Fig. 6 and Table 1. They show that given specific BMC definitions and the particular scenario the simulation was run under, the centralized BMC is the best solution. However, out of caution,

Table 1 **BMC concept evaluation: killed TBM vs launched interceptors**

BMC concept	Killed TBMs	Launched interceptors	Ratio (launched/killed)
Centralized	28.7	31.4	1.09
Delegated	21.7	30.9	1.42
Distributed	14	24.2	1.73

we prefer to confine this statement to the Middle East arena, mainly because scenarios for other regions were not evaluated. According to these results, the centralized BMC scored more killed TBMs, for a lower price for each TBM destroyed.

To evaluate the sensitivity of the achieved results to various parameters, a sensitivity analysis that relates to one of the parameters only, was performed. The evaluated parameter was *detection time*, and the evaluated BMC was the centralized BMC concept. The results are shown in Fig. 7.

From the results that are presented in the graph, one can clearly see that there is a certain time up to which the number of killed TBMs and launched interceptors is more or less stable, and from that point there occurs a steep trend of the curve downward. These results hint that there are obvious relations among the processes that should be further investigated.

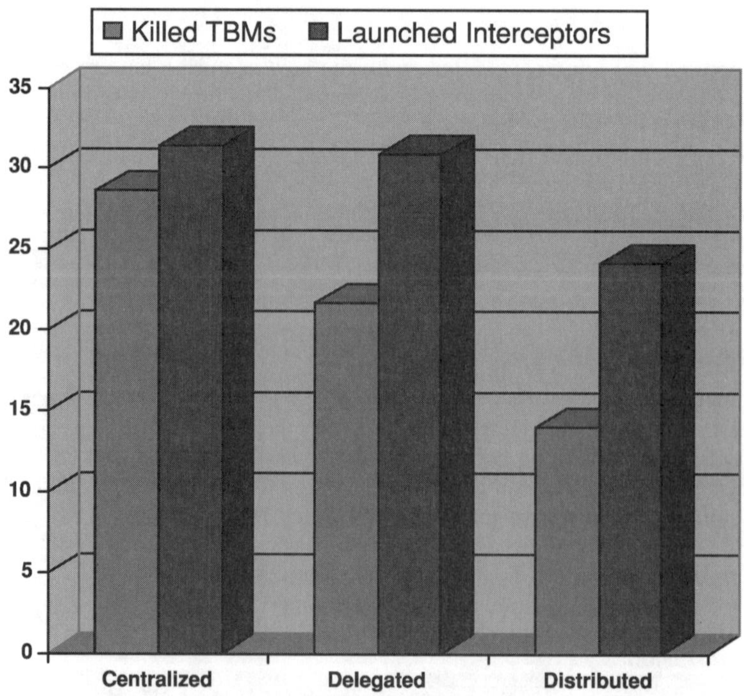

Fig. 6 BMC concept evaluation: killed TBM vs launched interceptors.

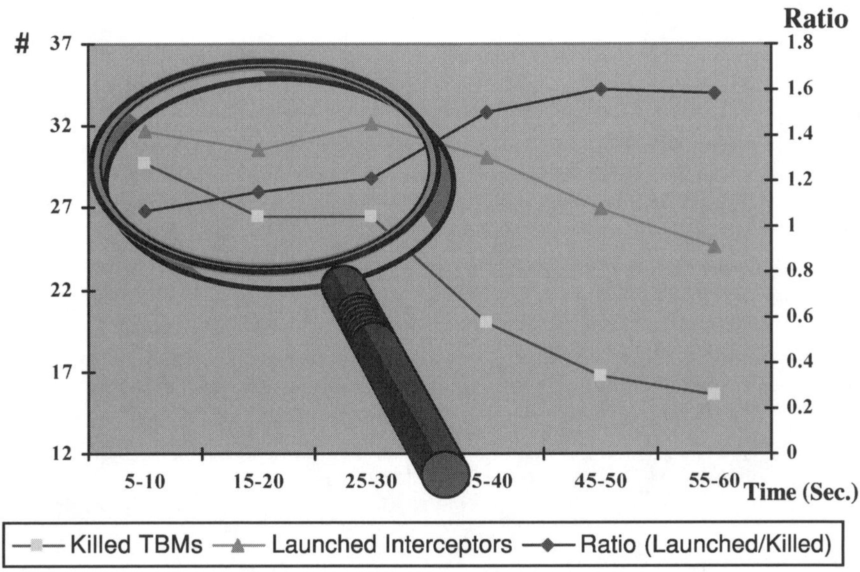

Fig. 7 Sensitivity analysis results.

V. Summary

BMC is an integral and important part of the ATBM weapon system. It can be implemented in many ways, and the range of solutions changes according to the needs and the resources at hand. The important thing in defining a BMC is to exactly formulate the problems the system, including the BMC, will have to face. Actually this part is the most difficult one. Once this obstacle has been removed, the solutions are only technical details.

It is important to remember that the BMC is not the leading part of the weapon system and in no way should it dictate solutions. On the other hand it cannot be ignored during the weapon system's development phases and it requires the same attention as any other part of the system.

The importance of the BMC is in its being a vital contributor to the execution of the mission. Therefore it is important to integrate the BMC with the entire system's elements in such a way that it will be able to monitor all the processes and intervene when necessary.

And last, but not least, is the human role in battle management. The level of human involvement is not a matter of fashion but is dependent on timing constraints and the required level of automation of the system. However we do believe that the time has not yet come and that technology has not reached the level of maturity that human operators can be taken out of the loop. On the contrary, the more complicated weapon systems are, and the more unexpected things may happen in war, the greater is the human operator's contribution to the success of the mission.

IV. Guidance and Control in Theater Ballistic Missile Defense

Chapter 11

Antiballistic Missile Interception Guidance

M. Guelman*
Technion—Israel Institute of Technology, Haifa, Israel

Nomenclature

$\boldsymbol{a}_M$	= missile interceptor acceleration
$\boldsymbol{a}_M^*$	= missile optimal acceleration vector
$\boldsymbol{a}_T$	= target acceleration
c	= ballistic missile engine exhaust velocity
E	= elliptic integral of the second kind
$\boldsymbol{E}$	= complete elliptic integral of the second kind
F	= elliptic integral of the first kind
$\boldsymbol{F}$	= complete elliptic integral of the first kind
$G(s)$	= missile transfer function
$\boldsymbol{G}$	= set of all transfer functions that impose zero miss distance to proportional navigation guidance
J	= performance index of optimality
$K(s)$	= controller transfer function
k	= performance index weighting factor
m	= ballistic missile mass
N	= proportional navigation constant
N'	= effective proportional navigation constant
$\boldsymbol{R}$	= interceptor-target distance vector
$\boldsymbol{R}_M$	= interceptor position vector
$\boldsymbol{R}_T$	= target position vector
T	= ballistic missile engine thrust
t_f	= flight time (finite time)
$\boldsymbol{V}_M$	= interceptor velocity vector
$\boldsymbol{V}_T$	= target velocity vector
V_C	= closing velocity
y	= normal position
X_M, Y_M, Z_M	= interceptor three dimensional coordinates

Copyright © 2000 by the American Institute of Aeronautics and Astronautics, Inc. All rights reserved.

*Professor, Faculty of Aerospace Engineering and Head, Asher Space Research Institute.

X_T, Y_T, Z_T	= target three dimensional coordinates
z_{m0}	= zero effort final range vector
γ	= path angle
δ	= missile velocity to line of sight angle
Δ_0	= interception duration
μ_0	= missile-target maneuver ratio
θ	= line of sight angle
$\boldsymbol{\lambda}_R, \boldsymbol{\lambda}_V$	= adjoint vectors
τ	= time-to-go
τ_1	= missile time constant
σ	= system output
ζ	= damping ratio
ω	= frequency
ω_n	= natural frequency
$\boldsymbol{\omega}_M$	= interceptor flight direction turning rate vector

Subscripts

c	= commanded value
m	= measured value
f	= final value
0	= initial value

Superscript

$\cdot$	= time differentiation

I. Introduction

BALLISTIC missiles have three phases of flight: boost, midcourse, and terminal. The boost phase occurs while the missile's fuel is still burning as it rises from its launcher and the guidance system is active. In the midcourse phase, which occurs in space, the flight is ballistic according to Kepler's laws. The terminal phase occurs as the missile reenters the Earth's atmosphere.

At the boost phase the ballistic missile is a large, visible target and dynamically has a very definite behavior pattern, without any random maneuvers. Once the midcourse is initiated the ballistic missile engines are cut off. During reentry they may have the capability to maneuver. Achieving a maneuvering capability lower in the atmosphere is not particularly challenging, as the Persian Gulf War SCUD missiles demonstrated. To counter such maneuvers a defensive interceptor must also be highly maneuverable. Achieving effective intercept capability requires either an interceptor with more maneuvering capability or shifting to interceptors designed to intercept higher in the atmosphere or outside the atmosphere.

In this chapter a review will be made of interceptor missile guidance. Different guidance laws, from classical (proportional navigation) to optimal, and differential games guidance laws will be discussed, as well as their application to ballistic missile interception.

II. Guidance Systems

Guidance is the process of modifying the trajectory of a vehicle in motion to reach a prespecified target. The target is, in the most general sense, a set of states (position, velocity) either fixed in time or time varying.

Every missile guidance system consists of a sensing system (navigation system), processing (guidance) system, and an actuating (control) system. The function of the navigation system involves knowing the present state with respect to the target itself. The function of the guidance system is to determine the commands to the control system to reach the target. The control system function is to implement the commands to achieve the ordered flight path.

The operation of the guidance system is based on the principle of feedback. The guidance system makes corrective adjustments of the vehicle motion control forces (aerodynamic, propulsive) when a guidance error is present. The guidance system closes the loop through the pursuit kinematics. Guidance systems are essentially nonlinear and operate only for a finite time.

The guidance law establishes a relationship between the commands (control variables) and the measured state (state variables and time):

$$\text{control variables} = G_L(\text{state variables, time})$$

In general the guidance process in antiballistic missile systems is divided into phases. There is a midcourse phase, from launch until the missile's seeker locks on the ballistic missile target, and a terminal phase, from the seeker's lock-on until interception. The system requirements vary from phase to phase. In midcourse guidance, the essential requirement is to achieve lock-on and generally inertial guidance is employed. To implement inertial guidance, either an external system tracks the target and provides target position and velocity updates to the interceptor missile, or a future target behavior is assumed. When an external tracking system is employed, the interceptor missile modifies its trajectory according to the updated information.

Once lock-on is achieved, terminal guidance is initiated and a specific terminal guidance law is implemented.

Terminal guidance has already been a research subject for more than half a century. At the beginning, guidance methods were developed on an intuitive basis. Later on, mathematical methods were employed for the synthesis of guidance laws.

Proportional navigation (PN) is the most commonly used method for missile guidance. A vast amount of literature exists on the subject (see e.g., Ref. 1 and the references therein). Solutions of PN[2,3] indicate that for the case of ideal dynamics, i.e., no delays exist between the line of sight (LOS) rate and the applied acceleration, capture can be assured from almost any initial state. When actual dynamics are considered, it is known that PN guidance (PNG) tends to diverge at the vicinity of the interception,[4–7] i.e., the LOS rate diverges, and correspondingly so does the required missile acceleration. This divergence may severely affect the miss distance. As such, it constitutes a major issue in missile design.

In the late 1960s new guidance laws, based on optimal control theory, were developed. Further extensions of guidance laws were developed later on, based on differential game theory.[8,9]

The basic difference in philosophy between missile guidance laws based on optimal control theory and those based on differential game theory is in the assumptions

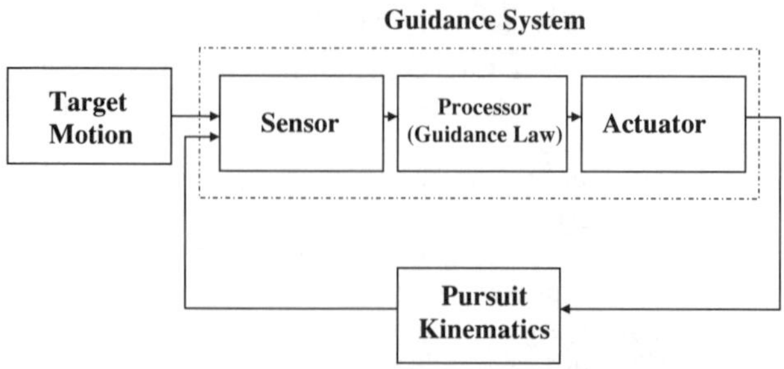

Fig. 1 Guidance system block diagram.

made by the guidance laws about the target's future trajectory and maneuvering capabilities. Optimal control theory assumes that the target's future maneuver strategy is completely defined, either in open-loop or closed-loop form. The feedback nature of missile guidance laws (see Fig. 1) allows the missile to correct for inaccurate predictions of target maneuvers. Optimal control theory guidance laws for intercept missiles are generally based on the application of linear quadratic optimal control theory to a linear constant coefficient missile. The difference between the various guidance laws depends on the model employed to derive the guidance law. The model uses various assumptions on availability of target acceleration information, enforcement of zero final miss and/or the airframe/autopilot response of the missile. In all cases the resulting optimal guidance law is a modified form of proportional navigation.

In contrast the differential game approach makes no assumption on future target maneuvers, but instead takes into consideration the target's maneuvering capabilities. The guidance law then guides the missile, so as to minimize the potential effects of the target's intelligent use of its maneuvering capabilities.

The advantages of optimal and differential game guidance laws are their ability to achieve small miss distances, their smaller energy requirements, and their ability to impose final constraints, such as final interception direction. However, optimal and differential game guidance laws require precise model knowledge, are extremely sensitive to model errors, and increase measurement requirements for estimation. In addition, optimal guidance laws need assumptions on future target behavior and differential game guidance laws, even though they *do not require assumptions on the target's future maneuvering strategy* (only target maneuvering capability), are extremely difficult to implement.

In recent years much effort was invested to tailor different guidance laws to intercept ballistic missiles at different phases of their flight. Clearly, different requirements are imposed at boost-phase interception than those imposed for interception during reentry.

Some of the basic characteristics of various guidance laws used for ballistic missile interception will now be described in more detail.

III. Proportional Navigation

The general formulation of a three-dimensional PN interception problem is rather complicated. However, assuming that the lateral and longitudinal maneuver

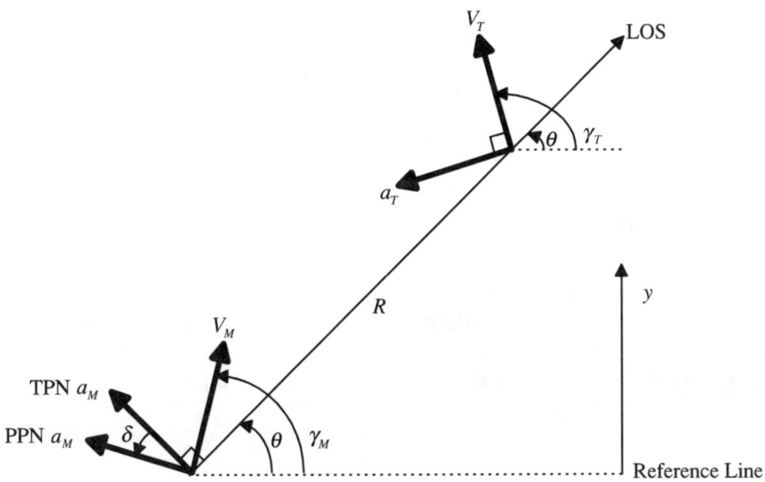

Fig. 2 Proportional navigation geometry.

planes are decoupled by means of roll control, one can deal with the equivalent two-dimensional problem in quite a realistic manner. In addition to this basic assumption, we shall also assume that the gravitational component of the total missile lateral acceleration is negligible.

The preceding assumptions enable us to formulate a general planar intercept missile-target geometry as depicted in Fig. 2.

The figure describes a missile employing PN to intercept a maneuvering target. It could be either true proportional navigation (TPN), where the maneuver acceleration is perpendicular to the instantaneous LOS, or pure proportional navigation (PPN), where the maneuver acceleration is perpendicular to the instantaneous velocity vector.

In both forms of proportional navigation the missile's acceleration is defined by

$$a_M = N V_M \dot{\theta} \tag{1}$$

where N is the navigation constant and $\dot{\theta}$ the LOS angular rate.

An *ideal* missile pursuing a nonmaneuvering target according to the PPN guidance law, with

$$N > \frac{V_M + V_T}{V_M}$$

and

$$V_M > V_T$$

will reach the target for all but a finite number of possible initial conditions at launch.[2] Moreover, the missile will arrive at the target along a straight line direction of which $\theta = \theta_f$ is determined by the initial conditions.

This result was further extended for the case of a maneuvering target showing that an ideal missile pursuing a maneuvering target according to the PPN guidance law, with

$$N > \frac{V_M + V_T}{V_M} \qquad V_M > \sqrt{2}V_T$$

will reach the target from almost any initial state.[3]

A. Proportional Navigation Linearized System

When *actual dynamics* are considered, it is known that PNG tends to diverge at the vicinity of the interception,[4] i.e., the LOS rate diverges, and correspondingly so does the required missile acceleration. This divergence may severely affect the miss distance. As such, it constitutes a major issue in missile design.

The kinematic equations of motion modeling the geometry given in Fig. 2 are

$$\dot{R} = V_T \cos(\theta - \gamma_T) - V_M \cos\delta \tag{2}$$

$$R\dot{\theta} = V_T \sin(\theta - \gamma_T) - V_M \sin\delta \tag{3}$$

$$\delta = \gamma_M - \theta \tag{4}$$

Under the admissible assumptions that the deviations from collision course are small and the closing velocity V_C is constant, we can write

$$\dot{R} = V_T \cos(\theta - \gamma_T) - V_M \cos\delta \triangleq -V_C \approx \text{const} \tag{5}$$

$$R = V_C \cdot \tau \tag{6}$$

where τ, the time-to-go, is given by

$$\tau = t_f - t, \qquad t_f = R_0/V_C \tag{7}$$

The commanded missile acceleration, under the linearization assumptions, generated by the PN control law, is

$$a_C = N'V_C\dot{\theta}_m \tag{8}$$

where $\dot{\theta}_m$ is the measured LOS rate and N' is the effective PN constant given by

$$N' = \begin{cases} NV_M \cos\delta / V_C & \text{for PPN} \\ NV_M/V_C & \text{for TPN} \end{cases} \tag{9}$$

The seeker dynamics are modeled by the transfer function $G_1(s)$:

$$G_1(s) = \frac{\dot{\theta}_m(s)}{\dot{\theta}(s)} \tag{10}$$

The missile's flight control dynamics are described by the transfer function $G_2(s)$

$$G_2(s) = \frac{a_M(s)}{a_c(s)} \tag{11}$$

From Eqs. (8), (10), and (11), the overall closed loop dynamics between the LOS rate and the actual missile acceleration is described by the transfer function

$$\tilde{G}(s) = N'V_C G_1(s) G_2(s) = N'V_C G(s) \tag{12}$$

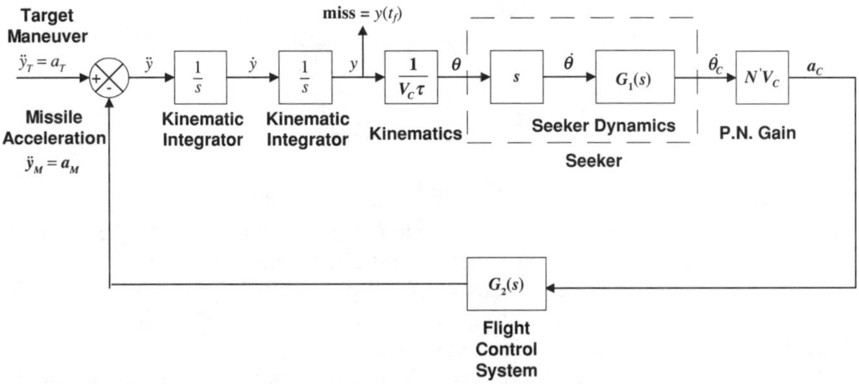

Fig. 3 Proportional navigation linearized system block diagram.

It is assumed that $G(s) = G_1(s) \cdot G_2(s)$ is asymptotically stable. A block diagram describing the system is given in Fig. 3.

In this linear time-varying system, missile acceleration a_M is subtracted form target acceleration a_T to form a relative acceleration $\ddot{y}$. A double integration yields the relative normal position y (see Fig. 2), which at the end of the engagement is the miss distance $y(t_f)$.

Dividing the relative normal position y by the range given in Eq. (6) yields the geometric LOS angle θ. It is assumed that θ is a small angle.

The missile seeker is represented in Fig. 3 as an ideal differentiator with an additional transfer function $G_1(s)$, representing the LOS measurement and noise filtering dynamics. The seeker generates a LOS rate command $\dot{\theta}_c$ that is multiplied by the PN gain $N' \cdot V_C$ to form a missile maneuver acceleration command $\dot{a}_C$, with N' being the effective PN constant. The flight control system, whose dynamics are represented by the transfer function $G_2(s)$, attempts to adequately maneuver the missile so as to follow the desired acceleration command.

B. Zero Miss Distance Proportional Navigation

The following problem was addressed in Refs. 11 and 12: Determine the set of all possible strictly proper missile transfer functions $G(s)$ such that the miss distance becomes zero for all flight times and all possible initial conditions and target maneuvers. That is, find the following class:

$$G = \{G(s) : y(t_f) \equiv 0 \qquad \forall t_f, \forall y_T(t)\} \tag{13}$$

For miss distance analysis the method of adjoints is utilized.[14,15] The adjoints technique is based on the system impulse response and can be used to analyze miss distance as a function of flight time caused by any initial condition or target maneuver. The general expression for the miss distance is given by[14]

$$y(t_f) = L^{-1}\{Q(s) \cdot y_T(s)\} \tag{14}$$

where

$$Q(s) \triangleq \exp\left(N' \int_{\infty}^{s} \frac{G(\sigma)}{\sigma} \mathrm{d}\sigma\right) \tag{15}$$

$$G(s) = G_1(s)G_2(s) \tag{16}$$

$$y_T(s) = L\{y_T(t)\} \tag{17}$$

In the preceding expressions, L denotes the Laplace transform and $y_T(t)$ denotes the system input, which can be either an initial condition or a target maneuver. $G(s)$ represents the LOS measurement and flight control dynamics of the PNG loop (see Fig. 3) and is assumed to be *asymptotically stable* with $G(0) = 1$.

In Ref. 12 the following theorem was proven.

Theorem. $G(s) \in \boldsymbol{G}$ if and only if $G(s)$ is biproper; i.e., the degree of the numerator equals the degree of the denominator.

The set $\boldsymbol{G}$ contains all of the transfer functions $G(s)$ that impose zero miss distance (ZMD) to PNG systems.

In Ref. 6 the existence of a strong relationship between system stability and miss distance was conjectured. In Ref. 12, the concept of finite-time global absolute asymptotic stability (FT-GAAS) was introduced.

Definition. A time-varying system $\dot{x} = f(x, t)$ is finite-time global, absolute asymptotic stable in the interval $J_{t^*} = [t_0, t^*] \subseteq J_{t_f}$ if there exists $P > 0$ such that $\|x(t)\|_P$ is a nonincreasing (decreasing) function of time $\forall x(t_0)$, $\forall t \in J_{t^*}$.

By employing the circle criterion,[16,17] an analytical expression relating system parameters and the time up to which the PNG system is FT-GAAS was given.

By employing the circle criterion, it was shown in Ref. 11 and 12 that FT-GAAS in the interval $J_t \triangleq [t_0, t]$ is assured, provided that the time-to-go $\tau = t_f - t$ satisfies

$$\tau \geq \tau_0 \triangleq -N' \min_{\omega \neq 0} Re[H(j\omega)] \tag{18}$$

where

$$H(j\omega) = \frac{G(j\omega)}{j\omega}$$

is assumed to be minimal, and $G(s)$ is assumed to be asymptotically stable with $G(0) = 1$.

The class of $G(s)$ for which divergence of the PNG system state variables is avoided, i.e., when $\tau_0 = 0$ is of special importance. This is the class of transfer functions that by assuring asymptotic stability also assure a *zero miss*. Denote such a class by

$$\boldsymbol{S} \triangleq \{G(s) : \tau_0 = 0\} \tag{19}$$

Now, it can be shown that $\tau_0 = 0$ if and only if

$$H(s) = \frac{G(s)}{s}$$

is positive real, i.e., $\boldsymbol{S} = \{PR\}$. Furthermore, $\boldsymbol{S} = \{PR\} \subseteq \boldsymbol{G}$. The physical consequence of $\boldsymbol{S} \subseteq \boldsymbol{G}$ is that if a combination of the state variables of the PNG system, e.g., LOS rate, missile maneuver acceleration, and missile commanded acceleration are kept bounded until the end of interception, no miss will occur.

C. Bounded Acceleration

The linear model presented previously is based implicitly on the assumption of nonlimited missile maneuverability. Actually, every real missile system is subject to maneuverability saturation caused by aerodynamic or structural constraints. To complete the guidance model description in this case, a new variable, the required missile maneuver acceleration a_R, is introduced. The nonlinear relationship between the actual and required missile maneuver is defined by

$$a_M = a_{M_{\max}} \operatorname{sat}\left\{\frac{a_R}{a_{M_{\max}}}\right\} \tag{21}$$

where

$$\operatorname{sat}(x) \triangleq \begin{cases} x & \text{if } x \leq 1 \\ 1 & \text{if } |x| > 1 \end{cases} \tag{22}$$

This limit is at the output of the guidance channel.

In a conventional PNG system, infinite missile acceleration is required near to interception ($t \rightarrow t_f$). This means that saturation is always reached, and miss distance will be greater than predicted by linear analysis.

In the previous section were characterized a set of PN-based guidance systems, in which an infinite acceleration is *avoided.* This is the class of systems yielding zero miss distance (ZMD), provided there is no missile acceleration saturation.

To avoid missile saturation and consequently achieve ZMD, it is necessary to find some bound μ on the required missile-target maneuver ratio μ_r defined as

$$\mu_r \triangleq \frac{\sup_{t\in[0,t_f]} |a_M(t)|}{\sup_{t\in[0,t_f]} |a_T(t)|} \tag{23}$$

If μ is found to be smaller than the a priori known missile-target maneuver ratio μ_0, no saturation will occur.

In Ref. 13 was proven that if

$$\operatorname{Re} H(j\omega) = \operatorname{Re}\frac{N'G(j\omega)}{j\omega} \geq 0 \;\forall\omega \in \Re \tag{24}$$

that is, $H(s)$ is positive real, then

$$\|a_M\|_\infty \leq \frac{N'}{N'-2}\|a_T\|_\infty \;\forall a_T \in L^\infty[0, t_f] \tag{25}$$

In view of the preceding discussion, the design guidelines sufficient for a PN-based system, to avoid output acceleration saturation, are as follows.

Design Guideline 1: Given flight control dynamics $G_1(s)$ and seeker dynamics $G_2(s)$, design a controller $K(s)$ such that $G(s) = K(s)G_1(s)G_2(s)$ is a phase lead network with a maximal phase lead not exceeding 180°.

Design Guideline 2: Given the missile-target maneuver ratio μ_0, choose N' such that $N'/(N'-2) \geq \mu_0$, or equivalently $N' \geq \frac{2\mu_0}{\mu_0 - 1}$.

From guideline 2 it is obvious that the smaller μ_0 is, the larger N' should be chosen.

D. Numerical Example

The design process proposed is illustrated using a third-order model of $G(s)$. The flight control dynamics are assumed a second-order transfer function with damping ζ and natural frequency ω_n, and the seeker LOS measurement dynamics are modeled by a single time lag. As a result, it is obtained

$$G_1(s)G_2(s) = \frac{1}{(\tau_1 s + 1) \cdot \left(s^2/\omega_n^2 + 2\zeta s/\omega_n + 1\right)} \tag{26}$$

with

$$\tau_1 = 0.3\,\text{s}, \qquad \zeta = 0.5, \qquad \omega_n = 10\,\text{rad/s} \tag{27}$$

Missile-target maneuver ratio is assumed to be

$$\mu_0 = 2 \tag{28}$$

According to design guideline 1, a controller $K(s)$ is to be designed such that $G(s) = K(s)G_1(s)G_2(s)$ satisfies $0 \leq \angle G(s) \leq 180\,\text{deg}$.

Considering the following proportional plus derivative (PD) ideal controller,

$$K(s) = \prod_{i=1}^{3} \left(\tau_{Z_i} s + 1\right) \tag{29}$$

a straightforward computation shows that $\tau_Z = 0.23$ satisfies the phase lead requirement. With controller (29) the resulting PN-based guidance law will ensure zero miss distance. Because $K(s)$ is a PD controller, noise amplification problems might arise. A realistic controller is suggested:

$$K(s) = \prod_{i=1}^{3} \frac{\left(\tau_{Z_i} s + 1\right)}{\left(\tau_{P_i} s + 1\right)} \tag{30}$$

It is apparent that with this type of a controller, design guideline 1 cannot be accomplished, because Eq. (13) is not satisfied and hence $H(s) \notin \{PR\}$. Nonetheless, if the additional lag is not too large, acceleration saturation can still be prevented.

Let $i = 1$, $\tau_{P_i} = \tau_P$, and $\tau_{Z_i} = \tau_Z$. if τ_P is small enough, the phase lag will occur at high frequencies, higher than the typical missile operating frequencies. Thus, no substantial degradation of performance is expected. The value $\tau_p = 0.05$ is a reasonable choice.

The controller (30) is an "actual" controller, and the resulting PN-based guidance law will be called "actual" ZMD-PNG.

After designing the appropriate controller, according to design guideline 2, it is required that $N' \geq 4$.

The performance of the guidance loop is evaluated in three cases: PNG, "ideal" ZMD-PNG, and "actual" ZMD-PNG.

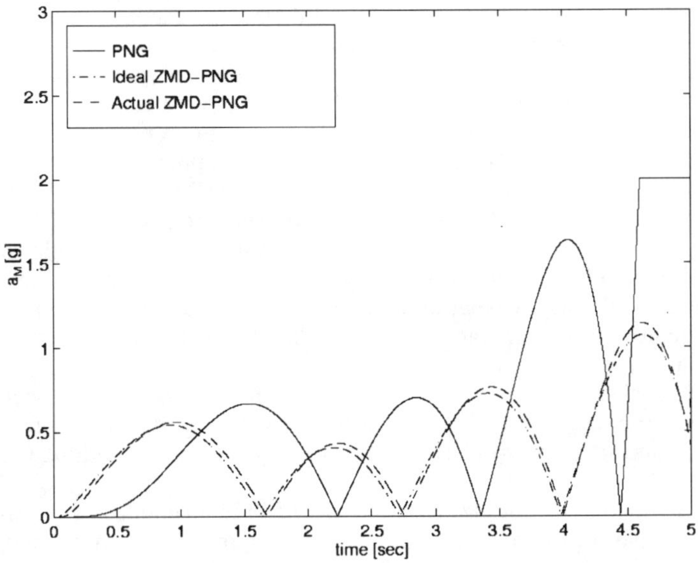

Fig. 4 Maneuver acceleration comparison for a sinusoidal target maneuver.

As a representative case a sinusoidal ("weave") target maneuver[18] is considered, satisfying

$$a_T = a_{T_0} \sin(\omega_T t) \tag{31}$$

Let $a_{T_0} = 1\,\text{g}$, $\omega_T = 2.5\,\text{rad/s}$, $t_f = 4\,\text{s}$. Figure 4 depicts the absolute value of missile acceleration for the three cases considered. Notice that in the case of PNG, the acceleration saturates. However, ZMD-PNG does not saturate in either the "ideal" or "actual" cases.

IV. Three Dimensional Minimum Energy Guidance

The common assumption in works on optimal guidance for interception of airborne maneuvering targets has been that evasive maneuvers are generated by accelerations normal to the velocity vector. Velocity magnitude was considered constant. In general, a performance index of optimality was defined as a linear combination of energy and final miss.[10] For a target moving at a constant velocity magnitude, it can be shown that the optimal cost (the value acquired by the optimality index for the optimal control) is a monotonic decreasing function of the interception duration. This result in turn implies that the absolute minimum is reached at infinite time, corresponding to a zero control acceleration. Hence there is no optimal solution for a free final time. On the basis of this observation a *fixed final time* was imposed also for the case of a maneuvering target. The selection of this final fixed time became then a subject of major importance.

Another basic element in the actual implementation of optimal guidance laws is that aerodynamically controlled interceptors can apply maneuvering accelerations normal to the velocity vector only. The component along the velocity vector results from a prescribed thrust profile and drag. This uncontrolled acceleration component affects the time-to-go.

Different methods were proposed to compute this unknown time-to-go. The simplest method defines time-to-go as the ratio between range and range rate. This method neglects the path curvature and leads to an erroneous estimate of the time-to-go, for engagement scenarios, other than pure head-on or tail chase, with an initially negative range rate. Another approach[18] makes use of the fact that one of the interceptor acceleration components is not under control. Time-to-go is obtained by equating the acceleration component along the uncontrolled direction to the actual applied acceleration. These estimates are approximate even while considering a completely deterministic situation. Furthermore they do not ensure the optimality of the commanded acceleration obtained under a fixed final time condition.

When considering interception of a ballistic missile, the constant velocity assumption is no longer valid because of the typically significant and growing acceleration during the boost phase, or the growing deceleration during the reentry phase.

Using as optimality index the required energy for interception at the boost phase, it is shown that the optimal cost has an absolute minimum for finite interception duration.[19] Therefore, the problem of interception of an accelerating target has an optimal solution for a *free final time*.

An interceptor M with velocity $\boldsymbol{V}_M$ is to control its acceleration vector $\boldsymbol{a}_M$ in order to intercept an accelerating target T as depicted in Fig. 5.

The interceptor equations of motion are defined by

$$\dot{\boldsymbol{R}}_M = \boldsymbol{V}_M \tag{32}$$

$$\dot{\boldsymbol{V}}_M = \boldsymbol{a}_M \tag{33}$$

The target equations of motion are given by

$$\dot{\boldsymbol{R}}_T = \boldsymbol{V}_T \tag{34}$$

$$\dot{\boldsymbol{V}}_T = \boldsymbol{a}_T, \qquad \boldsymbol{a}_T = \boldsymbol{a}_T(t) \tag{35}$$

It is required to find the interceptor acceleration $\boldsymbol{a}_M$ such that for any engagement initiated at $\boldsymbol{R}_{M_0}, \boldsymbol{R}_{T_0}, \boldsymbol{V}_{M_0}, \boldsymbol{V}_{T_0}, \boldsymbol{a}_{T_0}$, interception is achieved:

$$\boldsymbol{R}_M(t_f) = \boldsymbol{R}_T(t_f) \tag{36}$$

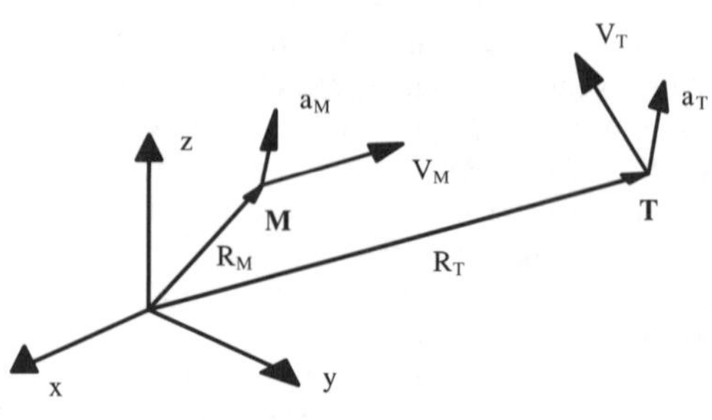

Fig. 5 Interception geometry.

while the performance index defined by

$$J = \frac{1}{2}\int_{t_0}^{t_f} a_p^2 \,\mathrm{dt} \tag{37}$$

is a minimum.

A. Optimal Acceleration

Define interceptor–target relative coordinates

$$\dot{\boldsymbol{R}} = \dot{\boldsymbol{R}}_M - \dot{\boldsymbol{R}}_T = \boldsymbol{V}_M - \boldsymbol{V}_T = \boldsymbol{V} \tag{38}$$

$$\dot{\boldsymbol{V}} = \dot{\boldsymbol{V}}_M - \dot{\boldsymbol{V}}_T = \boldsymbol{a}_M - \boldsymbol{a}_T(t) \tag{39}$$

Applying the maximum principle the Hamiltonian of the system is formed,

$$H = \boldsymbol{\lambda_R} \cdot \boldsymbol{V} + \boldsymbol{\lambda_V} \cdot (\boldsymbol{a}_M - \boldsymbol{a}_T) - \tfrac{1}{2}a_M^2 \tag{40}$$

with adjoint vectors $\boldsymbol{\lambda_R}$, $\boldsymbol{\lambda_V}$ defined by,

$$\dot{\boldsymbol{\lambda}}_{\boldsymbol{R}} = 0, \qquad \boldsymbol{\lambda_R}(t_f) = \boldsymbol{\lambda}_{\boldsymbol{R}f} \quad \text{(const)} \tag{41}$$

$$\dot{\boldsymbol{\lambda}}_{\boldsymbol{V}} = -\boldsymbol{\lambda_R}, \qquad \boldsymbol{\lambda_V}(t_f) = 0 \tag{42}$$

The Hamiltonian is maximum with respect to $\boldsymbol{a}_M$ for

$$\boldsymbol{a}_M^* = \boldsymbol{\lambda_V} \tag{43}$$

and integrating the state and adjoint equations along an optimal trajectory,

$$\boldsymbol{a}_M^* = \frac{3(t - t_f)}{\Delta_0^3} z_{m_0} \tag{44}$$

with z_{m_0} the zero effort final range,

$$z_{m_0} = -\frac{\Delta_0^3}{3}\boldsymbol{\lambda}_{\boldsymbol{R}f} = \boldsymbol{R}_0 + \Delta_0 \boldsymbol{V}_0 - \int_{t_0}^{t_f}\left[\int_{\sigma_0}^{\sigma} \boldsymbol{a}_T(\tau)\,\mathrm{d}\tau\right]\mathrm{d}\sigma \tag{45}$$

$\boldsymbol{R}_0$, $\boldsymbol{V}_0$ are respectively the initial relative range and velocity and Δ_0 the interception duration,

$$\Delta_0 = t_f - t_0 \tag{46}$$

The optimal acceleration vector $\boldsymbol{a}_M^*$ has a constant inertial direction, as defined by z_{m_0} and linearly decreasing amplitude with time, becoming zero at $t = t_f$.

Furthermore, introducing the optimal acceleration from Eq. (44) into the index of optimality (37) and integrating,

$$J = \frac{3z_{m_0}^2}{2\Delta_0^3} \tag{47}$$

B. Cost Absolute Minimum for a Ballistic Missile in the Boost Phase

For a ballistic missile in the boost phase, thrust is axially applied along the missile velocity vector. In a first-order approximation, at high altitudes, drag effects can be neglected. Under this assumption it follows that

$$a_T = \frac{T}{m} \tag{48}$$

$$\dot{m} = -\frac{T}{c} \tag{49}$$

where T, m, and c are the target thrust, mass, and engine exhaust velocity, respectively.

For a target with constant thrust, as is generally the case, differentiating Eq. (48) and introducing into Eq. (49) we obtain,

$$\dot{\boldsymbol{a}}_T = \frac{a_T^2}{c}\mathbf{1}_{V_T} \tag{50}$$

with $\mathbf{1}_{V_T}$ the target velocity unit vector.

Integrating the target acceleration from initial conditions $t = t_0$, $a_T = a_{T_0}$,

$$\boldsymbol{a}_T = \frac{1}{\sigma_0 - (t - t_0)}\boldsymbol{V}_{c_0} \tag{51}$$

is obtained, where $\boldsymbol{V}_{c_0} = c\mathbf{1}_{V_T}$ and $\sigma_0 = c/a_{T_0}$.

For this case

$$z_{m_0} = \boldsymbol{R}_0 + \Delta_0\boldsymbol{V}_0 - \left[\Delta_0 + \sigma_0\left(1 - \frac{\Delta_0}{\sigma_0}\right)\ln\left(1 - \frac{\Delta_0}{\sigma_0}\right)\right]\boldsymbol{V}_{c_0} \tag{52}$$

The interception cost is

$$J = \frac{3}{2\Delta_0^3}\left\{\boldsymbol{R}_0 + \Delta_0\boldsymbol{V}_0 - \left[\Delta_0 + \sigma_0\left(1 - \frac{\Delta_0}{\sigma_0}\right)\ln\left(1 - \frac{\Delta_0}{\sigma_0}\right)\right]\boldsymbol{V}_{c_0}\right\}^2 \tag{53}$$

The cost J is a continuous function of Δ_0 in the interval $(0, \sigma)$. Examining the slope of the function J at both ends of the interval, a condition for the existence of an *absolute minimum* in the interval can be established. This condition is

$$\frac{c\left(c - \boldsymbol{V}_0 \cdot \mathbf{1}_{V_T}\right)}{a_{e_0}} > \boldsymbol{R}_0 \cdot \mathbf{1}_{V_T} \tag{54}$$

In practical cases of boost-phase interception of a ballistic missile, this condition is always satisfied. Figure 6 shows the cost as a function of the interception duration Δ_0 for given initial conditions of relative range and velocity, and target acceleration. The cost is calculated for values of interception times up to the cutoff time t_c. The absolute minimum is reached for interception time $\Delta_0 = \Delta_0^*$.

When solving the optimal interception for a free end time, with time-independent final state conditions, the optimal interception duration can be obtained from the necessary condition $H_f = 0$. From Eqs. (40–43) at $t = t_f$,

$$H_f = \boldsymbol{\lambda}_{Rf} \cdot \boldsymbol{V}_f = 0 \tag{55}$$

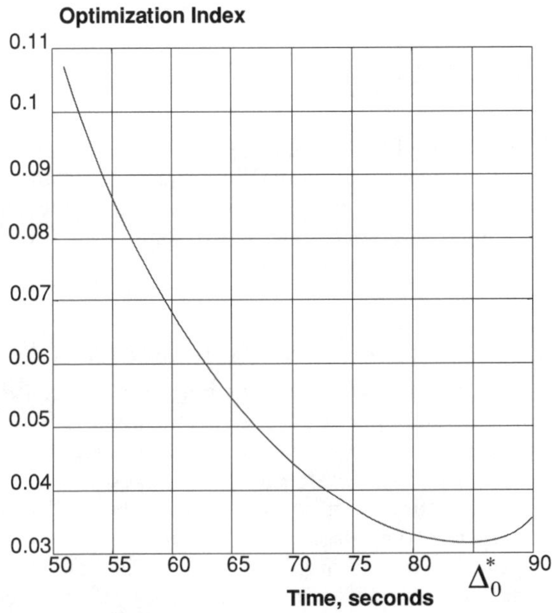

Fig. 6 Cost function dependence on interception time.

is obtained. Because the optimal acceleration direction is defined by z_{m_0}, collinear with constant vector $\boldsymbol{\lambda}_{Rf}$ [Eq. (46)] it follows that the acceleration direction corresponding to the absolute energy minimum is normal to the final relative velocity.

By adequate manipulations, it can be shown[19] that for a ballistic missile in the boost phase, Eq. (50) is equivalent to

$$a_3 \ln^2\left(1 - \frac{\Delta_0}{\sigma_0}\right) + a_2 \ln\left(1 - \frac{\Delta_0}{\sigma_0}\right) + a_1 = 0 \tag{56}$$

where

$$a_1 = \left[3\boldsymbol{R}_0 + \Delta_0\left(\boldsymbol{V}_0 - 3\boldsymbol{V}_{c_0}\right)\right] \cdot \left[\boldsymbol{R}_0 + \Delta_0\left(\boldsymbol{V}_0 - \boldsymbol{V}_{c_0}\right)\right] \tag{57}$$

$$\begin{aligned} a_2 = {} & -\left[(\sigma_0 - \Delta_0)\left[3\boldsymbol{R}_0 + \Delta_0\left(\boldsymbol{V}_0 - 3\boldsymbol{V}_{c_0}\right)\right]\right. \\ & \left. + (3\sigma_0 - \Delta_0)\left[\boldsymbol{R}_0 + \Delta_0\left(\boldsymbol{V}_0 - \boldsymbol{V}_{c_0}\right)\right]\right] \cdot \boldsymbol{V}_{c_0} \end{aligned} \tag{58}$$

$$a_3 = (\sigma_0 - \Delta_0)(3\sigma_0 - \Delta_0)c^2 \tag{59}$$

The solution of Eq. (56) provides Δ_0^* the absolute minimum of J as given in Eq. (51).

The well-known procedure to obtain the feedback optimal acceleration is to replace the initial values $\boldsymbol{R}_0$, $\boldsymbol{V}_0$, $\boldsymbol{V}_{T_0}$, and $\boldsymbol{a}_{T_0}$ as well as time for their current values. The optimal guidance law becomes then a function of the current system state and time to interception, and is defined by

$$a_M^* = -\frac{3}{\Delta^2}\left[R + \Delta V - \left(\Delta + \frac{c}{a_T}\left(1 - \frac{a_T\Delta}{c}\right)\ell n\left(1 - \frac{a_T\Delta}{c}\right)\right)V_{c_0}\right] \tag{60}$$

The actual implementation of the optimal feedback acceleration requires estimation of the relative range and velocity, target flight direction, and thrust acceleration, as well as the constant parameter c, the ballistic missile engine exhaust velocity. Time to go Δ is computed at each step, as the solution of Eq. (56), using the estimated variables and the constant parameter c.

V. Optimal Guidance with Accelerations Normal to Velocity Vector

To derive optimal guidance laws when employing optimal control theory solutions for the linear quadratic systems, the engagement was described employing approximate linear equations in a Cartesian reference frame. This reference frame was attached to the LOS with no constraints on the control accelerations. Because in actual systems accelerations can be only partially controlled, only accelerations normal to LOS were considered for implementation. The basic assumption underlying this approach is that the acceleration along the LOS only affects the interception time. The interception itself is only affected by the accelerations normal to the LOS. The acceleration component along the LOS was indirectly introduced by solving on-line for the time-to-go.

When studying PN in Sec. III, it was indicated that when applying accelerations normal to the LOS (TPN) there are strong limitations in the capture region. This is in contrast to the case when accelerations are applied normal to the velocity vector (PPN). In the case of PPN, capture can be assured from almost any initial state. Following this result, there is a clear interest in deriving optimal guidance laws with accelerations normal to the velocity vector.

The interceptor equations of motion are given by Eqs. (32) and (33) with the control acceleration $\boldsymbol{a}_M$ defined by

$$\boldsymbol{a}_M = \boldsymbol{\omega}_M \times \boldsymbol{V}_M \tag{61}$$

with $\boldsymbol{\omega}_M$ being the interceptor's flight direction turning rate. The acceleration is so defined as to take into account the following constraint:

$$\boldsymbol{a}_M \cdot \boldsymbol{V}_M = 0 \tag{62}$$

i.e., the interceptor acceleration vector is normal to its velocity vector.

Thus the problem is defined as follows: Determine the interceptor turning rate $\boldsymbol{\omega}_M$ such that for any engagement initiated at $\boldsymbol{R}_{M_0}$, $\boldsymbol{R}_{T_0}$, $\boldsymbol{V}_{M_0}$, and $\boldsymbol{V}_{T_0}$ interception is achieved, whereas the performance index J, defined by

$$J = kt_f + \frac{1}{2}\int_0^{t_f} \omega_P^2 \,\mathrm{d}t \tag{63}$$

is minimized.

The performance index is a weighted sum of the final time and the integral of the turning rate squared. The integral term in the index J is in fact equivalent to the integral of the squared acceleration, since interceptor velocity remains constant, and represents the expended maneuvering energy. For the case $k = 0$, performance index (63) is equivalent to the performance index defined in Eq. (37).

It should be remarked that there are no interceptor acceleration constraints. By adjusting the weighting coefficient k, the highest normal acceleration encountered along the trajectory can be controlled. Furthermore the evader is free to maneuver, but its future trajectory is assumed known to the interceptor.

A. Optimal Control

Employing the maximum principle it was shown that the optimal turning rate vector is given by[20]

$$\boldsymbol{\omega}_M^* = \boldsymbol{\lambda}_R \times \boldsymbol{V}_M \tag{64}$$

with $\boldsymbol{\lambda}_R$ a constant vector.

Furthermore, for given initial conditions, $\boldsymbol{\omega}_M^* \forall t$ has a fixed direction in space, which is normal to the plane defined by the constant vector $\boldsymbol{\lambda}_R$ and the initial interceptor velocity vector $\boldsymbol{V}_{M_0}$. The entire interception trajectory lies in this inertially fixed plane, the *trajectory plane*, and thus the results derived for the planar case[21] can be used to obtain the three-dimensional optimal solution.

The coordinate systems used to present the three-dimensional guidance solution are shown in Fig. 7. Without loss of generality, the origins of the coordinate systems are chosen to be at the initial location of the interceptor. The $\hat{X}$ axis of the reference coordinate system is aligned with the initial interceptor vector $\boldsymbol{V}_{M_0}$. To define the trajectory plane, let φ denote the inclination of the trajectory plane relative to the $\hat{X}$–$\hat{Y}$ plane as shown in Fig. 7. In that plane, a coordinate system is defined by $(\hat{x}, \hat{y})$, with the same origin as the reference system, and with $\hat{x} = \hat{X}$.

The variables of the planar solution are depicted in Fig. 8, showing also the constant vector $\boldsymbol{\lambda}_R$, which is oriented at a constant angle θ_f relative to $\hat{x}$. γ_M is the interceptor flight-path angle in the trajectory plane, while its location in that plane is denoted by (x_M, y_M). Because the origin of the coordinate system $(\hat{x}, \hat{y})$ is chosen at the initial location of the interceptor and $\hat{x}$ points along $\boldsymbol{V}_{M_0}$, the initial interceptor flight-path angle in the trajectory plane is $\gamma_M(0) = 0$.

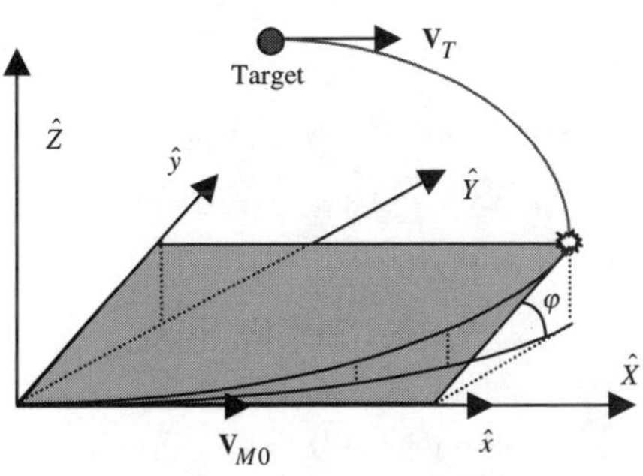

Fig. 7 Interception trajectory plane in three-dimensional space.

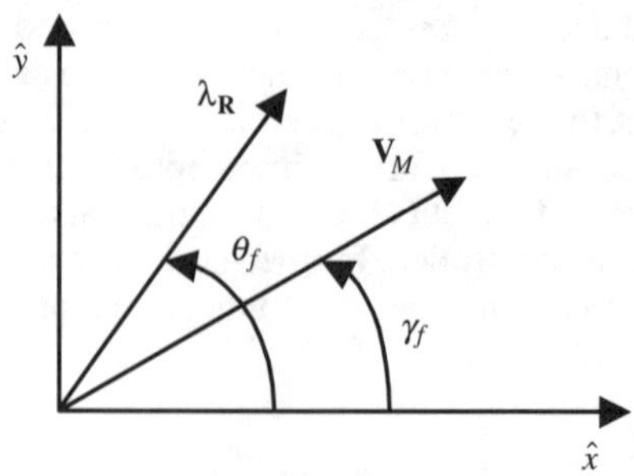

Fig. 8 Planar interception geometry and constant vector λ_R.

The optimal acceleration amplitude and sign are defined by[21]

$$a_M^* = \left[\frac{k V_M [\cos(\theta_f - \gamma_M) - \cos(\theta_f - \gamma_{M_f})}{\dot{R}_f} \right]^{\frac{1}{2}} \tag{65}$$

$$\text{sign}(a_M^*) = \text{sign}\left[\sin\left(\theta_f - \gamma_{M_f}\right)\right] \tag{66}$$

where

$$\dot{R}_f = \left[V_M \cos\left(\theta_f - \gamma_{M_f}\right) + V_{T_f} \cos(\theta_f - \gamma_T(t_f))\right] \tag{67}$$

with V_{T_f} the magnitude of the projection of the target velocity onto the trajectory plane at interception and γ_{T_f} the angle between this projection and $\hat{x}$.

The optimal guidance law depends on the current value of only one state variable γ_M, and three unknown parameters: the interception time t_f, the final flight-path angle γ_{M_f}, and the angle θ_f. Furthermore, the optimal acceleration a_M^* is zero at t_f. As was shown in Ref. 21, the motion of the interceptor can be analytically integrated.

Integrating from

$$t = 0, \qquad \gamma_M(0) = 0, \qquad x_M(0) = 0, \qquad y_M(0) = 0$$

to

$$t = t_f, \qquad \gamma_M(t_f) = \gamma_{M_f}, \qquad x_M(t_f) = x_{M_f}, \qquad y_M(t_f) = y_{M_f}$$

the following is obtained:

$$x_{M_f} = V_M(A \cos\theta_f + B \sin\theta_f) \tag{68}$$

$$y_{M_f} = V_M(A \sin\theta_f + B \cos\theta_f) \tag{69}$$

where constants A and B given by

$$A = t_f - 2C[\boldsymbol{E} \cos(\psi_f) - E(\alpha, \cos\psi_f)] \tag{70}$$

$$B = 2C\sqrt{\sin^2(\theta_f/2) - \sin^2\psi_f)} \tag{71}$$

final time t_f given by

$$t_f = C[\boldsymbol{F}(\cos\psi_f) - F(\alpha, \cos\psi_f)] \tag{72}$$

F is the elliptic and $\boldsymbol{F}$ are the complete elliptic integral of first kind; E is the elliptic and $\boldsymbol{E}$ is the complete elliptic integral of the second kind.

The constants in the preceding equations are

$$\psi_f = \frac{\theta_f - \gamma_{M_f}}{2} \tag{73}$$

$$\alpha = \sin^{-1} \frac{\cos(\theta_f/2)}{\cos \psi_f} \tag{74}$$

$$C = \text{sign}(a_M^*)\sqrt{\frac{V_M}{k}\left[V_M \cos(\theta_f - \gamma_{M_f}) - V_{T_f} \cos(\theta_f - \gamma_{T_f})\right]} \tag{75}$$

Note that because V_{T_f}, γ_{T_f} as well as C are functions of t_f, Eq. (72) is implicit in t_f.

The interceptor coordinates at time t_f expressed in the three-dimensional coordinate frame $(\hat{X}, \hat{Y}, \hat{Z})$ are given by

$$X_{M_f} = x_{M_f} \tag{76a}$$

$$Y_{M_f} = y_{M_f} \cos \varphi \tag{76b}$$

$$Z_{M_f} = y_{M_f} \sin \varphi \tag{76c}$$

With the evader motion assumed to be perfectly known, to achieve capture at $t = t_f$,

$$X_{M_f} = X_T(t_f) \tag{77a}$$

$$Y_{M_f} = Y_T(t_f) \tag{77b}$$

$$Z_{M_f} = Z_T(t_f) \tag{77c}$$

where $X_T(t_f)$, $Y_T(t_f)$, $Z_T(t_f)$ are the target three-dimensional coordinates at the final time t_f.

Equations (77a–77c) are three, nonlinear algebraic equations that depend on the unknowns t_f, θ_f, γ_{M_f}, and φ. Because, as earlier stated, t_f is given only implicitly, Eqs. (72) and (77) are four implicit nonlinear algebraic equations for the four unknowns.

Let us now summarize the three-dimensional guidance law application: Eqs. (65) and (66) provide the control amplitude and sign, respectively, the required constants t_f, θ_f, γ_{M_f}, and φ are obtained numerically, solving Eqs. (72) and (77).

B. Numerical Example of Application

A target is moving along a circular path at a constant velocity and a constant rate of turn. The target trajectory is confined to the $\hat{X}$–$\hat{Z}$ plane, its rate of turn is 4 deg/s and $\boldsymbol{V}_{T_0}$ is parallel to $\hat{X}$. The interceptor/target velocity ratio is set to $V_M/V_T = 1.5$, and the weight k in the performance index J is set to $k = 1$. The origin of the reference system is defined at the initial location of the interceptor and points along $\boldsymbol{V}_{M_0}$.

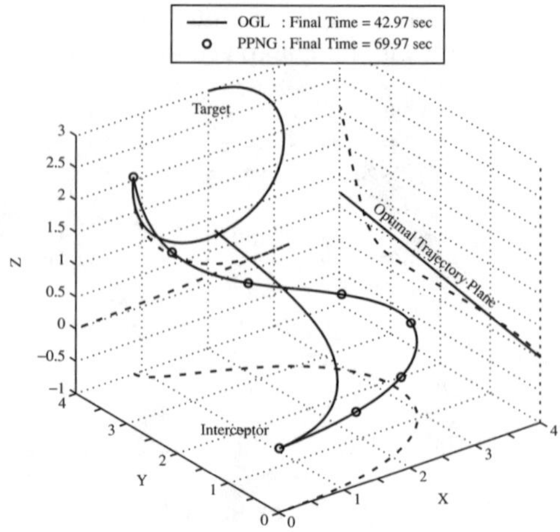

Fig. 9 Optimal guidance law and PPN trajectories for a maneuvering evader.

For comparison purposes, pure proportional navigation guidance (PPNG) for the preceding example is also presented.

The interceptor and target trajectories for the example are presented in Fig. 9, showing also the interception times. The projection of the optimal interceptor trajectory on the $\hat{Y}$–$\hat{Z}$ plane is also drawn and clearly shows that this trajectory is restricted to one plane. The interceptor-to-target acceleration ratios as a function of time are shown in Fig. 10. The performance indices are normalized by the value of J obtained by the optimal guidance law. The optimal interception occurs at an earlier time than the PPNG interception. This result is obtained even though the magnitudes of acceleration for the two solutions are of comparable size, as can be seen in Fig. 10.

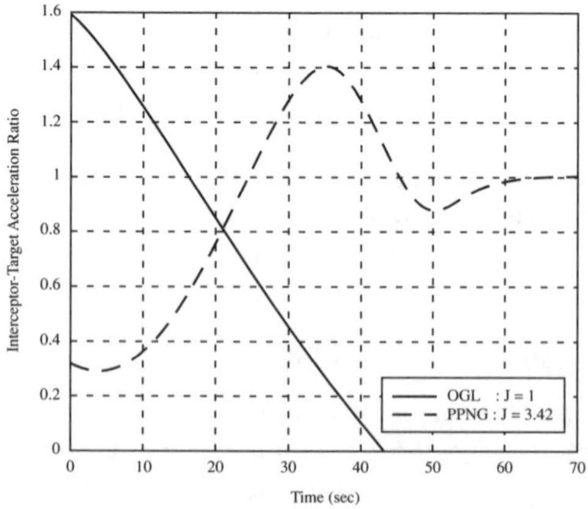

Fig. 10 Optimal guidance law and PPN accelerations for a maneuvering evader.

VI. Summary

In this chapter a review of guidance systems was presented. Classical and modern guidance laws able to intercept ballistic missiles at boost or reentry phases were discussed. Both two- and three-dimensional interception geometries, as well as constraints on the interceptor acceleration direction, were considered. Numerical results of representative cases were presented for various guidance laws.

References

[1]Shneydor, N., "Proportional Navigation Guidance-A Survey," Rafael Rept. MT/P/013/30/84, May 1984.

[2]Guelman, M., "A Qualitative Study of Proportional Navigation," *IEEE Transactions on Aerospace and Electronic Systems*, Vol. AES-7, No. 4, July 1971, pp. 637–643.

[3]Guelman, M., "The Closed Form Solution of Proportional Navigation," *IEEE Transactions on Aerospace and Electronic Systems*, Vol. AES-12, pp. 472–482, July 1976.

[4]Zarchan, P., *Tactical and Strategic Missile Guidance*, Progress in Astronautics and Aeronautics, Vol. 124, AIAA, Washington, DC, 1990.

[5]Shinar, J., "Divergence Range of Homing Missiles," *Israel Journal of Technology*, Vol. 14, July 1976, pp. 47–55.

[6]Guelman, M., "The Stability of Proportional Navigation Systems," AIAA Paper 90-3380-CP, July 1990.

[7]Rew, D.Y., Tahk, M.J., and Cho, H., "Short Time Stability of Proportional Navigation Guidance Loop," *IEEE Transactions on Aerospace and Electronic Systems*, Vol. 32, No. 4, July 1996, pp. 1107–1115.

[8]Tanaka, T., and Hirofumi, E., "Hyperstable Range In Homing Missiles," AIAA Paper 90-3381-CP, July 1990.

[9]Gutman, S., "On Optimal Guidance for Homing Missiles," *Journal of Guidance and Control*, Vol. 2, No. 4, 1979, pp. 296–300.

[10]Anderson, G.M., "Comparison of Optimal Control and Differential Game Intercept Missile Guidance Laws," *Journal of Guidance, Control, and Dynamics*, Vol. 4, No. 2, 1981.

[11]Gurfil P., Jodorkovsky, M., and Guelman, M., "Finite Time Stability Approach to Proportional Navigation Systems Analysis," *Journal of Guidance, Control, and Dynamics*, Vol. 21, No. 6, 1998, pp. 853–861.

[12]Gurfil, P., Jodorkovsky, M., and Guelman, M., "Simple Guidance Law against Highly Maneuvering Targets," *Proceedings of the 38th AIAA Guidance, Navigation and Control Conference*, AIAA, Reston, VA, 1998, pp. 570–580.

[13]Gurfil, P., Jodorkovsky, M., and Guelman, M., "Design of Non Saturating Guidance Systems," *Journal of Guidance, Control, and Dynamics*, Vol. 23, No. 4, 2000, pp. 693–700.

[14]Zarchan, P., "Complete Statistical Analysis of Nonlinear Missile Guidance Systems-SLAM," *Journal of Guidance and Control*, Vol. 2, No. 1, 1979, pp. 71–78.

[15]Sandberg, I.W., "Some Results on the Theory of Physical Systems Governed by Nonlinear Functional Equations," *Bell Systems Technology Journal*, Vol. 44, No. 5, 1965, pp. 871–898.

[16]Zames, G., "On Input-Output Stability of Time-Varying Nonlinear Feedback Systems-Part II: Conditions Involving Circles in the Frequency Plane and Sector Nonlinearities," *IEEE Transactions on Automatic Control*, Vol. AC-11, 1966, pp. 465–476.

[17]Zarchan, P., "Proportional Navigation and Weaving Targets," *Journal of Guidance, Control, and Dynamics*, Vol. 18, No. 5, 1995.

[18]Hough, M.E., "Optimal Guidance and Nonlinear Estimation for Interception of Decelerating Targets," *Journal of Guidance, Control, and Dynamics*, Vol. 18, No. 2, 1995, pp. 316–324.

[19]Guelman, M., and Golan, O.M., "Minimum Energy Guidance for Boost Phase Ballistic Missile Interception," *American Control Conference*, Vol. 6, Seattle, WA, June 21–23, 1995.

[20]Guelman, M., Idan, M., and Golan, O.M., "Three Dimensional Minimum Energy Guidance," *IEEE Transactions on Aerospace and Electronic Systems*, Vol. 31, No. 2, April 1995.

[21]Guelman, M., and Shinar, J., "Optimal Guidance Law in the Plane," *Journal of Guidance, Control, and Dynamics*, Vol. 7, No. 4, 1984, pp. 471–477.

Chapter 12

Improved Methodology for Theater Missile Defense End-Games

Joseph Z. Ben-Asher*
WALES Ltd., Ramat-Gan, Israel
and
Isaac Yaesh†
Israeli Military Industries, Ramat Hasharon, Israel

Nomenclature

A = state matrix
a = miss distance cost factor
B = control matrix
b = terminal lateral relative velocity cost factor
c = terminal missile acceleration cost factor
D = disturbance matrix
d = estimated value of target acceleration
h = normalized time-to-go
N' = proportional navigation gain
n = noise of the time-to-go estimator
n_c = missile commanded acceleration
n_L = missile acceleration
n_T = target acceleration
$\mathcal{O}()$ = order of magnitude
P = Riccati matrix
S = inverse Riccati matrix
t = elapsed time
t_{go} = time-to-go
t_f = final time
u = control function
V_c = closing velocity

Copyright © 2000 by the American Institute of Aeronautics and Astronautics, Inc. All rights reserved.

*Special Consultant; also Associate Professor, Aerospace Engineering, Technion–Israel Institute of Technology. Senior Member AIAA.

†Head, Department of Control Simulations and Aerodynamics, Advanced Systems Division.

V_e = target velocity
V_p = missile velocity
w = unknown part of the disturbance function
x = state
Y_e = target separation from line-of-sight
Y_p = missile separation from line-of-sight
y = relative separation
α = scale factor of time-to-go estimator
β = bias of time-to-go estimator
γ = target control effort cost factor
γ_{e_0} = nominal flight-path angle of target
γ_e = perturbed flight-path angle of target
γ_{p_0} = nominal flight-path angle of missile
γ_P = perturbed flight-path angle of missile
θ = feedforward term of the control function
τ = actual time-to-go
τ_{meas} = estimated time-to-go
ξ = augmented state variable

I. Introduction

A. Motivation and Objectives

GUIDANCE applications in ground-to-air–based theater missile defense (TMD) systems are characterized by high requirements in terms of small miss distances against fast moving and possibly maneuvering targets. On the other hand, modern defense systems are typically equipped with highly sophisticated subsystems, both onboard the intercepting missiles and as part of the supporting systems (e.g., radar systems), enabling good estimates of the target's flying parameters. Guidance methods that exploit such real-time measurements are more likely to become candidates for TMD applications, whereas simple proportional navigation–based guidance methods will usually fall short with respect to satisfying the tough requirements.

Advanced methods based on one-sided optimization problems and on differential game problems are explored in Ref. 1. In this chapter, we will present this approach and its applicability to end-game guidance applications. This will be accomplished by introducing a representative guidance scheme that uses the target's acceleration estimates to improve the end-game performance against possible target maneuvers. Additionally, this particular scheme is developed with low sensitivity to time-to-go (i.e., time to interception) errors. This is a rather typical situation in TMD scenarios where time-to-go, being dependent on the future behavior of the target, is subject to some uncertainty while the current target's acceleration is continuously estimated.

It should be emphasized that we elaborate here on one *specific* candidate from the set of possible end-game guidance schemes, and this choice is by no means claimed to be the best. In practice, one should design a guidance system in accordance with its own specific requirements. However, the lessons learned here with respect to design considerations, such as optimality criteria and sensitivity reduction, as well as the optimization and simulation approaches, are of a general type and may serve as guidelines for improved methodology.

B. Historical Background

Since the first successful test of the Lark missile[2] in December 1950, proportional navigation (PN) has come to be widely employed by homing missiles. Under this scheme the missile is governed by

$$n_c = N' V_c \dot{\lambda} \tag{1}$$

where n_c is the missile's normal acceleration, $\dot{\lambda}$ is the change rate of the line-of-sight (the dot represents time derivative), V_c is the closing velocity and N' is the so-called navigation constant ($N' > 2$).

In the mid-1960s it was realized that PN with $N' = 3$ is, in fact, an optimal strategy for the linearized problem,[3] when the cost J is the control effort, as follows:

$$J = \int_0^{t_f} n_c^2(t)\,\mathrm{d}t \tag{2}$$

subject to $y(t_f) = 0$, where y is the relative interceptor–target separation and t_f is the collision time (the elapsed time from the beginning of the end-game until interception). For this case, $\dot{\lambda}$ may be expressed as follows, where the derivation is given in Eq. (18):

$$\dot{\lambda} = \frac{y + \dot{y} t_{\text{go}}}{V_c (t_{\text{go}})^2}, \qquad t_{\text{go}} \equiv t_f - t \tag{3}$$

Hence

$$n_c = \frac{3(y + \dot{y} t_{\text{go}})}{t_{\text{go}}^2} \tag{4}$$

In cases where target maneuvers are significant, extensions of the PN law have been developed such as augmented proportional navigation (APN, see Ref. 4) where the commanded interceptor's acceleration n_c depends on the target acceleration n_T, so that

$$n_c = N' V_c \dot{\lambda} + \frac{N'}{2} n_T \tag{5}$$

It was also realized that when the transfer function relating the commanded and actual accelerations n_c and n_L, respectively, has a significant time lag (which is typical for aerodynamically controlled missiles at high altitudes, e.g., the interceptor described in Sec. III.A) the APN law can lead to a significant miss distance. To overcome this difficulty, the minimum effort guidance law (MEL, see Ref. 2) was proposed whereby J [Eq. (2)] is minimized, subject to state equation constraints that include the missile's dynamics of the form

$$\frac{n_L}{n_c} = \frac{1}{1 + Ts} \tag{6}$$

where s is the Laplace transformed differentiation operator and T is the missile's time lag (which depends on the flight conditions at the end-game).

The resulting guidance law easily overcomes the large time-lag problem, but is strongly dependent on the time constant and the time-to-go, namely,

$$n_c = \frac{N'(y + \dot{y}t_{go})}{t_{go}^2} + \frac{N'}{2}n_T - Kn_L \tag{7}$$

The gains N' and K are defined as follows:

$$N' = \frac{6h^2(e^{-h} - 1 + h)}{2h^3 + 3 + 6h - 6h^2 - 12he^{-h} - 3e^{-2h}} \tag{8}$$

and

$$K = \frac{T^2}{t_{go}^2}(e^{-h} + h - 1) \tag{9}$$

where

$$h = \frac{t_{go}}{T}$$

Improved guidance schemes can be obtained with the appropriate selection of a cost function that replaces J of Eq. (2). We will demonstrate this claim with a scheme that reduces the sensitivity to time-to-go estimation errors. To this end, we next present the preliminary assumptions that render this derivation feasible and realizable.

C. Mathematical Modeling

We shall make the following assumptions:

1) The end-game is two-dimensional and gravity is compensated independently.

2) The speeds of the pursuer (the missile) P and the evader (the target) E are constant during the end-game (approximately true for short end-games).

3) The trajectories of P and E can be linearized around their collision course.

4) The pursuer is more maneuverable than the evader.

5) The pursuer can measure the target's and its own acceleration in addition to the relative separation and velocity, and has an estimate of the time-to-go (may be subjected to errors).

We assume that the collision condition is satisfied (Fig. 1), namely

$$V_p \sin(\gamma_{p_0}) - V_e \sin(\gamma_{e_0}) = 0 \tag{10}$$

where V_e and V_p are the pursuer's and evader's velocities and γ_{p_0}, γ_{e_0}, the pursuer's and evader's nominal heading angles, respectively. In this case, the nominal closing velocity V_c is given by

$$V_c = -\dot{R} = V_p \cos(\gamma_{p_0}) - V_e \cos(\gamma_{e_0}) \tag{11}$$

and the (nominal) terminal time is given by

$$t_f = \frac{R}{V_c} \tag{12}$$

where R is the nominal length of the line-of-sight.*

*R can be obtained from a laser range finder—an onboard active device—or similar devices.

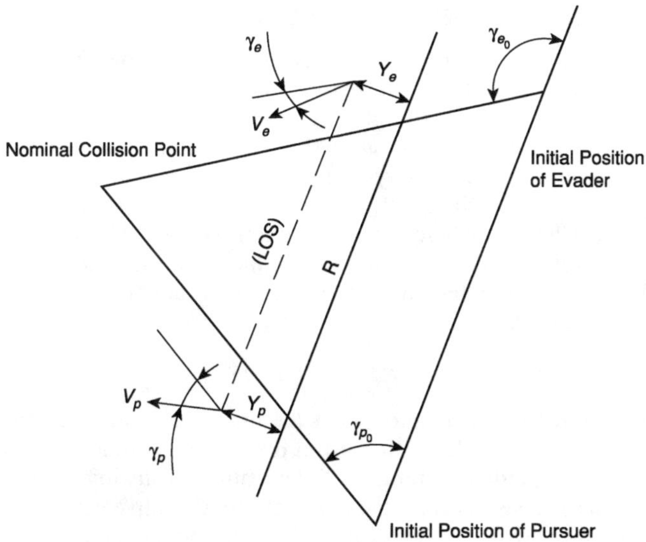

Fig. 1 Problem geometry.

If we allow Y_e, Y_p to be the separation (see Fig. 1) of the pursuer and the evader, respectively, from the nominal line-of-sight, and let y be the relative separation (namely $y \equiv Y_e - Y_p$), we obtain the following dynamic equation:

$$\dot{y} = \dot{Y}_e - \dot{Y}_p = V_e \sin\left(\gamma_{e_0} + \gamma_e\right) - V_p \sin\left(\gamma_{p_0} + \gamma_p\right) \tag{13}$$

where γ_p, γ_e are the deviations from the base line of the pursuer's and evader's headings, respectively, as a result of control actions applied. If these deviations are small enough, we may use small angles approximation to obtain

$$\sin\left(\gamma_{p_0} + \gamma_p\right) \approx \sin\left(\gamma_{p_0}\right) + \cos\left(\gamma_{p_0}\right)\gamma_p \tag{14}$$

$$\sin\left(\gamma_{e_0} + \gamma_e\right) \approx \sin\left(\gamma_{e_0}\right) + \cos\left(\gamma_{e_0}\right)\gamma_e \tag{15}$$

Substituting the results into Eqs. (10) and (13) we find [using Eq. (10)] that $\dot{y}$ becomes

$$\dot{y} = \dot{Y}_e - \dot{Y}_p = V_e \cos\left(\gamma_{e_0}\right)\gamma_e - V_p \cos\left(\gamma_{p_0}\right)\gamma_p \tag{16}$$

We can also find an expression for the line-of-sight (LOS) angle and its rate of change. Recall that λ is the LOS angle, and, without loss of generality, let $\lambda(0) = 0$. We observe that $\lambda(t)$ is

$$\lambda(t) = \frac{y}{R} \tag{17}$$

hence

$$\dot{\lambda}(t) = \frac{\mathrm{d}}{\mathrm{d}t}\left(\frac{y}{R}\right) = \frac{y}{V_c(t_f - t)^2} + \frac{\dot{y}}{V_c(t_f - t)} \tag{18}$$

and we have thus obtained Eq. (3).

D. Sensitivity to Time-to-Go Estimation Errors

The effect of the time-to-go estimation error has been shown in Ref. 4 to cause significant degradation in the performance of the optimal guidance law. In the following section we present a straightforward approach for mitigating this effect.

The idea follows from the observation that the terminal relative lateral velocity $\dot{y}(t_f)$ represents also the sensitivity of the miss distance with respect to uncertainty in the time-to-go estimate. To show that this is so, we can use the results (see e.g. Ref. 1, Chap. 3) where the interception problem with terminal velocity constraints was solved, and where it was assumed that the guidance system had a negligible time lag. For the case of zero terminal conditions (game-theoretic optimal *rendezvous*) we have

$$y(t) = c_1 t_{\text{go}}^2 + c_2 t_{\text{go}}^3 = c_1(t_f - t)^2 + c_2(t_f - t)^3$$

where $y(t)$ is the relative separation, t_f is the final time, and c_1, c_2 are constants of integration. Notice that this differs from the game-theoretic optimal *interception* problem. In the guidance literature "interception" is distinguished from "rendezvous." The latter considers also the terminal lateral relative velocity (in addition to the miss distance) whereas the former minimizes only the miss distance.

Recalling that $y(t_f)$ is the miss distance, we can evaluate the effect of small variation in t_f as follows:

$$y(t + \Delta t_f) = y(t_f) + \partial y(t)/\partial t_f|_{t=t_f} \Delta t_f + O\left(\Delta t_f^2\right) \approx \partial y(t)/\partial t_f|_{t=t_f} \Delta t_f$$

It is now clear why optimal rendezvous is less sensitive to uncertainty in t_f than optimal interception, because

$$\partial y(t)/\partial t_f|_{t=t_f}\} = \begin{matrix} 0 & \text{for rendezvous} \\ c_1 & \text{for intercept} \end{matrix}$$

where, in general, $c_1 \neq 0$.

In this chapter the guidance system is a first-order lag (i.e., a single time-constant relates the commanded acceleration with the actual acceleration—a case that can be made more elaborate if required). We formulate a linear quadratic differential game problem with a cost the includes the adversaries' control efforts and miss distance, as well as *a* weighted combination of the terminal lateral velocity and the pursuer's acceleration. (The control effort of the evader is introduced for methodological reasons to bound the evasive maneuvers against which we design our system.) The latter is included for the purpose of relaxing the terminal acceleration requirements. The differential game approach rather than the one-sided optimization method is preferred because of its more general character and the fact that as $\gamma \rightarrow \infty$ nonmaneuvering target results are obtained. However, the ideas pursued henceforth are valid for both formulations. Note that we do not assume, under this methodology, that the target is actually smart enough to play optimally. Rather, we design the system with guaranteed performance against various target maneuvers, the optimal being the worst-case scenario.

For this case, direct integration of the state-costate equations turns out to be very difficult, and so the problem will be solved by employing a Riccati equation formulation. In the present chapter, the results of Ref. 1 (Chap. 5) are extended so as to allow the measurement of the target's maneuvers by the pursuer. Therefore, the resulting guidance law is an improved version of the MEL having a reduced sensitivity to errors in the (active or passive) time-to-go measurements. The new guidance law of this chapter is compared using MATLAB® simulations to the APN and MEL laws in terms of sensitivity to errors in the time-to-go.

II. Problem Formulation and Analysis

A. Problem Formulation

Define

$$x_1 = y, x_2 = \frac{\mathrm{d}y}{\mathrm{d}t}, \qquad x_3 = -V_p \cos\left(\gamma_{p_0}\right)\frac{\mathrm{d}\gamma_p}{\mathrm{d}t} \tag{19}$$

$$u = -V_p \ \cos\left(\gamma_{p_0}\right)\frac{\mathrm{d}\gamma_{p_c}}{\mathrm{d}t}, \qquad w = V_e \ \cos\left(\gamma_{e_0}\right)\frac{\mathrm{d}\gamma_e}{\mathrm{d}t} \tag{20}$$

where x_3 is the pursuer's actual acceleration and u is the corresponding command. The problem then has the following state-space representation:

$$\dot{x} = Ax + Bu + D(w + d)$$
$$A = \begin{bmatrix} 0 & 1 & 0 \\ 0 & 0 & 1 \\ 0 & 0 & -\frac{1}{T} \end{bmatrix} B = \begin{bmatrix} 0 \\ 0 \\ \frac{1}{T} \end{bmatrix} D = \begin{bmatrix} 0 \\ 1 \\ 0 \end{bmatrix} \tag{21}$$

In Eq. (21) d is the estimated value of the normal acceleration of the evader, which is known in advance and is assumed (for simplicity) to be constant, and w is the unknown part of the normal acceleration of the evader that "plays" as the adversary in the following minimax problem:

$$\min_u \max_w J = \frac{a}{2}x_1^2(t_f) + \frac{b}{2}x_2^2(t_f) + \frac{c}{2}x_3^2(t_f) + \frac{1}{2}\int_0^{t_f} u^2(t) - \gamma^2 w^2(t)\,\mathrm{d}t \tag{22}$$

We note that w can be thought to reflect evasive maneuvers or the error in the estimation of the normal acceleration of the evader. The coefficient a weights the miss distance and is always positive. The coefficients b and c weight the terminal velocity and acceleration, respectively, and are nonnegative in this study. The former is used to obtain the desired sensitivity reduction to time-to-go errors, whereas the latter can be used to control the terminal acceleration. The constant γ penalizes evasive maneuvers, and therefore, by assumption 4 of Sec. I.C, is required to be $\gamma > 1$.

Notice that in the guidance literature other possible formulations are found; e.g., hard bounding the control actions rather than penalizing them in the cost. The basic ideas concerning the terminal cost components, however, are widely applicable.

B. Optimal Feedback Solution

The theory of linear-quadratic differential games is covered in many textbooks (e.g. Ref. 3, Chap. 10 and Ref. 1, Chap. 2) and we shall not try to cover it here. The solution to our problem can be obtained by solving the following Riccati equation:

$$-\dot{P} = PA + A^T P - PBB^T P + \gamma^{-2} PDD^T P \tag{23}$$

where the terminal conditions are

$$P(t_f) = \begin{bmatrix} a & 0 & 0 \\ 0 & b & 0 \\ 0 & 0 & c \end{bmatrix}$$

and the optimal pursuer strategy includes state feedback as well as feedforward of the target maneuvers (Ref. 1, Chap. 2). It is of the form

$$u = -B^T P x - B^T \theta$$
$$\frac{d\theta}{dt} = -[A^T + P(\gamma^{-2} D D^T - B B^T)]\theta - PDd, \qquad \theta(t_f) = 0 \tag{24}$$

For the interested reader, the detailed solution is given in the Appendix to this chapter.

III. Numerical Results

A. Interception Conflict Description, Guidance Laws, and Error Sources

In this section, we consider a numerical example that illustrates the merits of the reduced- sensitivity guidance law. We analyze the effect on the miss distance of a 3-g constant acceleration target maneuver and of a 1-deg heading error. The end-game is assumed to take 3 s, and the time-constant T is taken to be 0.5 s. The conflict is assumed to be a head-on or tail-chase, with a closing velocity of 3000 m/s. All of the numerical values are typical to end-games of TMD scenarios. The effect of three guidance laws will be analyzed: 1) augmented proportional navigation (APN)—Eq. (5), 2) minimum effort guidance law (MEL)—Eq. (7), and 3) reduced sensitivity guidance law (RSL) as developed in the previous section. In the implementation we will employ the following parameters (with the appropriate units): a = 10,000, b = 1000, c = 1000, and $\gamma = 12$.

Notice that the LOS change rate $\dot{\lambda}$ is assumed to be exactly measured and is not affected by possible errors in the time-to-go estimation. Therefore, unlike the MEL and the RSL, the performance of the APN will not depend on these errors. Two possible types of errors can corrupt the time-to-go estimation. These are multiplicative (i.e., scale factor) and additive (i.e., bias or noise) errors.

In other words,

$$\tau_{\text{meas}} = \alpha\tau + \beta + n \tag{25}$$

where α, β, and n denote the scale factor, bias error and noise, respectively. The analysis of the effect of the noise error is outside the scope of this work. In the sequel the results of a thorough analysis of the effect of bias errors β in the range of [0, 0.5] s will be described. Similar results can be obtained for scale-factor errors. All of the aforementioned guidance laws will be considered, namely, the MEL, RSL, and APN. Notice that all three guidance laws use target acceleration measurements. This is in contrast to Ref. 1 (Chap. 5) where a version of the RSL was introduced that did not use such measurements.

The effect of a time-to-go estimation error, which varies between 0–0.5 s on the interceptor's performance, is computed for the three guidance laws and two error sources (constant target maneuvers and heading error). Thus in the feedback gain calculation the measured time-to-go as given in Eq. (25) will be used where α is equal to 1 and n is zero. The comparison among the three guidance laws is made by examining the following important variables: 1) maximum commanded interceptor acceleration and miss distance caused by target acceleration and 2) maximum commanded interceptor acceleration and miss distance caused by initial heading error.

We note that the APN guidance law was included in the comparison because it is well known and widely applied in practice. However, the APN guidance law exhibits a divergence some time before the conflict end. Therefore, it may use very large accelerations that become unbounded at t_f, possibly resulting in a very small miss distance that may not be achieved in practice because of maneuver limits of the pursuer. To make the comparison to the other two guidance laws (namely MEL and RSL) more equitable, we chose to include a hard limiter of 15 g on the commanded pursuer's acceleration in our simulations. This limit is reasonable, considering the 3-g maneuvers we take for the target.

B. Simulation Results: Miss Distance and Maximum Accelerations

To allow for a clear comparison, we classify the simulation results according to their error sources (i.e., target acceleration and heading error). The results are illustrated by comparing the graphs for the three guidance laws.

1. *Step of 3 g in Target Acceleration*

The RSL law results in Fig. 2 obviously have a lower sensitivity to the time-to-go estimation error than MEL, with considerably lower miss-distance values. APN is completely insensitive to the time-to-go estimation error and exhibits miss-distance

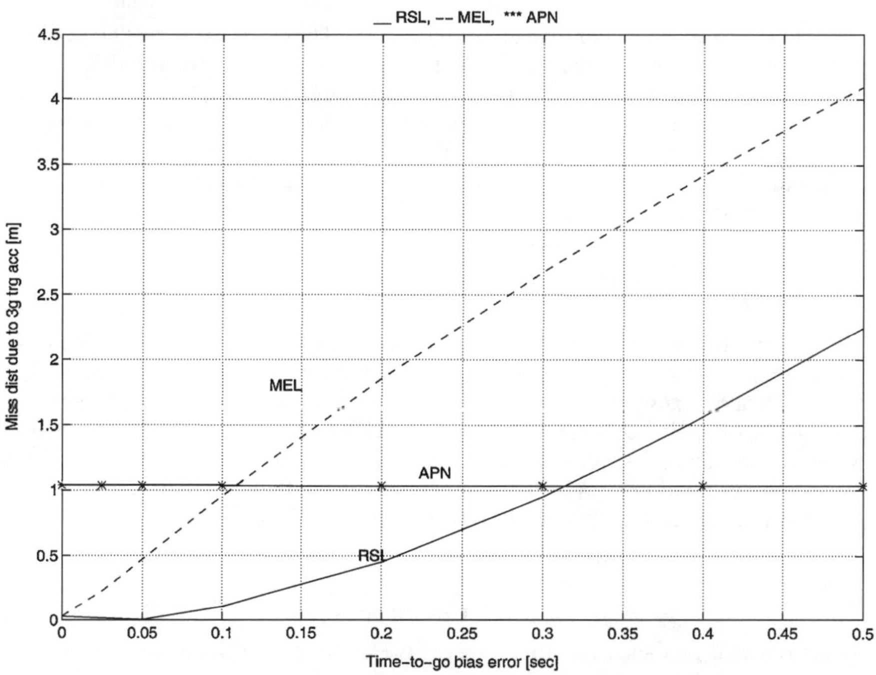

Fig. 2 Miss distance caused by target maneuver.

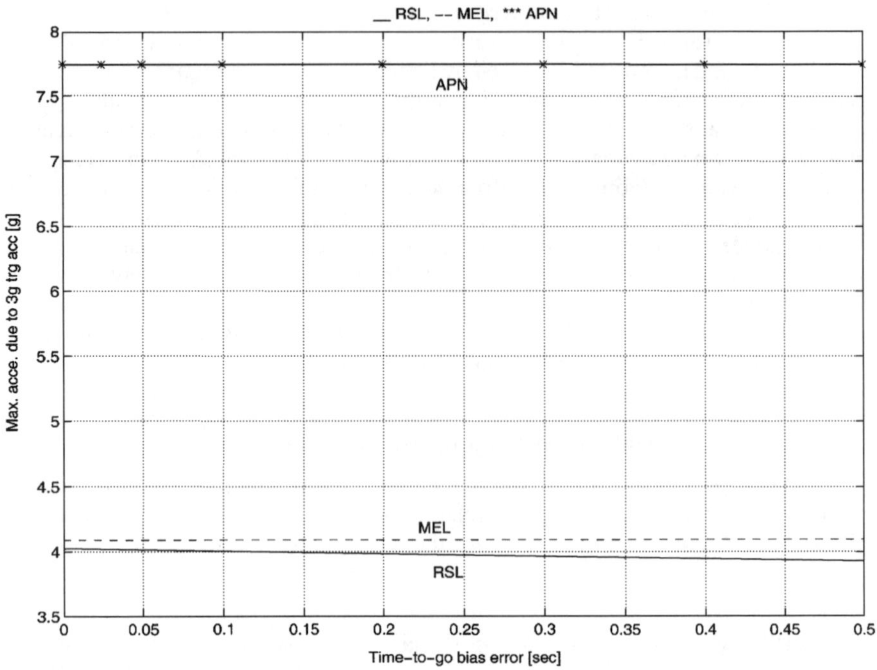

Fig. 3 Maximum acceleration caused by target maneuver.

values that are even smaller than those of the RSL. Thus, it may seem at first glance that the best choice is to use the APN guidance law. This impression appears to be wrong if the maximum accelerations used throughout the interception conflict are compared (see Fig. 3). This comparison shows that the APN uses nearly as twice as much acceleration as RSL. MEL uses accelerations almost as small as RSL but with considerably more sensitivity to time-to-go estimation error in the miss distance. Thus RSL seems to be the best choice if both miss distance and interceptor maneuvers are taken into account.

2. *Heading Error of 1.0 Deg*

For this case the RSL performance is the most impressive. The MEL has a miss distance (Fig. 4) that is almost linear with the time-to-go estimation error, with a miss distance of about 8 m for an estimation error of 0.2 s. In fact MEL is worse than APN for estimation errors larger than 0.03 s. The RSL, on the other hand, shows a very low sensitivity, which leads to a miss distance of about 0.3 m for a time-to-go estimation error of 0.2 s, and less than 2 m with errors as large as 0.5 s. The required accelerations are still larger with the RSL (Fig. 5).

IV. Conclusions

An optimal guidance law that reduces the effect of the time-to-go estimation error was developed and compared to two other well-known guidance schemes.

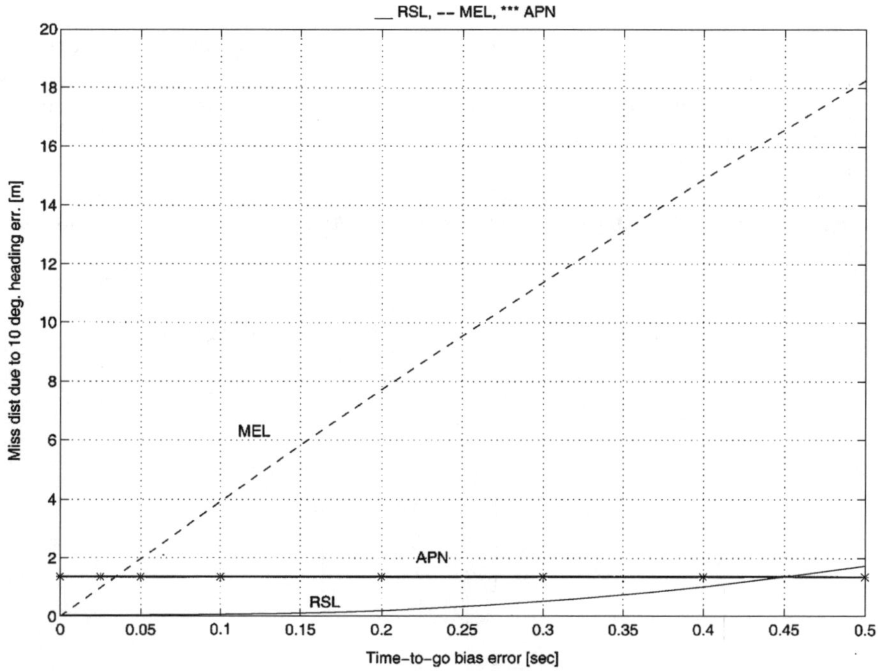

Fig. 4 Miss distance caused by heading error.

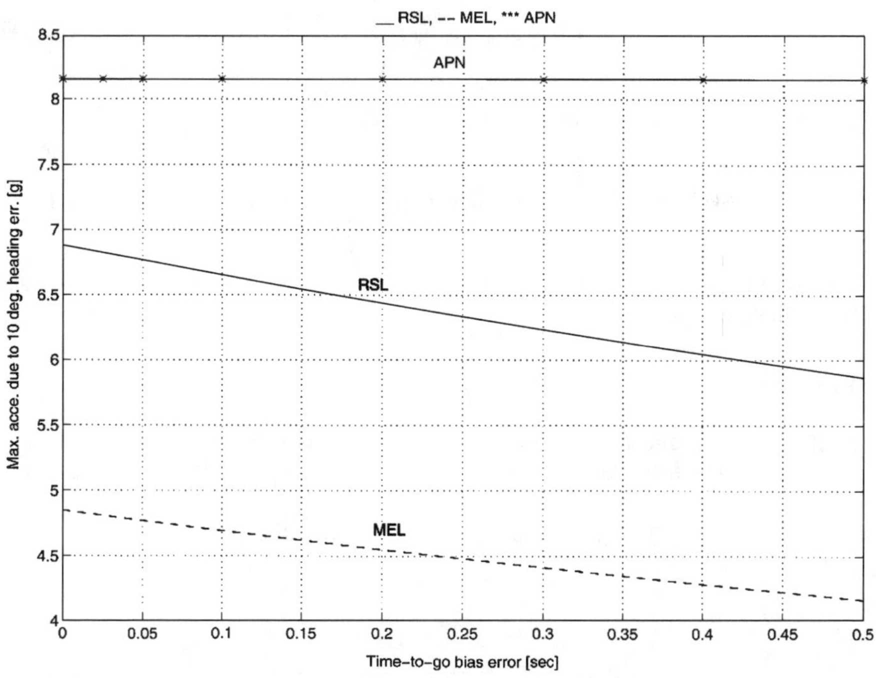

Fig. 5 Maximum maneuver caused by heading error.

The lessons learned are as follows.

1) Differential games and optimal control theory are rich sources for new practical guidance schemes.

2) Employing quadratic costs facilitates the derivation and, in many cases, may lead to closed-formed formulae for the control via analytical solutions of the Riccati equation

3) Weighting the terminal velocity and acceleration may improve the guidance performance by reducing the sensitivity to time-to-go errors and by limiting the terminal maneuver.

Appendix: Analytical Solution of the Riccati Equation

Let

$$S \equiv P^{-1} \tag{A1}$$

and define

$$S = \begin{bmatrix} S1 & S2 & S3 \\ S2 & S4 & S5 \\ S3 & S5 & S6 \end{bmatrix} \tag{A2}$$

Thus

$$\dot{S} = AS + SA^T - BB^T + \gamma^{-2}DD^T \tag{A3}$$

and

$$S(t_f) = \begin{bmatrix} a^{-1} & 0 & 0 \\ 0 & b^{-1} & 0 \\ 0 & 0 & c^{-1} \end{bmatrix}$$

Equation (A3) can be rewritten explicitly as

$$\dot{S} = \begin{bmatrix} -2S2 & -S4 - S3 & -S5 + S3/T \\ & -2S5 - 1/\gamma^2 & -S6 + S5/T \\ & & 2S6/T + 1/T^2 \end{bmatrix} \tag{A4}$$

Because the equation for $\dot{S}_6$ is independent of the others, the solution for $S6$ can be obtained easily:

$$S6(t) = -\frac{1}{2T} + e^{2h}\left(\frac{1}{2T} + \frac{1}{c}\right) \tag{A5}$$

where $h = \tau/T$ and $\tau = t_f - t$. We can now continue to solve sequentially for $S5, \ldots, S1$. The following results have been obtained by MAPLE symbolic code:

$$S5(t) = -\frac{1}{2} - \frac{1}{2}e^{2h} - \frac{Te^{2h}}{c} + \frac{e^h(c+T)}{c} \tag{A6}$$

$$S4(t) = \tau + \frac{T}{2}e^{2h} + \frac{T^2}{c}e^{2h} - 2Te^h - \frac{2T^2}{c}e^h - \frac{\tau}{\gamma^2} + \frac{3T}{2} + \frac{T^2}{c} + \frac{1}{b} \tag{A7}$$

$$S3(t) = -\frac{T}{2} + \frac{T}{2}e^{2h} + \frac{T^2e^{2h}}{c} - e^h\tau - \frac{e^hT\tau}{c} - \frac{T^2e^h}{c} \tag{A8}$$

$$S2(t) = -\frac{\tau^2}{2} - \left(\frac{T^2}{2} + \frac{T^3}{c}\right)e^{2h} - \frac{T^2c + 2T^3}{2c}$$
$$+\left(T^2 - \frac{2T^3}{c} + T\tau + \frac{T^2\tau}{c}\right)e^h + \frac{\tau^2}{2\gamma^2} - T\tau - \frac{T^2\tau}{c} - \frac{\tau}{b} \tag{A9}$$

$$S1(t) = \frac{\tau^3}{3} + \left(\frac{T^3}{2} + \frac{T^4}{c}\right)e^{2h} - \left(2T^2\tau - \frac{2T^4}{c} + \frac{2T^3\tau}{c}\right)e^h$$
$$-\frac{\tau^3}{3\gamma^2} + T\tau^2 + T^2\tau + \frac{T^4 + 2T^3\tau}{c} + \frac{T^2\tau^2}{c} + \frac{\tau^2}{b} + \frac{1}{a} \tag{A10}$$

The feedback gains can now be obtained by inverting S and by using Eqs. (A1) and (A2). Because of the complexity of the results, this stage is best performed numerically, rather than symbolically.

For the case of $d = 0$ the formulae (A5–A10) are sufficient to compute the controller. For $d \neq 0$, the equation for θ in Eq. (24) has to be solved. To this end we rewrite Eq. (24) as

$$u = -B^T Px - B^T PS\theta \tag{A11}$$

and

$$\frac{\mathrm{d}(S\theta)}{\mathrm{d}t} = \frac{\mathrm{d}S}{\mathrm{d}t}\theta + S\frac{\mathrm{d}\theta}{\mathrm{d}t} = (AS + SA^T - BB^T + \gamma^{-2}DD^T)\theta$$
$$+ S(-A^T\theta + PBB^T\theta - \gamma^{-2}PDD^T\theta - PDd)$$
$$= A(S\theta) - Dd, \qquad S\theta(t_f) = 0 \tag{A12}$$

For a given d (including a constant one) Eq. (A12) can be backward integrated to obtain $\theta(t), t \in [0, t_f]$.

To this end we define

$$\xi = S\theta \tag{A13}$$

Because

$$\frac{\mathrm{d}\xi}{\mathrm{d}t} = A\xi - Dd, \qquad \xi(t_f) = 0 \tag{A14}$$

we readily obtain

$$\xi(t) = \int_t^{t_f} e^{A(t-\tau)}(Dd)\,\mathrm{d}\tau = e^{At}\int_t^{t_f} e^{-Az}(Dd)\,\mathrm{d}\tau \tag{A15}$$

hence,

$$\xi(t) = S(t)\theta(t) = \begin{bmatrix} -(t-t_f)^2/2 \\ t_f - t \\ 0 \end{bmatrix} d \tag{A16}$$

or in terms of the time-to-go $\tau = t_f - t$ we have

$$\xi(\tau) = S(\tau)\theta(\tau) = \begin{bmatrix} -\tau^2/2 \\ \tau \\ 0 \end{bmatrix} d \tag{A17}$$

The overall guidance law is then realized via Eq. (A11).

References

[1]Ben-Asher, J. Z., and Yaesh, I., *Advances in Missile Guidance Theory*, Vol. 180, Progress in Astronautics and Aeronautics, AIAA, Washington DC, 1998.

[2]Zarchan, P., *Tactical and Strategic Missile Guidance*, Progress in Astronautics and Aeronautics, AIAA, Washington DC, 1990, 1997.

[3]Bryson, A. E., and Ho, Y. C., *Applied Optimal Control*, Hemisphere, New York, 1975, Chap. 5.

[4]Nesline, W. N., and Zarchan, P., "A New Look at Classical vs Modern Homing Missile Guidance," *Journal of Guidance and Control*, Vol. 4, No. 1, 1981, pp. 878–880.

Chapter 13

Interception of Maneuvering Targets in Theater Missile Defense

Josef Shinar*

Technion—Israel Institute of Technology, Haifa, Israel

Nomenclature

$\mathbf{A}$	= system matrix, Eq. (10)
$\boldsymbol{a}$	= lateral acceleration
$\boldsymbol{a}^c$	= lateral acceleration command
$\boldsymbol{a}_x$	= longitudinal acceleration
$\mathbf{B}$	= pursuer's control matrix, Eq. (10)
B	= time-varying matrix, Eq. (A7)
$\mathbf{C}$	= evader's control matrix, Eq. (10)
C	= time-varying matrix, Eq. (A8)
$\boldsymbol{D}$	= constant vector, Eq. (13)
D_0, D_1	= regions of the normalized game space, Fig. 2
f	= frequency of measurements
$\boldsymbol{H}$	= variational Hamiltonian
J	= cost function
M	= normalized miss distance
M_1	= normalized lethal radius of the warhead
N'	= effective navigation ratio
$\boldsymbol{P}$	= probability of interception avoidance with incorrect bias
$\boldsymbol{P}_s$	= probability of interception avoidance without bias
$\boldsymbol{Q}$	= probability of interception avoidance with correct bias
t	= time
t_{go}	= time-to-go
$\boldsymbol{u}$	= normalized pursuer control
V	= velocity
$\boldsymbol{v}$	= normalized evader control
W	= normalized zero effort miss distance to the TBM's target, Eq. (31)

Copyright © 2000 by the American Institute of Aeronautics and Astronautics, Inc. All rights reserved.

*Max and Lottie Dresher Professor of Aerospace Performance and Propulsion, Faculty of Aerospace Engineering. Fellow AIAA.

$\mathbf{X}$ = vector of state variables
X = coordinate in the direction of the initial line of sight
$\mathbf{X}_i$ = state variable, $i = 1, 2, \ldots, n$
Y = distance of lateral separation
$\mathbf{Z}$ = dimensional zero effort miss distance, Eq. (16)
Z = normalized zero effort miss distance, Eq. (18)
α = normalized longitudinal acceleration, Eq. (53)
β = normalized maneuverability rate of change, Eq. (45)
$\mathbf{\Gamma}$ = dimensional rate of change of optimal trajectories, Eq. (A18)
Γ = normalized rate of change of optimal trajectories, Eq. (26)
γ = dummy variable, Eq. (19)
ε = target/interceptor time constant ratio, Eq. (15)
η = ratio of *lethal radius* and guaranteed miss distance, Eq. (38)
θ = normalized time-to-go, Eq. (17)
ν = interceptor/target speed ratio, Eq. (28)
μ = interceptor/target maneuverability ratio, Eq. (14)
σ = line-of-sight angle
ϕ = aspect angle
τ = time constant
Δt_{est} = estimation delay

Subscripts

B = biased
E = evader (TBM)
d = TBM destination
F = final
max = maximum
P = pursuer (interceptor)
0 = initial condition

Superscripts

b = biased
c = center, compensated (belongs to DGL/C)
T = transposed
0 = belongs to DGL/0
1 = belongs to DGL/1
α = for variable speed model
β = for variable maneuverability ratio model
$*$ = optimal

I. Introduction

THE very notion of theater missile defense (TMD) was created as one of the lessons learned from the events of the Persian Gulf War. It came to redefine the priorities set earlier by the more ambitious Strategic Defense Initiative (SDI) and started an accelerated international development effort to meet the threat of tactical ballistic missiles (TBMs) encountered in that war. As a result of this effort we see today, ten years later, several emerging TMD systems (Arrow, PAC-3, THAAD, etc.) to be deployed in the next decade. All of them succeeded to demonstrate the potential of intercepting reentering TBMs with excellent homing accuracy. In recent flight tests performed against nonmaneuvering targets direct hits were achieved.[1–3] Therefore, one may believe that the threat of using TBMs, probably equipped with nonconventional warheads as a terror weapon, will be eliminated by the time of the deployment of these defense systems.

In analyzing the *less than perfect* homing performance of the Patriot PAC-2 system in the Gulf War, two additional (not yet openly spelled out) lessons can be learned. The first (trivial) one is that no weapon system can be effective against a threat that has not been properly defined. It is well known that the characteristic of the Al-Hussein missiles, used against Israel and Saudi Arabia, were not included in the operational requirement that initiated the PAC-2 modifications introduced in the original Patriot system. The Patriot PAC-2 system in the Gulf War performed exactly as it was designed, but (unfortunately) the *target was wrong*. The second lesson learned from the disintegration of most of the Al-Hussein missiles is that "the unexpected can (and according to Murphy's law, will indeed) happen."

Currently known TBMs have been aimed to hit static targets and were not designed to maneuver. As a consequence, they are *supposed* to fly highly predictable trajectories. Nevertheless, because of their high reentry velocity they have a substantial aerodynamic maneuvering potential in the lower atmosphere, comparable to that of the interceptors. Moreover, this great maneuverability potential can be easily materialized by a rather modest technical effort, within the reach of many rogue countries.

At higher altitudes, where neither the reentry vehicles nor the interceptor missiles have any aerodynamic maneuver potential, another situation can occur. It is not unrealistic to assume that the designer of the reentry vehicle of a future TBM may trade off a part of the warhead for a simple, rocket-motor–based maneuvering device and a certain amount of propellant. (It has to be remembered that something quite similar happened with the Al-Hussein missiles built from the original SCUDs.) If such a device creates a sufficient level of lateral acceleration, it can provide a nonzero probability of interception avoidance and consequently an unacceptable leakage.[4]

It seems reasonable that the successful development and the subsequent deployment of the earlier-mentioned TMD systems can motivate the development of a new generation of TBMs with presently unknown maneuvering characteristics. Experience has shown that from the definition of an operational requirement it takes 12–15 years to develop and deploy a guided missile system. Therefore, one should make an effort to anticipate future threats and start adequate actions to meet them long before they actually appear. Otherwise, the disappointing and frustrating experience of the Gulf War can be repeated.

The objective of this chapter is to report the results of a multiyear investigation that has been performed at the Faculty of Aerospace Engineering in the Technion—Israel Institute of Technology and has been motivated by the lessons learned from the Persian Gulf War. This investigation has concentrated on analyzing future interception scenarios against highly maneuverable reentry vehicles, beyond the horizon of the ongoing TMD development projects. At the outset, both analytical and simulation studies were used to evaluate different guidance and estimation schemes against highly maneuvering generic TBM-type targets. It was concluded that currently used guidance and estimation methods are unable to guarantee the same "hit-to-kill" homing accuracy against maneuvering threats, which had been demonstrated in flight against ballistic targets.

Having analyzed the origin of the deficiencies in the currently used methods, the subsequent effort was aimed at developing a new approach for guidance law synthesis that corrects these shortcomings and has the potential of an improved homing accuracy. The most critical deficiency has its origin in the conservative mindset of the guided missile community. All known missile guidance laws used at the present were developed based on a linearized kinematic (constant speed) model and a linear quadratic optimal control concept (with unbounded control).[5] Thus, the limited maneuver potential of the interceptor has not been explicitly taken into account in these guidance laws. Moreover, the optimal control concept requires knowing the current and future target maneuvers. For the sake of simplicity, in most cases constant target maneuvers have been assumed. The information on the current target maneuver, because it cannot be directly measured, has been obtained from an estimator. The guidance law implementation has been based on the common practice of applying the separation theorem associated with the certainty equivalence principle. For the analysis of future TMD scenarios against highly maneuverable reentry vehicles neither the optimal control formulation nor the application of the certainty equivalence principle are appropriate. These points are elaborated in some detail in Secs. II and VI.

The structure of this chapter is the following. In the next section the TMD scenario is formulated as a linear zerosum pursuit-evasion game, followed by the analytical solution of its mathematical model. In Sec. III the results of the first analytical investigations are summarized. It is followed by the summary of extensive simulation studies performed during the last seven years and the lessons that indicate the necessary guidance law improvements are stated. In Sec. V the extension of the linearized kinematic model is outlined. In Sec. VI an improved guidance law, which compensates the inherent estimation delay in a realistic scenario with noise corrupted measurements, is presented.

Because of the comprehensive nature of this chapter, an effort was made to keep the mathematics to the minimal necessary level and to orient readers who are interested in details to available publications.

II. Problem Formulation

A. General

Future TMD scenarios can be characterized by the following features.

1) Missile defense systems deployed in the region will be able to intercept and destroy nonmaneuvering reentry vehicles, flying on predictable ballistic trajectories.

2) Some of the reentry vehicles may have a large maneuvering potential, leaving only a marginal advantage for the interceptor missiles.

3) These maneuverable reentry vehicles can perform random maneuvers, rendering their trajectory unpredictable.

Keeping these features in mind, it is clear that such a scenario cannot be formulated as an optimal control problem. The eventual maneuvers of the reentry vehicles are independently controlled and as a consequence they cannot be predicted. It means that future target maneuver time history (or strategy) cannot be known, rendering the optimal control formulation inadequate. The mathematical framework for analyzing a system controlled by two independent agents is in the realm of dynamic noncooperative game theory.[6] The very concepts of game theory are based on the assumption that the players have no knowledge of the other's control strategy. Because a future TMD scenario of intercepting a maneuverable target clearly has this feature, it has to be formulated as a two-person differential game, or more specifically as a zero-sum pursuit-evasion game. The game solution provides simultaneously the optimal interceptor guidance law (the optimal pursuer strategy), the "worst" target maneuver (the optimal evader strategy) and the resulting guaranteed miss distance (the *value* of the game). Although such a formulation and solution concepts date back to the 1950s, (see the seminal book by Rufus Isaacs[7]) and was repeatedly endorsed,[8,9] the missile community has failed to recognize the potential involved in it.

B. Mathematical Modeling

The pursuit–evasion game model of the terminal phase of a future TMD interception is based on the following set of simplifying assumptions.

1) The game starts when the interceptor missile (the pursuer) P is "locked" on the approaching reentry vehicle (the evader) E.

2) The interception engagement takes place in a plane.

3) Both missiles have constant velocities V_j and bounded lateral accelerations:

$$|\boldsymbol{a}_j| \leq (\boldsymbol{a}_j)\text{max} \qquad (j = E, P)$$

4) The trajectories of both missiles can be linearized along the initial line of sight.

5) Maneuvering dynamics of both missiles are approximated by first-order transfer functions with the respective time constants τ_E and τ_P.

6) The maneuvering of the reentry vehicle does not limit its capability to hit its assigned surface target if the interception fails.

In Fig. 1 a schematic view of the end-game geometry is shown. Note that the respective velocity vectors of the missiles are generally not aligned with the reference line of sight. The aspect angles ϕ_P and ϕ_E are, however, small. Thus, the approximations $\cos(\phi_i) \approx 1$ and $\sin(\phi_i) \approx (\phi_i)$, $(i = P, E)$, are uniformly valid and coherent with assumption 4. Moreover, based on assumptions 3 and 4, the final time of the interception can be computed for any given initial conditions of the end-game:

$$t_f = \arg\left\{X_f = X_0 - \int_{t_0}^{t_f} [V_E + V_P]\,\mathrm{d}t = 0\right\} \tag{1}$$

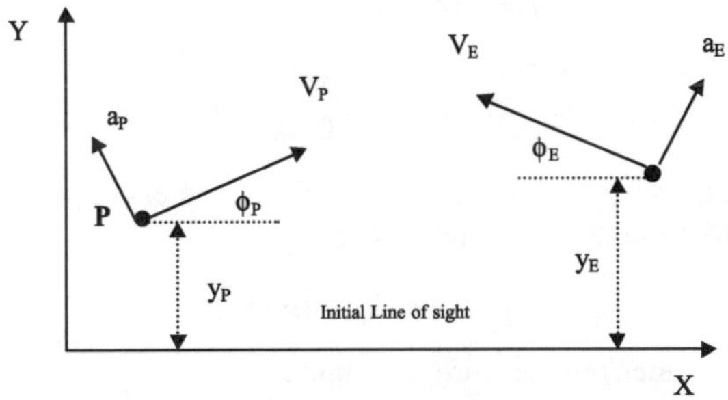

Fig. 1 End-game geometry.

allowing to define the time-to-go by

$$t_{go} \overset{\Delta}{=} t_f - t \tag{2}$$

The equations of motion perpendicular to the initial line of sight and the respective initial conditions are written, based on assumptions 3–5, as follows:

$$y(t) \overset{\Delta}{=} y_E(t) - y_P(t) = x_1 \tag{3}$$

$$\frac{dx_1}{dt} = x_2; \qquad x_1(0) = 0 \tag{4}$$

$$\frac{dx_2}{dt} = x_3 - x_4; \qquad x_2(0) = V_E\phi_{E_0} - V_P\phi_{P_0} \tag{5}$$

$$\frac{dx_3}{dt} = [(\boldsymbol{a}^c)_E - x_3]/\tau_E; \qquad x_3(0) = 0 \tag{6}$$

$$\frac{dx_4}{dt} = [(\boldsymbol{a}^c)_P - x_4]/\tau_P; \qquad x_4(0) = 0 \tag{7}$$

where $(\boldsymbol{a}^c)_E$ and $(\boldsymbol{a}^c)_P$ are the commanded lateral accelerations of E and P respectively.

$$(\boldsymbol{a}^c)_E = (\boldsymbol{a}_E)_{\max} \boldsymbol{v}; \qquad |\boldsymbol{v}| \le 1 \tag{8}$$

$$(\boldsymbol{a}^c)_P = (\boldsymbol{a}_P)_{\max} \boldsymbol{u}; \qquad |\boldsymbol{u}| \le 1 \tag{9}$$

The nonzero initial conditions $V_E\phi_{E_0}$ and $V_P\phi_{P_0}$ represent the respective initial velocity components not aligned with the initial (reference) line of sight. By assumption 5 these components are small compared with the components along the line of sight.

The set of equations (4–7) can be rewritten in a compact form as a linear, time dependent, vector differential equation

$$\frac{d\boldsymbol{X}}{dt} = \mathbf{A}(t)\boldsymbol{X} + \mathbf{B}(t)\boldsymbol{u} + \mathbf{C}(t)\boldsymbol{v}; \qquad \boldsymbol{X}(t_0) = \boldsymbol{X}_0 \tag{10}$$

with the state vector

$$\boldsymbol{X}^T = (x_1, x_2, x_3, x_4) = \left(y, \frac{dy}{dt}, \boldsymbol{a}_P, \boldsymbol{a}_E\right) \tag{11}$$

The natural cost function of the game is the miss distance

$$\boldsymbol{J} = |\boldsymbol{D}^T \boldsymbol{X}(t_f)| = |x_1(t_f)| \tag{12}$$

where

$$\boldsymbol{D}^T = (1, 0, 0, 0) \tag{13}$$

The problem involves two nondimensional parameters of physical significance: the pursuer/evader maximum maneuverability ratio

$$\mu \overset{\Delta}{=} (\boldsymbol{a}_P)_{\max}/(\boldsymbol{a}_E)_{\max} \tag{14}$$

and the ratio of evader/pursuer time constants

$$\varepsilon \overset{\Delta}{=} \tau_E/\tau_P \tag{15}$$

The transformation

$$Z(t) = D^T \Phi(t_f, t)X(t) \tag{16}$$

where $\Phi(t_f, t)$ is the transition matrix of the original homogeneous system, reduces the vector equation (10) to a scalar one. It is easy to see from Eqs. (12), (13), and (16) that the new state variable is the zero-effort miss distance. For the sake of generality, nondimensional variables are defined. The independent variable is the normalized time-to-go

$$\theta \triangleq (t_f - t)/\tau_P; \qquad \theta(t = 0) = t_f/\tau_P = \theta_0 \tag{17}$$

and the nondimensional state variable is the normalized zero-effort miss distance. For the present problem, described by Eqs. (4–7), it is

$$Z(\theta) \triangleq \boldsymbol{Z}(t)/\tau_P^2(\boldsymbol{a}_E)_{\max} = \left\{x_1 + x_2(\tau_P\theta) + x_3\tau_E^2\psi(\theta/\varepsilon) - x_4\tau_P^2\psi(\theta)\right\}/\tau_P^2(\boldsymbol{a}_E)_{\max} \tag{18}$$

where

$$\psi(\gamma) \triangleq e^{-\gamma} + \gamma - 1 \tag{19}$$

The definition (18) imbeds the assumption of perfect information, meaning that all of the original state variables (x_1, x_2, as well as the lateral accelerations x_3 and x_4) are known to both players. Using the nondimensional variables the normalized game dynamics becomes

$$\frac{dZ}{d\theta} = \mu\psi(\theta)\boldsymbol{u} - \varepsilon\psi(\theta/\varepsilon)\boldsymbol{v}; \qquad Z(\theta_0) = Z_0 \tag{20}$$

with the following normalized initial conditions

$$Z(\theta_0) \triangleq Z_0 = \left(V_E\phi_{E_0} - V_P\phi_{P_0}\right)/\tau_P^2(\boldsymbol{a}_E)_{\max} \tag{21}$$

and with the control constraints

$$|\boldsymbol{u}| \leq 1; \qquad |\boldsymbol{v}| \leq 1 \tag{22}$$

The nondimensional pay-off function of the game is the normalized miss distance

$$J = |Z_f| = |Z(\theta = 0)| \tag{23}$$

to be minimized by the pursuer and maximized by the evader.

C. Perfect Information Game Solution

The general solution of the family of perfect information linear differential games with bounded controls is presented in the Appendix to this chapter, in a dimensional form. Its application to the model described by Eqs. (4–7) and (20–23) was published long ago[10] and is briefly repeated. The necessary conditions of optimality determine the candidate optimal control strategies of the players as

$$\boldsymbol{u}^*(Z, \theta) = \boldsymbol{v}^*(Z, \theta) = \text{sign}\,\{Z(\theta)\}; \qquad Z(\theta) \neq 0 \tag{24}$$

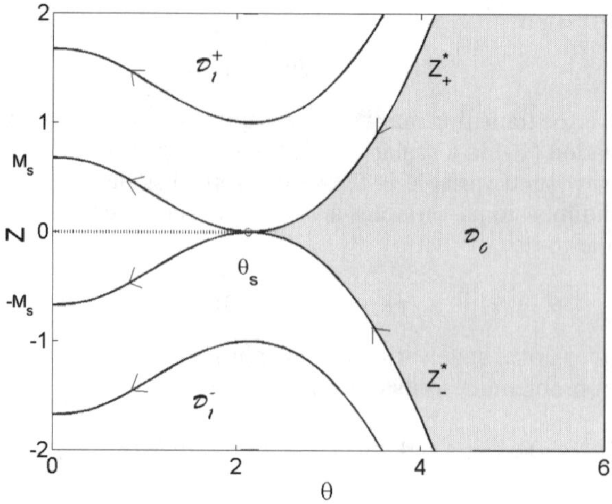

Fig. 2 Game space decomposition.

Substituting Eqs. (23) into (21) yields along candidate optimal trajectories

$$\frac{dZ^*}{d\theta} = \Gamma(\theta)\,\text{sign}\{Z(\theta)\} \tag{25}$$

where

$$\Gamma(\theta) = \mu\psi(\theta) - \varepsilon\psi(\theta/\varepsilon) \stackrel{\Delta}{=} \Gamma^1(\theta, \mu, \varepsilon) \tag{26}$$

By integrating Eq. (25) backward (starting at $\theta = 0$), a family of *regular* optimal trajectories is generated. Since this family does not fill the entire nondimensional game space (Z, θ), the game solution consists of decomposing it into two regions (see Fig. 2). In the regular region, denoted as D_1, the optimal strategies are of the "bang-bang" type given by Eq. (24) and the value of the game is a unique function of the initial conditions. The boundaries of this region are the pair of optimal trajectories $Z^*_+(\theta)$ and $Z^*_-(\theta)$, reaching tangentially the θ axis ($Z = 0$) at the normalized time-to-go θ_s, as shown in Fig. 2, where $\theta_s = \theta_s(\mu, \varepsilon)$ is nonvanishing solution of the equation $\Gamma(\theta) = 0$.

In the other region, enclosed by the boundaries $Z^*_+(\theta)$ and $Z^*_-(\theta)$, denoted as D_0, the optimal strategies are *arbitrary*. All of the trajectories starting in D_0 must go through the point ($Z = 0, \theta = \theta_s$), called the "*throat*," where D_0 terminates. As a consequence, the value of the game for the entire region of D_0, obtained by integrating $\Gamma(\theta)$ between $\theta = 0$ and $\theta = \theta_s$, is constant:

$$J^*_0 = \mu(1 - \varepsilon)\,\psi(\theta_s) - (\mu - 1)\,\theta_s^2/2 \stackrel{\Delta}{=} M_s(\mu, \varepsilon) \tag{27}$$

When a trajectory starting in D_0 reaches the throat, the evader must select the direction of its maximal maneuver (either to the right or to the left) and the pursuer has to follow it. Therefore, the optimal evasive maneuver that guarantees $M_s(\mu, \varepsilon)$ is a maximal maneuver in a fixed direction for the duration of at least $\theta_s(\mu, \varepsilon)$. The values of $\theta_s(\mu, \varepsilon)$ and $M_s(\mu, \varepsilon)$ are depicted in Figs. 3 and 4. These results are of great practical importance, because for the majority of cases the initial conditions

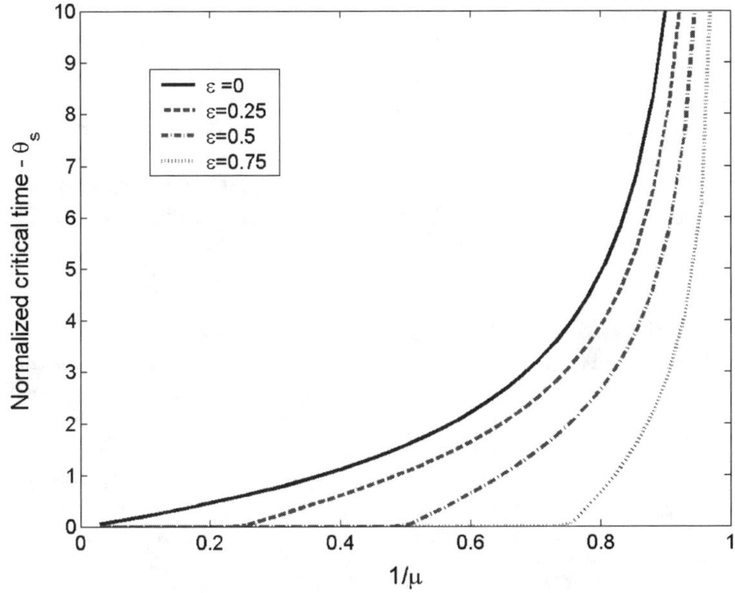

Fig. 3 Critical normalized time $\theta_s(\mu, \varepsilon)$.

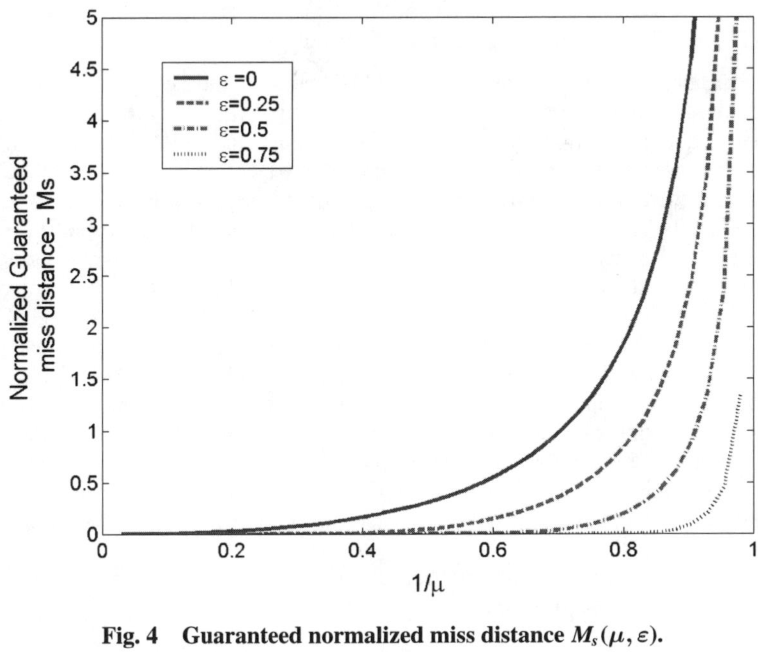

Fig. 4 Guaranteed normalized miss distance $M_s(\mu, \varepsilon)$.

of an interception are in D_0. Because in D_0 the optimal strategies are arbitrary, the interceptor can use there a linear guidance law or even a bang-bang type of strategy as Eq. (24).

In characterizing this game solution, denoted as DGL/1, two cases can be distinguished based on the value of the product $\mu\varepsilon$ (having the physical interpretation of the pursuer/evader agility ratio). If the inequality $\mu\varepsilon < 1$ is satisfied, neither θ_s nor M_s (the guaranteed normalized miss distance for D_0) are zero. This includes, as a particular case, the game model of *ideal* evader dynamics ($\tau_E = \varepsilon = 0$), solved first by Gutman[11] (denoted in the sequel as DGL/0). In this particular case the term multiplying x_3, the actual lateral acceleration of the evader in Eq. (18), vanishes and the implementation of the guidance law becomes simpler. There is no need to know the evader's lateral acceleration, because it becomes a control variable.

However, if $\mu\varepsilon \geq 1$, both θ_s and the corresponding M_s are zero. It means that for the majority of all practically important initial conditions a direct hit is guaranteed against any feasible evasive maneuver. This robust hit-to-kill accuracy (the desirable outcome in antiballistic missile defense) is based on the assumption of perfect information, i.e., accurate knowledge of all of the state variables, including the actual lateral acceleration of the evader. Unfortunately, this result remains only theoretical, because in reality guidance laws are implemented in a noise-corrupted environment, rendering the information structure imperfect.

III. First Analytical Studies

A. Game Solution with Constrained Evader

One important difference between the TMD scenario and a classical interception engagement is that the basic objective of the reentry vehicle is to hit an assigned surface target. To accomplish this goal, its maneuvering options are not entirely free. In mathematical terms, this fact imposes a trajectory constraint on the maneuverable reentry vehicle. In the model presented in Sec. II.B, the effect of this constraint has been eliminated by assumption 6. To evaluate the usefulness of the perfect information pursuit-evasion game solution of Sec. II.C in an actual TMD scenario, the first analysis was oriented to study the effect of this trajectory constraint on the guaranteed outcome of the interception.[12]

In this analysis the origin of the coordinate system is located at the assigned surface target, and its X axis is aligned with the initial line of sight. For sake of simplicity a point-defense scenario is considered. The engagement starts ($t = 0$) when the interceptor is launched. Assumptions 2–4 in Sec. II.B are adopted, but 5 is modified. Because of the apparent difficulty (at least, at that time) in measuring target acceleration directly, it was decided to assume ideal evader dynamics[10] (the worst case for the pursuer), expressed by setting $\tau_E = 0$. Of course, assumption 6 was not used.

The time needed for the reentry vehicle to reach its destination after an interception failure at t_f is given by

$$t_d = (V_P/V_E)t_f \triangleq \nu\, t_f \tag{28}$$

The trajectory constraint of the reentry vehicle is expressed by

$$|y_E(t_f) + y_1(t_f)\,t_d| \le (\boldsymbol{a}_E)_{\max}\,(t_d)^2/2 \tag{29}$$

where

$$y_1 \triangleq \frac{\mathrm{d}y_E}{\mathrm{d}t} \tag{30}$$

This constraint leads to define, in addition to Eq. (18) with $\tau_E = 0$, a second nondimensional state variable

$$W(\theta) \triangleq [y_E + \tau_P(\theta + \theta_d)y_1]/\tau_P^2(\boldsymbol{a}_E)_{\max} \tag{31}$$

where

$$\theta_d \triangleq t_d/\tau_P \tag{32}$$

The solution of the new game (with two state variables) is an order of magnitude more complex than the original one and is presented in detail in two papers.[12,13] Here only the main result is quoted.

The solution indicates that the trajectory constraint (29) becomes active only if

$$\theta_d \le (\sqrt{2} + 1)\,\theta_s \tag{33}$$

where θ_s is defined in the unconstrained game with $\tau_E = 0$. As long as Eq. (33) is not satisfied, the solutions of the two games coincide. If Eq. (33) is satisfied, the solution of the game with constraint depends on $(\theta_s)^d$, the nonvanishing solution of

$$(\sqrt{2} - 1)\theta_d = \mu\psi(\theta) \tag{34}$$

replacing θ_s of the unconstrained game and the guaranteed miss distance becomes

$$(M_s)^d = \int_0^{(\theta_s)^d} [\mu\psi(\theta) - \theta]\,\mathrm{d}\theta \tag{35}$$

Obviously, $(\theta_s)^d \le \theta_s$ and as a consequence $(M_s)^d \le M_s$. In Figs. 5 and 6 the values of $(\theta_s)^d$ and $(M_s)^d$ are plotted, for different values of μ, as a function of θ_d. Even though for $\mu \le 1$ the theoretical value of $(\theta_s)^d$ is infinite, in reality it becomes bounded because of the finite duration of the game ($\theta_0 = 50$ in this example). The relationship between the actual normalized miss distance (denoted as M) and the value of M_s is plotted in Fig. 7 as the function of θ_0/θ_s, both for the unconstrained and the constrained game with the fixed parameters ($\mu = 1.3$, $\nu = 1.0$). Based on the solution of the game with trajectory constraint it was possible to show that for realistic TMD scenarios the inequality (33) is generally not satisfied and the trajectory constraint remains inactive. Thus, further investigations concentrated on the unconstrained version of the game.

B. Stochastic Analysis

The nonzero miss distance, guaranteed in the previous deterministic analysis (35), may or may not be satisfactory for an effective defense, depending on the

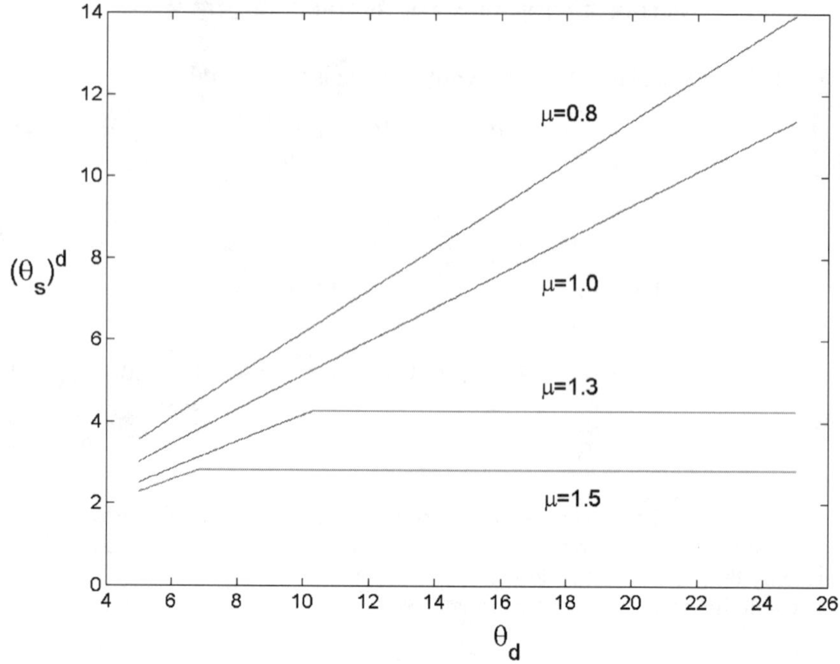

Fig. 5 Results of the perfect information game with constraint: normalized critical time-to-go $(\theta_s)^d$.

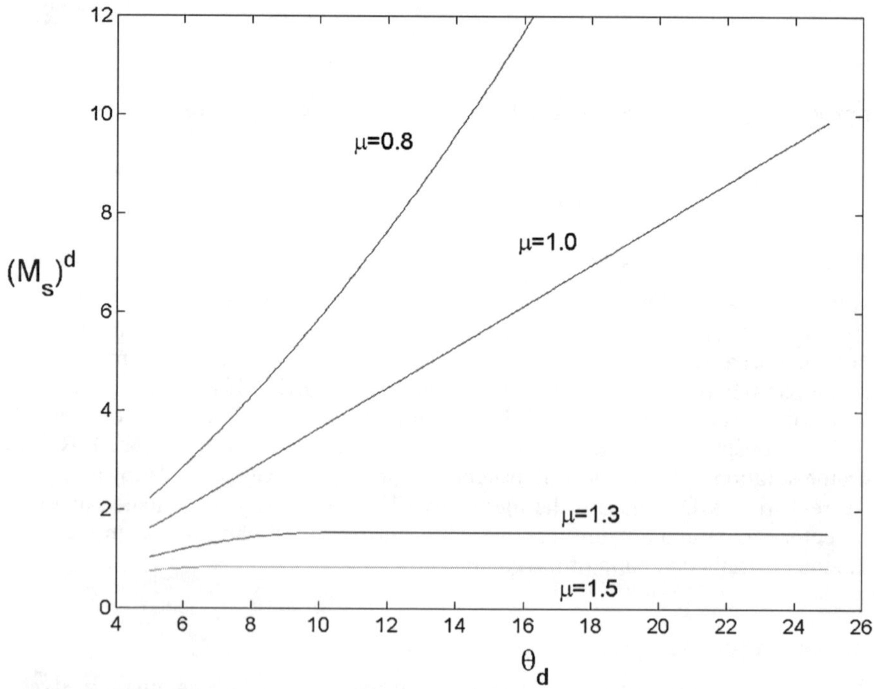

Fig. 6 Results of the perfect information game with constraint: normalized guaranteed miss distance $(M_s)^d$.

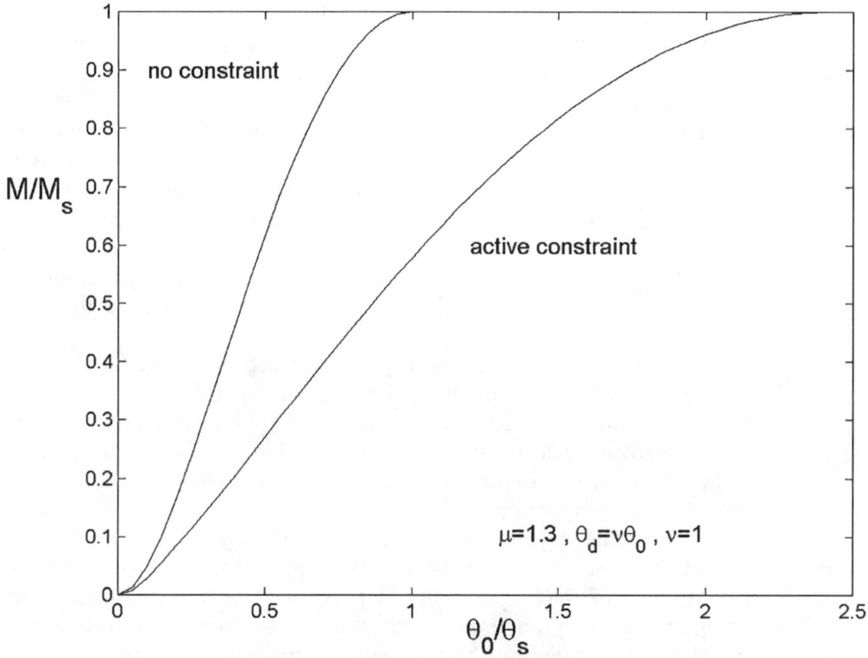

Fig. 7 Effect of the constraint on the guaranteed miss distance.

lethal radius of the interceptor's warhead. In this case a stochastic analysis[14] formulating the problem as an imperfect information game is required. In such an analysis the cost function J is the probability of successful interception avoidance. It is defined via a lethality function $\Phi\{|Z_f|\}$, depending on the relationship between the normalized lethal radius of the warhead M_1 and the normalized miss distance $|Z_f|$. The simplest model for such a lethality function, used in an earlier paper,[14] is

$$\begin{aligned} \Phi[|Z_f|] = 1 \qquad &\Leftarrow \qquad |Z_f| \geq M_1 \\ \Phi[|Z_f|] = 0 \qquad &\Leftarrow \qquad |Z_f| \leq M_1 \end{aligned} \tag{36}$$

Using this definition the cost function is

$$J = E\{\Phi[|Z_f|]\} \tag{37}$$

to be minimized by the defense system and maximized by the TBM designer (and/or operator). The most important parameter in such formulation is the ratio of the lethal radius of the interceptor's warhead and the miss distance guaranteed by the perfect information game solution:

$$\eta \triangleq M_1/M_s \tag{38}$$

In the following stochastic analysis it is assumed from the outset that $\eta < 1$. The destruction of a maneuvering threat cannot be guaranteed, but the actual miss distance in most cases will be smaller than the value predicted by the perfect information game solution, because in a realistic TMD scenario the TBM has no information on the interceptor and cannot perform optimal evasive maneuvers in the deterministic sense. Most probably, it will execute random maneuvers, because nonmaneuvering or maneuvering in a fixed direction will result in a predictable trajectory followed by certain interception and destruction. Based on the results of the perfect information game solution, the following intuitive guidelines for the structure of the random maneuvers have been established.

1) A maneuvering sequence should cover the entire interception range of the defense system using maximum lateral acceleration without violating the constraint.

2) It must have a *small* number of randomly timed direction changes (switches).

3) The duration of each maneuver should be of the order of θ_s.

In summary, the parameters of a *pure* (deterministic) evasive strategy are the switching distances from the designated target. The random selection of the parameters creates the *mixed strategy* (a probability distribution over the set of admissible pure strategies) for the designer or the operator of the TBM.

In such a situation the defense system, in spite of having perfect information, must select the time for launching the interceptor randomly, covering the entire feasible domain of interception altitudes. (Otherwise, the designer of the TBM, knowing the interception range, can plan a deterministic optimal evasion.) Although by implementing such a random strategy the destruction of a maneuvering TBM cannot be always guaranteed, the actual miss distance in most cases will be smaller than the value predicted by the *perfect information* (deterministic) game solution, because the interception altitude becomes a random variable.

The best launch direction in a perfect information scenario is toward the predicted collision point ($Z_0 = 0$). In the imperfect information scenario of interest ($\eta < 1$ and random TBM maneuvers) a nonzero initial bias, based on a presumed continuous maneuver, can be considered. The magnitude of this bias and its direction can be random. Moreover, the guidance law also can include a compatible time-varying bias

$$\boldsymbol{u}^b = \text{sign}\{Z - Z^b - (\theta)\} \tag{39}$$

replacing Eq. (24). Thus, the defense also applies a mixed strategy.

The analysis of the imperfect information game with mixed strategies is illustrated by the following example. It is assumed that the random maneuver sequence of the TBM that satisfies the guidelines 1–3 is of the random telegraph type (frequently used in missile analysis[15]), characterized by a single parameter λ. In such a stochastic process the average duration between two subsequent direction changes (switches) is $1/\lambda$, and the probability that there will be no switch during a given period of time Δt is equal to $\exp\{-\lambda \Delta t\}$. This probability is independent of any past event.

In the first part of the example it is assumed that the interceptor implements the unbiased guidance law of DGL/0, the initial conditions of the end-game are in D_0 and the random maneuver sequence of the TBM starts before the *throat*

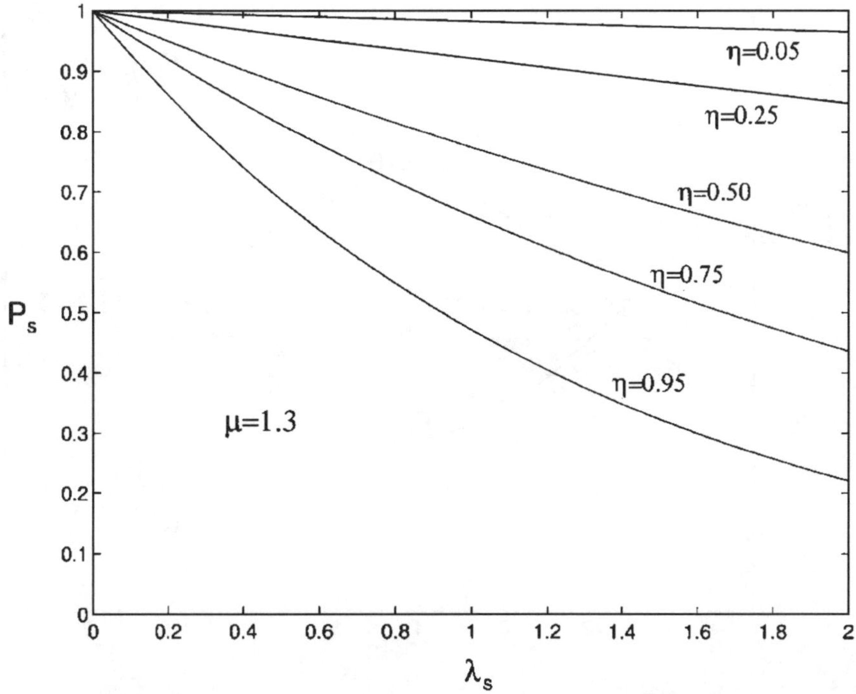

Fig. 8 Value of the imperfect information game without bias.

$(Z = 0, \theta = \theta_s)$ is reached. In this case the maneuver direction of the TBM is by definition optimal and the probability of successful interception avoidance $\boldsymbol{P}_s$ is the function of the engagement parameters μ, η, and λ. This probability is plotted for $\mu = 1.3$ in Fig. 8 as a function of $\lambda_s \triangleq \lambda\, \theta_s(\mu)$. From this figure two important conclusions can be drawn.

1) The interest of the TBM is to use a λ_s as small as possible. Because practical considerations eliminate $\lambda_s = 0$ (a constant maneuver), a limit value of $(\lambda_s)_{\min}$ has to be established.

2) The probability of a defense failure with a deterministic guidance law is unacceptably large, in spite of the inherent information advantage, even for high values of $\eta < 1$.

The probability of a defense failure can be reduced by using a bias either in the initial launch direction or/and in the guidance law, as already indicated. If $0.5 < \eta < 1$, then it is easy to find a bias that guarantees that every second TBM will be intercepted and destroyed, or that two interceptors fired against the same TBM with different biases guarantee the protection of a defended site. Not being able to measure (or estimate) the accelerations of the TBM, the bias must be selected by random guessing. The objective of the bias in the guidance law is to achieve a successful interception with certainty if the TBM maneuvers in the correctly assumed direction, and to maximize its probability even if a direction change occurs.

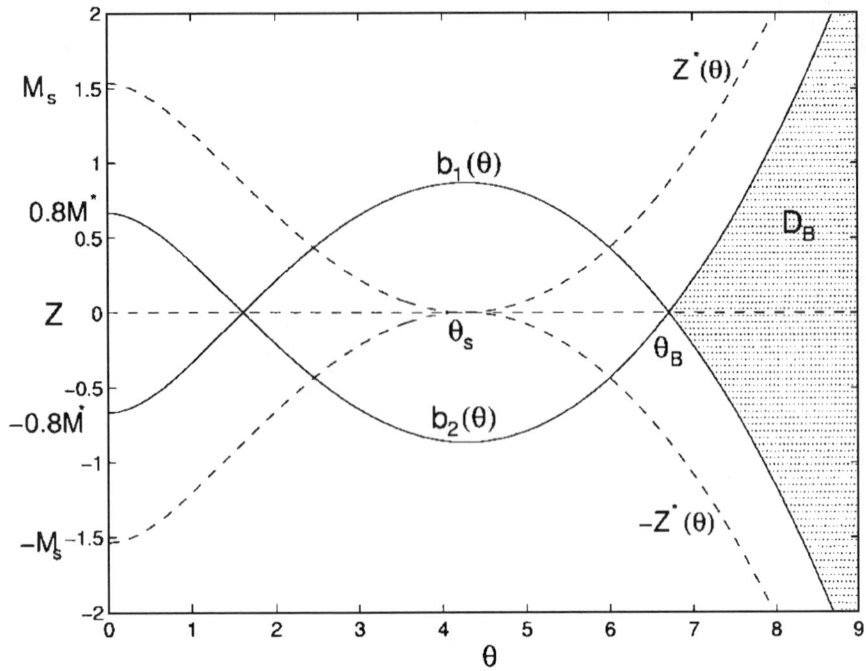

Fig. 9 Biased switching lines $b_1(\theta)$ and $b_2(\theta)$ in the imperfect information game.

By selecting the following time-varying bias[14]

$$Z^b(\theta) = \pm [|Z_+^*(\theta) - 0.8M_1|] \tag{40}$$

two biased switch lines, parallel to the boundaries of the minimal tube, are obtained. They intersect each other twice on the θ axis as can be seen in Fig. 9. The last time to select the sign of the bias is $\theta_B > \theta_s$. The ratio θ_B/θ_s can be computed as the function of η and μ. The existence of two biases of opposite sign requires defining two probability functions:

$\boldsymbol{P}(Z, \Theta) \triangleq$ the probability of interception avoidance if the direction of the TBM maneuver is such that the bias is incorrect

$\boldsymbol{Q}(Z, \Theta) \triangleq$ the probability of interception avoidance if the direction of the TBM maneuver is such that the bias is correct

Note that the values of $\boldsymbol{P}^b(Z, \theta) \triangleq \boldsymbol{P}(Z = 0, \theta_B)$ and $\boldsymbol{Q}^b \triangleq \boldsymbol{Q}(Z = 0, \theta_B)$ are not equal to each other ($\boldsymbol{P}^b > \boldsymbol{Q}^b$). If the bias is guessed randomly, the probability of interception avoidance is $[\boldsymbol{P}^b + \boldsymbol{Q}^b]/2$.

If the defense system can estimate the direction of the lateral accelerations of the TBM, a better result can be expected. If this information is obtained before θ_B, the interceptor can determine the direction of the correct bias and reduce the probability of interception avoidance to $\boldsymbol{Q}^b$. Assuming an ideal estimation, the value of $\boldsymbol{Q}^b$ is plotted in Fig. 10. It can be seen that for a given η, there exists a value of $\lambda_s = \lambda_s^*$ that maximizes $\boldsymbol{Q}^b$.

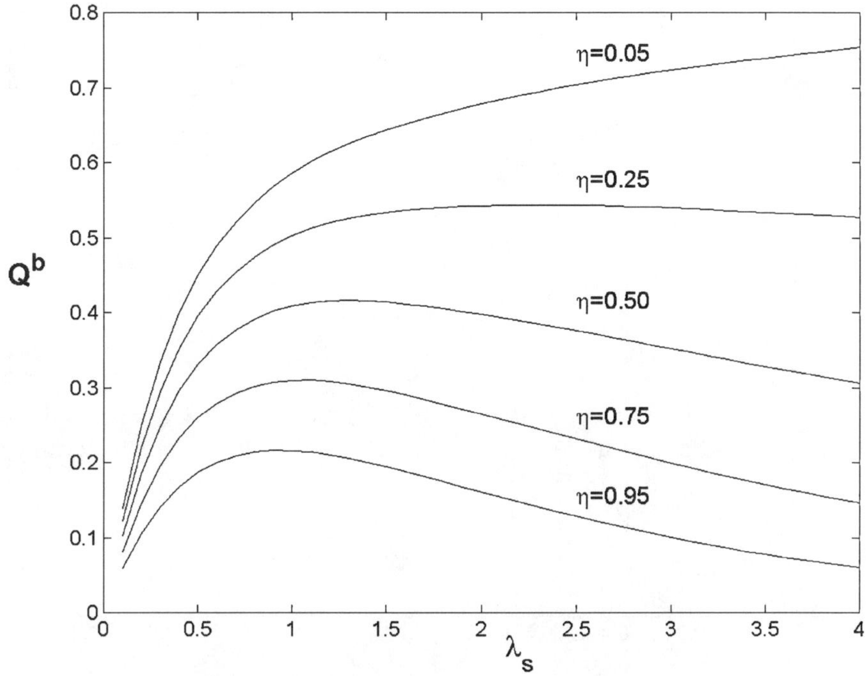

Fig. 10 Q^b **as a function of** λ_s **and** η **for** $\mu = 1.3$.

Unfortunately, the estimation of the target acceleration is never instantaneous. Any delay in identifying the correct direction of the target acceleration (because of the finite convergence time of the estimator) increases the probability of interception avoidance, though it always will remain lower than in the case of a random guess. In any case, the longer the estimation delay, the smaller is the (optimal) value of λ_s^*. This can be seen on Fig. 11 plotted for $\eta = 0.5$. In a set of numerical examples, worked out with $\mu = 1.3$ and $\eta = 0.54$ and summarized in Table 1, the following results were obtained.

This stochastic analysis has demonstrated the importance of having a warhead of substantial lethal radius (not relying on a direct hit) if highly maneuverable TBMs have to be intercepted and destroyed. Moreover, the need for an improved guidance law that guarantees very small miss distances has been reemphasized.

Table 1 Summary of numerical examples

Guidance strategy	Avoidance probability	Optimal λ_s
No bias	$\boldsymbol{P}_s = 0.92$	$\lambda_s^* = (\lambda_s)_{\min} = 0.3$
Random bias (no estimation)	$(\boldsymbol{P}^b + \boldsymbol{Q}^b)/2 = 0.48$	$\lambda_s^* = (\lambda_s)_{\min} = 0.3$
Correct bias (ideal estimation, $\Delta\theta_{\text{est}} = 0$)	$\boldsymbol{Q}^b = 0.39$	$1.0 < \lambda_s^* < 1.5$
Correct bias (estimation delay, $\Delta\theta_{\text{est}} = 5\theta_s$)	$\boldsymbol{Q}^b = 0.46$	$\lambda_s^* = 0.6$

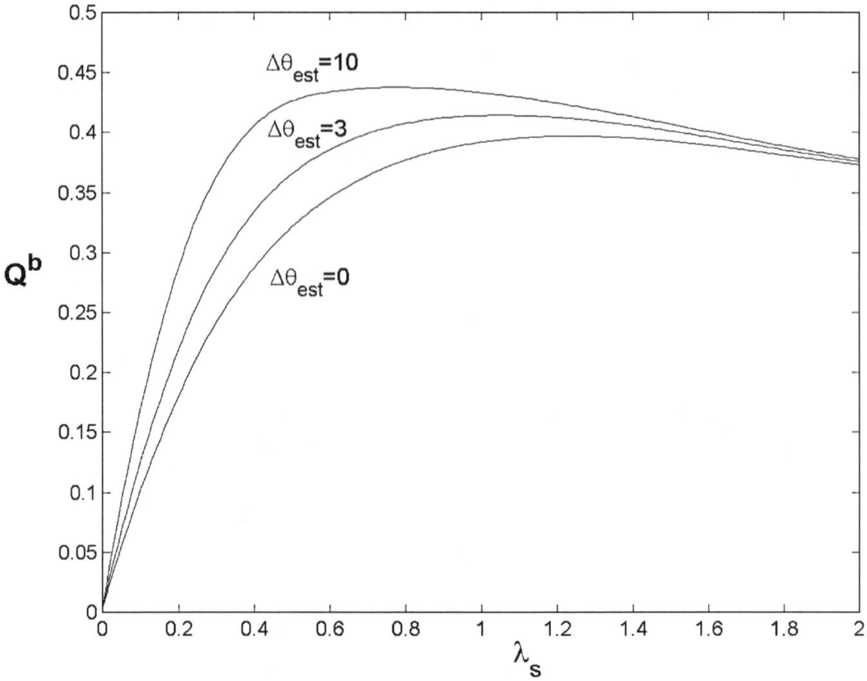

Fig. 11 Effect of estimation delay on $Q^b(\eta = 0.5, \mu = 1.3)$.

IV. Simulation Results

A. General Outline

Because a realistic interception environment is different from the simplified models used for analysis, it has been of common practice to evaluate guided missile performance by extensive simulations. The multiyear investigation performed at the Faculty of Aerospace Engineering in the Technion also included several simulation studies. Their results are summarized in this section. The earlier simulations were based on three-dimensional nonlinear kinematics, point-mass vehicle models with simplified control dynamics, assuming noise-free measurements. These studies concentrated on comparing guidance law performance against different TBM maneuvers expected in the future. The effect of noise corrupted measurements, requiring an estimator in the guidance system, were tested later in linearized two-dimensional Monte Carlo simulations.

B. First Simulations (1992–1996)

In the first simulation study, the interception of a high-speed reentering TBM with structural asymmetries was investigated.[12] Because of the asymmetries, high intensity lateral accelerations and roll rates were developed generating a barrel roll type of trajectory. Both the maneuverability and the roll rate varied during the reentry. The interceptor was a generic endoatmospheric guided missile of simplified (first order) control dynamics. The study evaluated four different guidance laws: 1) proportional navigation (PN) with effective navigation ratio of $N'=4$; 2) augmented proportional navigation (APN)[13] with the optimal gain of $N'=3$; 3) a guidance law derived using optimal control theory, assuming constant target lateral acceleration and compensating for own dynamics,[14] denoted as OGL, and 4) a semioptimal guidance law, similar to OGL, but without considering target maneuvers, denoted as SGL.

The conclusions drawn from the simulation results have shown that neither PN nor APN are adequate to intercept a maneuvering reentry vehicle. SGL does much better, but needs a very high maneuverability advantage ($\mu > 4$) to obtain small miss distances. OGL could achieve a similar performance with $\mu > 1.7$, if the assumption of noise-free measurements (or ideal estimation) were valid. Because it has been well known that such conditions are not realistic, the bottom line of this simulation study was, "Currently available guidance laws and estimation techniques are unable to guarantee a "hit-to-kill" accuracy in the interception of highly maneuvering tactical ballistic missiles expected in the future."[12]

In subsequent simulations[15] the guidance laws DGL/0 and DGL/1, derived from a differential game formulation, were also included in the evaluation. The results clearly confirmed the earlier conclusions of Anderson[8]: "Guidance laws derived using pursuit–evasion game concepts provide a better and more robust homing accuracy than guidance laws based on an optimal control."

It has to be pointed out that this first phase of simulation had merely an exploratory nature. The barrel roll type of TBM maneuvers, although successful in generating substantial miss distances, are nonoptimal. In spite of that, the main conclusions of the study have remained valid.

C. Comparison to Linear Analysis

The next phase of extensive simulations[16,17] was aimed to answer the following questions.

1) Are the conclusions of previous studies, derived on the basis of a simplified mathematical model, valid for the real world problem of intercepting highly maneuvering reentry vehicles expected in the future?

2) To what extent can linear guidance theory be used to predict the guaranteed miss distance in an actual real-world engagement between a guided missile and its highly maneuverable target?

In this new simulation study it was assumed that the reentry vehicle performs a random bang-bang type of maneuver using maximum available lateral acceleration, the optimal structure predicted by the game analysis. The study concentrated to identify the maximum miss distance generated by such evasive maneuvers by varying the (random) time between the direction change (switch) of the maneuver and the time of closest approach. As in the earlier simulations, several guidance laws were compared. This comparison clearly demonstrated the superiority of DGL/1 over all the others, as expected. In these simulations the implementation of OGL and DGL/1 included an information delay on the target maneuver as one of the parameters. The results indicated that the information delay caused a serious homing performance degradation of these guidance laws.

This study created an enhanced understanding "how key parameters in the models of the scenario affect the outcome of an engagement between a guided missile and a highly maneuvering target." At the same time it also indicated the limitations of the existing and currently used linear guidance theory. The sensitivity trends of the guaranteed miss distance with respect to the parameters of the interception in a realistic environment were found to be similar (although not identical) to the trends predicted by a linear model. In spite of the similarity in trends, it was realized that current linear guidance theory cannot predict accurately the miss distance in an actual real-world missile/target engagement. The main reason for this deficiency has been identified as the assumptions of the linearized model on constant velocities and constant lateral acceleration bounds. In this scenario the effects of nonlinear kinematics seemed to be secondary.

D. Simulation with Noisy Measurements

Guidance law implementation with noise corrupted measurements was studied by a set of Monte Carlo simulations, including a Kalman filter type of estimator in the guidance loop. Such an implementation, which has been the common practice in the missile guidance community, is based on the (unjustified) application of the certainty equivalence principle, proven to be valid for linear problems with unbounded control, quadratic cost and Gaussian noise. These simulations were carried out, for the sake of simplicity, using a planar linearized model of the interception end-game, as described by Eqs. (4–9).

Testing the homing performance of the guidance law implementation in a noisy environment yielded disappointing results. Simulation results indicated that the largest error source is the inherent delay in estimating the target acceleration, used in some of the guidance laws, such as OGL and DGL/1. It is of common experience that even if the accuracy and the convergence of a position estimate are satisfactory, the estimated acceleration is less precise and it converges much more slowly.

State variable estimation from noisy measurements for the implementation of perfect information guidance laws creates two types of errors: a (converged) steady-state estimation error and a (dynamic) delay. Because of the measurement noise, the estimated state is never the actual one. If the actual state variables are constant or vary slowly, the estimation error converges to a rather small value. The Kalman filter has the role of minimizing the root mean square average of this estimation error. However, if there is a sudden change in one of the variables, the estimation error of this variable becomes large and it may take a substantial time until the estimated state converges to its new value. This phenomenon can be clearly observed in Fig. 12. Because this dynamic effect seems to be dominant, the entire estimation process was roughly approximated by a simplified model, where the only imperfection is a pure time-delay Δt_{est} in the (otherwise ideal) measurement of the target acceleration. This model allows a deterministic analysis,[22] creating a preliminary insight on the performance degradation caused by noisy measurements.

The analysis of the estimation delay's effect was focused on DGL/1, which seemed to be an excellent guidance law in a noise-free environment. Because of the estimation delay the maneuvering evader can generate a nonzero miss distance even if $\mu\varepsilon \geq 1$, because DGL/1 is the optimal guidance law *only* for the perfect information game ($\Delta t_{\mathrm{est}} = 0$). For each value of $\Delta t_{\mathrm{est}} > 0$, there exists an optimal evader maneuver that maximizes the miss distance. This maneuver consists of an optimally timed direction change (switch) of the maximal lateral acceleration command (from left to right, or vice versa), as already used in earlier simulations.

In Fig. 13 the maximum normalized miss distance generated by the evader is plotted as a function of the normalized estimation delay ($\Delta\theta_{\mathrm{est}} = \Delta t_{\mathrm{est}}/\tau_P$) for

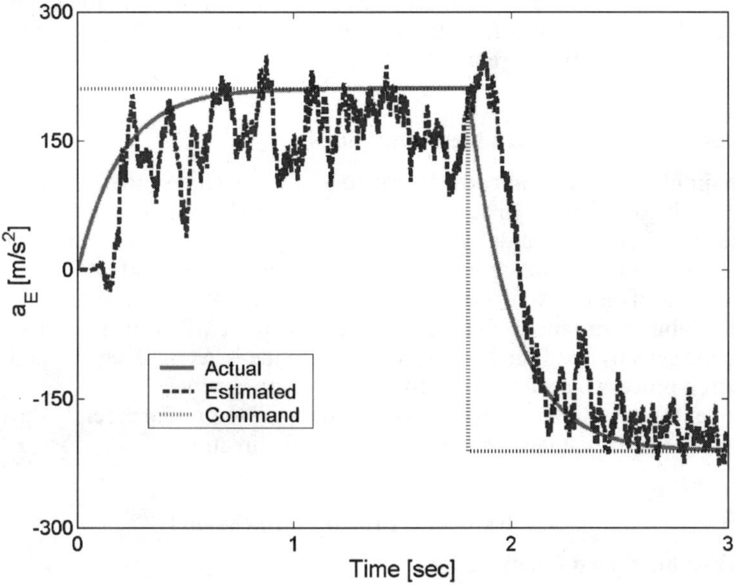

Fig. 12 Estimator performance.

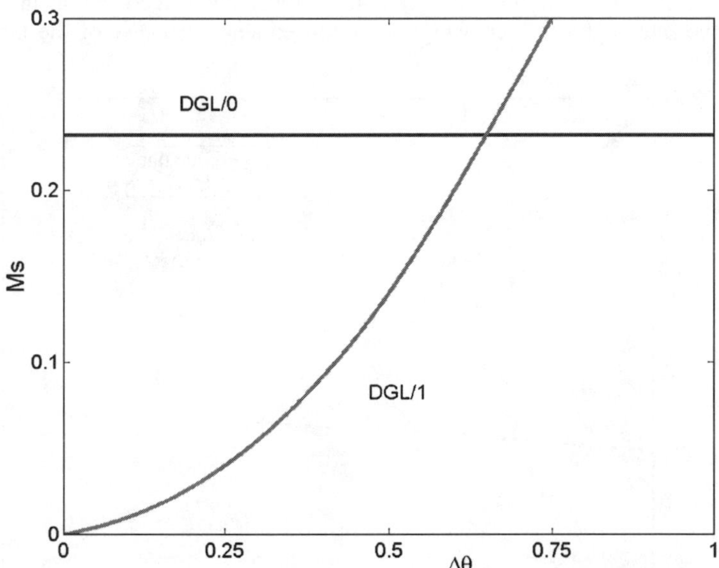

Fig. 13 Maximum normalized miss distance as a function of normalized estimation delay.

an example with $\mu = 2.25$ and $\varepsilon = 1$. The devastating performance degradation caused by the estimation delay is clearly observed. If the estimation delay is too long, it is better not to incorporate the target acceleration in the guidance law at all, i.e., to use DGL/0, where $\varepsilon = 0$ is assumed.

E. Lessons Learned from the Simulations

The simulation studies already described lead to conclude[23] that a new guidance law has to be developed. To achieve the satisfactory homing performance, which is needed for an effective defense against highly maneuverable reentry vehicles expected in the future, this guidance law must have two important features. 1) It has to be based on an extended linear model, which takes into account speed and maneuverability variations that occur in a realistic TMD scenario. 2) It has to reduce the sensitivity of the homing accuracy to the inherent delay created by the estimation process based on noise corrupted measurements.

The next two sections of this chapter are devoted to present recently developed concepts for guidance law improvements in both directions.

V. Extended Linear Game Model

A. Variable Speed Formulation

In the simulations described in Sec. III.B and III.C, the interception end-game took place between 16 and 28 km of altitude. Typical velocity profiles of the TBM and the interceptor are shown in Fig. 14. It can be seen that during the end-game the speed of the TBM remains almost unchanged, while the velocity of the interceptor is increasing. As a consequence, because of the larger air

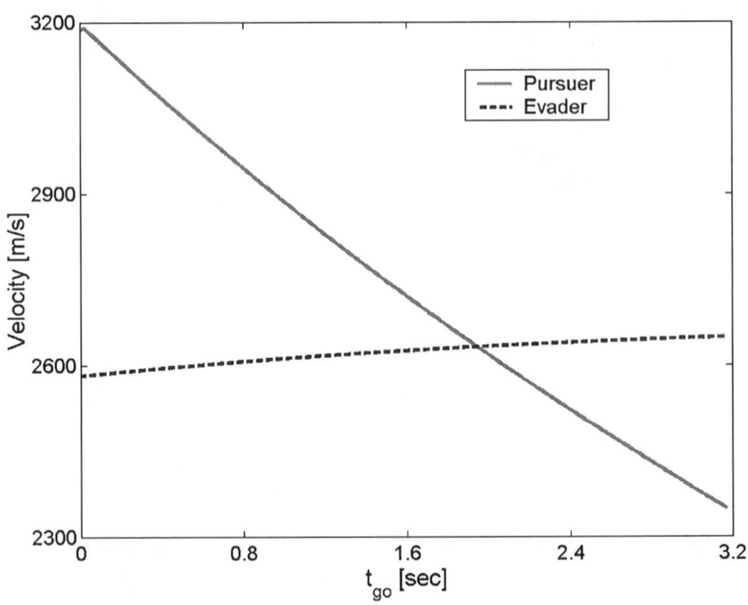

Fig. 14 End-game velocity/altitude profiles.

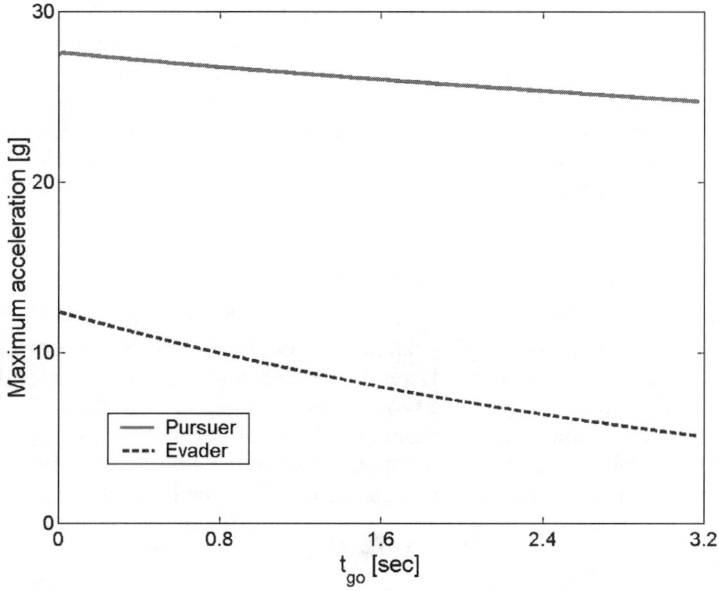

Fig. 15 Time histories of end-game maneuverability.

density in the lower altitudes, the maneuverability of the TBM is monotonically increasing.

The design of the generic interceptor (carried out by a group of students after the Persian Gulf War) has been aimed to keep the maneuverability in the end-game almost constant in spite of the increasing altitude and the resulting lower air density. The maneuverability profiles of both missiles are depicted in Fig. 15.

In such a scenario, assumption 3 of Sec. II is not valid. To use a more realistic model of the end-game this assumption has to be replaced by the following: The velocity and the maximum lateral acceleration of each missile on a nominal trajectory are known functions of the respective altitudes and can be expressed as the function of time.

For this time-varying model the vector of the state variables has to be enlarged:

$$\boldsymbol{X}^T = (x_1, x_2, x_3, x_4, x_5, x_6) = \left(y, \frac{\mathrm{d}y}{\mathrm{d}t}, \boldsymbol{a}_P, \boldsymbol{a}_E, \phi_P, \phi_E\right) \tag{41}$$

Thus, the original equations of motion (4), (6), and (7) remain valid, but Eq. (5) has to be rewritten as

$$\frac{\mathrm{d}x_2}{\mathrm{d}t} = x_4 - x_3 + \boldsymbol{a}_{xE}(t)x_6 - \boldsymbol{a}_{xP}(t)x_5; \qquad x_2(0) = V_{E_0}x_{6_0} - V_{P_0}x_{5_0} \tag{42}$$

where $\boldsymbol{a}_{xP}(t)$ and $\boldsymbol{a}_{xE}(t)$ are the respective longitudinal accelerations of the missiles, derived from the known velocity profiles.

Moreover, there are two new differential equations for x_5 and x_6.

$$\frac{\mathrm{d}x_5}{\mathrm{d}t} = x_4/V_p(t); \qquad x_{5_0} = \phi_{P_0} \tag{43}$$

$$\frac{\mathrm{d}x_6}{\mathrm{d}t} = x_3/V_E(t); \qquad x_{6_0} = \phi_{E_0} \tag{44}$$

Because the set of equations (4), (29), (6), (7), (30), and (31) can be cast in a vector form of Eq. (10), the structure of the game solution will be similar to the structure presented in Fig. 2. Of course, the transition matrix $\Phi(t_f, t)$ and the expression of the zero-effort miss distance are different. Moreover, the parameters of the solution θ_s and M_s strongly depend on the time varying velocity and maneuverability functions. This dependence is illustrated with two simple examples that were presented in a conference paper.[24]

B. Time-Varying Evader Maneuverability

As the first example an interception scenario with constant velocities ($\boldsymbol{a}_{xE} = \boldsymbol{a}_{xP} = 0$) but with a time-varying lateral acceleration bound is examined. Therefore, in this example Eqs. (42–44) are not needed, and the expression of the normalized zero-effort miss distance remains as it is stated in Eq. (18). For sake of simplicity it is assumed that the maneuverability of the pursuer $(\boldsymbol{a}_P)_{\max}$ remains constant and only the lateral acceleration bound of the evader varies in time. The data of Fig. 15 suggest that a linear approximation in the form of

$$(\boldsymbol{a}_E)_{\max}(t) = (\boldsymbol{a}_E)_{\max}(t_f)[1 - \beta(t_{go})/\tau_P] \tag{45}$$

where β is nondimensional constant, is appropriate.

In this case the nondimensional form of Eq. (A18) with respect to the normalized time-to-go θ is

$$\Gamma^\beta(\theta, \mu_f, \varepsilon) = \mu_f \psi(\theta) - \varepsilon\, \psi(\theta/\varepsilon)(1 - \beta\theta) \tag{46}$$

The nonvanishing solution of the equation $\Gamma^\beta(\theta, \mu_f, \varepsilon) = 0$ (if exists) provides the value of $\theta_s^\beta(\mu_f, \varepsilon, \beta) > 0$ and the normalized value of the game in the region D_0 is

$$M_s^\beta = \int_0^{\theta_s^\beta} \Gamma^\beta(\theta)\, \mathrm{d}\theta = M_s^\beta(\mu_f, \varepsilon, \beta) \tag{47}$$

In Fig. 16 the dependence of M_s^β on β and ε is depicted for $\mu_f = 1.285$.

For the case of constant μ, presented in Sec. II, the equation $\Gamma(\theta, \mu, \varepsilon) = 0$ does not have a nonvanishing solution for θ, if $\mu\varepsilon \geq 1$. It means that for these cases the value of the game in D_0 is zero (with the practical significance of a robust "direct hit" homing accuracy). Those values of μ_f having this property are depicted in Fig. 17 as a function of β for $\varepsilon = 0.5$. These analytical results provide an improved predictability of the miss distances in scenarios with time-varying maneuverability. This property was demonstrated by comparison to simulation results[17] presented in Table 2. Fixed parameters of the simulations were: $t_f = 3$ s, $(\boldsymbol{a}_P)_{\max} = 27.5\ g$, $\beta = 0.038$.

C. Time-Varying Pursuer Velocity

The next example is the end-game of an interception scenario with an accelerating interceptor $[\boldsymbol{a}_{xP}(t) > 0]$ against a constant speed reentering TBM $[\boldsymbol{a}_{xE}(t) = 0]$. Assuming constant interceptor acceleration $\boldsymbol{a}_{xP}(t) = \boldsymbol{a}_{xP}$, as suggested by Fig. 14,

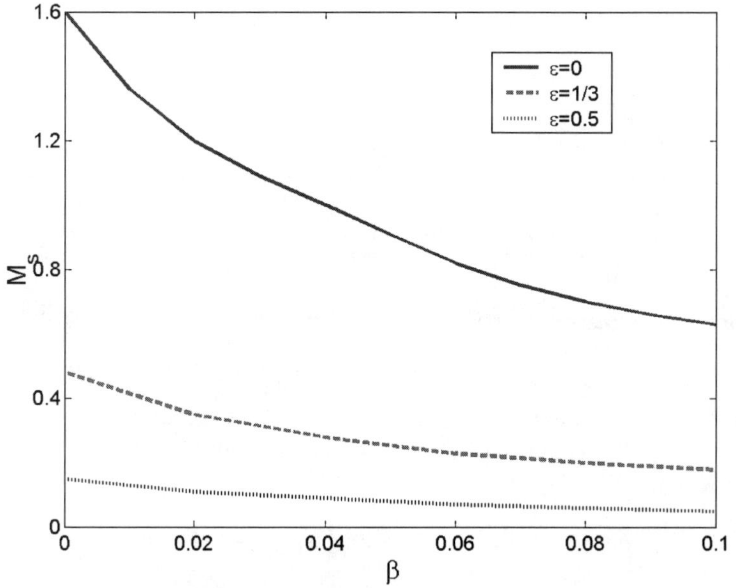

Fig. 16 Normalized guaranteed miss distance as a function of $\beta(\mu_f = 1.285)$.

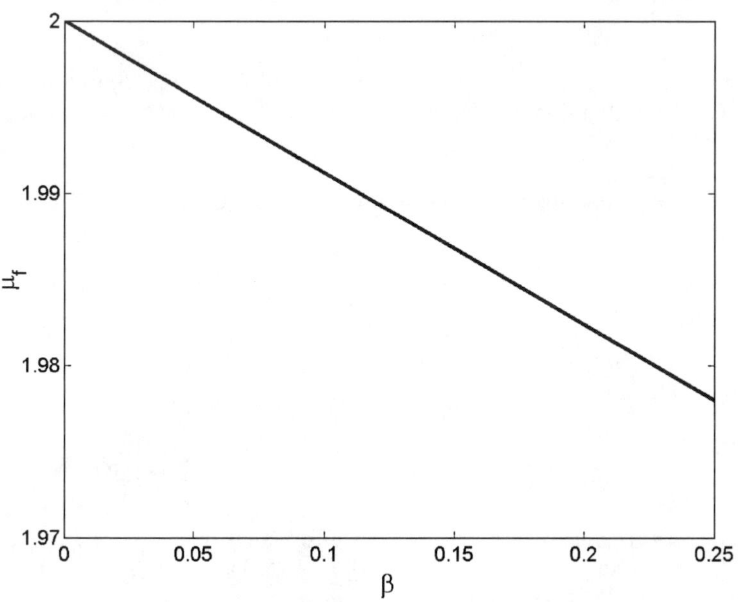

Fig. 17 The value of μ_f required for zero miss distance.

Table 2 Prediction comparison

τ_E, s	τ_P, s	$(\boldsymbol{a}_E)_{max}$, g	Guidance law	RS,[a] m	PL,[b] m	PE,[c] m
0.2	0.2	21.5	DGL/0	7.2	13.5	8.3
0.2	0.2	18.4	DGL/0	3.9	5.8	4.3
0.01	0.3	21.5	DGL/1	22.9	28.5	17.5
0.01	0.4	21.5	DGL/1	30.3	51.3	31.7

[a]RS = maximum miss distance in realistic simulation.
[b]PL = prediction of the original linear model.
[c]PE = prediction of the extended linear model.

the pursuer's velocity is a linear function of the time (or the time-to-go):

$$V_P(t) = V_{P_0} + \boldsymbol{a}_{xP}t = V_{P_f} - \boldsymbol{a}_{xP}(t_{go}) \tag{48}$$

For the sake of simplicity the maneuverability of both missiles assumed to be constant. Therefore, μ the pursuer/evader maneuverability ratio is a fixed parameter. The vector of the state variables in this case has five components:

$$X^T = (x_1, x_2, x_3, x_4, x_5) = \left(y, \frac{\mathrm{d}y}{\mathrm{d}t}, \boldsymbol{a}_P, \boldsymbol{a}_E, \phi_P,\right) \tag{49}$$

The relevant equations of motion are (4), (6), and (7), the rewritten form of Eq. (5)

$$\frac{\mathrm{d}x_2}{\mathrm{d}t} = x_4 - x_3 - \boldsymbol{a}_{xP}(t)x_5; \qquad x_2(0) = V_{E_0}\phi_{E_0} - V_{P_0}x_{5_0} \tag{50}$$

and Eq. (43).

Applying the transformation of the "terminal projection" (16) to this dynamic system a new expression of the normalized zero-effort miss distance is obtained:

$$Z^\alpha = Z^1 + \Delta Z^\alpha \tag{51}$$

where Z^1 is the normalized zero-effort miss distance for the constant speed model (18) and

$$\Delta Z^\alpha = -\alpha\left[I_3(\theta)x_3 + 0.5\theta^2 V_{P_f}x_5/\tau_P\right]/(\boldsymbol{a}_E)_{max} \tag{52}$$

where

$$\alpha = \boldsymbol{a}_{xP}\tau_P/\mathrm{V}_{P_f} \tag{53}$$

and

$$I_3(\theta) = \int_0^\theta \left\{\int_0^\theta \left\{\int_0^\theta [e^{-\theta}/(1-\alpha\theta)]\,\mathrm{d}\theta\right\}\mathrm{d}\theta\right\}\mathrm{d}\theta \tag{54}$$

The state variables that effect the zero-effort miss distance are $x_3 = \boldsymbol{a}_P$ and $x_5 = \phi_P$ only. Using the new definitions of Eqs. (53) and (54) the nondimensional expression of (A18) becomes for the present case

$$\Gamma^\alpha(\theta, \mu, \varepsilon) = \Gamma^1(\theta, \mu, \varepsilon) - \mu\alpha I_3(\theta) \tag{55}$$

where $\Gamma^1(\theta, \mu, \varepsilon)$ is the term for the constant speed model given in Eq. (26).

The nonvanishing solution of the equation $\Gamma^\alpha(\theta, \mu, \varepsilon) = 0$ provides $\theta_s^\alpha(\mu, \varepsilon, \alpha) > 0$ and the normalized value of the game in the region D_0 is

$$M_s^\alpha = \int_0^{\theta_s^\alpha} \Gamma^\alpha(\theta)\, d\theta = M_s^\alpha(\mu, \varepsilon, \alpha) \tag{56}$$

For $\alpha > 0$ the value of $\theta_s^\alpha(\mu, \varepsilon, \alpha)$ is smaller than $\theta_s(\mu, \varepsilon)$ and as the consequence $M_s^\alpha(\mu, \varepsilon, \alpha)$ will also be smaller than $M_s(\mu, \varepsilon)$. However, the main importance of the extended mode is a modified guidance law resulting from the modified normalized zero-effort miss distance

$$\boldsymbol{u}^* = \text{sign}\{Z^\alpha\} \tag{57}$$

Only by using this guidance law (an optimal strategy of the game in the entire game space and the unique one in D_1) it is guaranteed that the normalized miss distance will not be larger, whatever maneuver the TBM will perform, than the value predicted by Eq. (56). The effect of α, the normalized acceleration parameter defined by Eq. (53), on the guaranteed normalized miss distance is shown in Fig. 18 for two pairs of μ and ε.

The contribution of the previously outlined extended linear model is twofold. It leads to a modified guidance law (57) with a better homing accuracy and provides an improved capability to predict the miss distances expected in scenarios with time-varying interceptor velocities. These favorable features have been demonstrated by comparison to simulation outcomes[24] and examples are presented in Table 3. The constant parameters in the nonlinear, realistic, simulations were: $t_f = 3$ s, $(\boldsymbol{a}_P)_{\max} = 27.5\,g$, $(\boldsymbol{a}_E)_{\max} = 21.5\,g$, $\tau_E = 0.1$ s, $\tau_P = 0.1$ s, $V_{P_f} = 3150$ m/s, $\alpha = 0.016$.

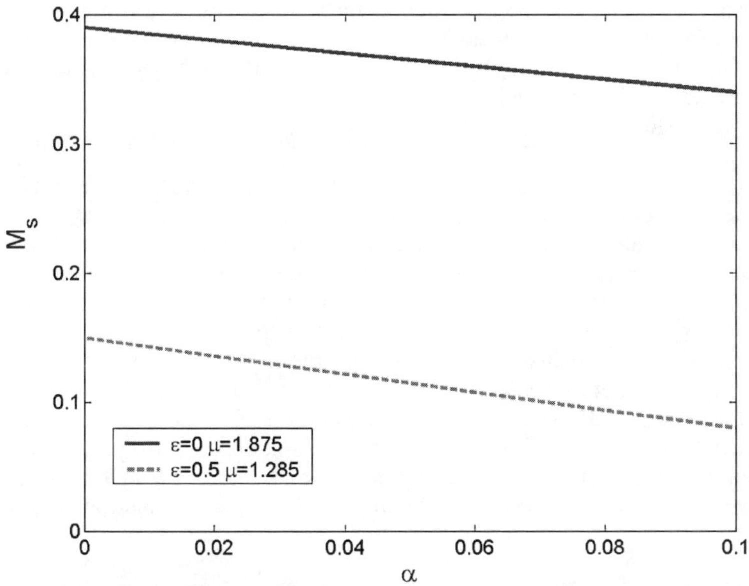

Fig. 18 Normalized guaranteed miss distance as a function of α.

Table 3 Maximum miss distance comparison, m

Evader model	Original guidance law, $\Delta Z^{\alpha} = 0$	Modified guidance law, $\Delta Z^{\alpha} \neq 0$
DGL/0	10.2	9.1
DGL/1	4.1	2.9

VI. Compensation of Estimation Delay

A. New Problem Formulation

In this section a new guidance law, denoted as DGL/C, is presented. Its objective is to reduce the sensitivity of the homing accuracy to the inherent delay created by the estimation process based on noise-corrupted measurements. By minimizing the effect of the estimation delay, this new guidance law has to provide an improved homing performance compared to both DGL/0 and DGL/1. Because the problem to be solved is a pursuit-evasion game with bounded controls, the classical certainty equivalence principle, which allows using the estimated state variables instead of the actual ones in the deterministic optimal control law, should not be used. Nevertheless, even if the certainty equivalence principle is not valid (as mentioned earlier, its validity was proven for linear quadratic Guassian optimal control problems with unbounded controls), a separate design of the estimator is allowed, but the optimization of the control law has to be based on the probability density function of the estimated state variables.[25] In other words, in the derivation of the guidance law the limitations of the estimation process have to be explicitly taken into account. As the first step in this direction the interception scenario of a maneuvering TBM is reformulated as a delayed information zero-sum pursuit-evasion game.

The reformulated problem can be stated as follows: Given the dynamic system (4–9), minimize the cost function (12), subject to the following set of available measurements of the pursuer

$$h_i(t) = x_i(t); \qquad i = 1, 2, 4; \qquad h_3(t) = x_3(t - \Delta t_{\text{est}}) \tag{58}$$

It is assumed that the evader has perfect information on all the state variables, as well as on the delay of the pursuer. In two recent papers[26,27] an intuitive approach, inspired by the ideas proposed by Petrosjan,[28] was used. It suggests creating, based on the available information at every point of the time, the *reachable set* of the evader, and to aim to the center of the convex hull of this reachable set. Simulation results, based on this intuitive approach demonstrated the substantial reduction of the maximum miss distance and the robustness of the new guidance law with respect to the target maneuver structure as can be seen in Fig. 19. At that time an analytical solution of the problem was not yet available. The guaranteed miss distance could be predicted only by deterministic simulations of the pure delay model of the interception. In the next part of this section a rigorous analytical solution of the delayed information zero-sum pursuit-evasion game formulation is presented.

B. Analytical Solution

The basic idea of the solution has been to replace the original normalized state variable $Z(\theta)$, defined in Eq. (18), by a new one, which is the center of the

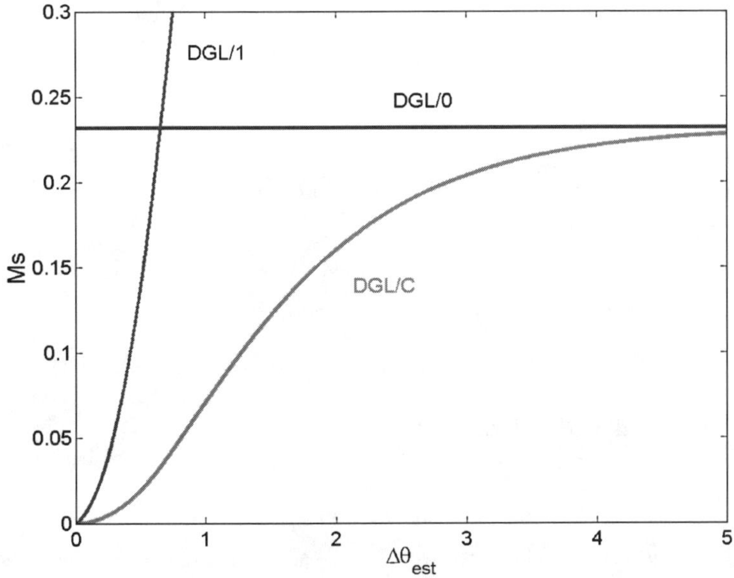

Fig. 19 Guaranteed normalized miss distance as a function of the normalized estimation delay for DGL/0, DGL/1, and DGL/C. μ = 2.25, ε = 1.

normalized uncertainty set (reachable set) created by the information delay. The original $Z(\theta)$ can be rewritten as

$$Z(\theta) = Z^0(\theta) + \Delta Z_E(\theta) \tag{59}$$

where

$$Z^0(\theta) = [x_1(\theta) + x_2(\theta)\theta\tau_P - \Delta Z_P(\theta)]/\tau_P^2(\boldsymbol{a}_E)_{\max} \tag{60}$$

and

$$\Delta Z_P(\theta) = \psi(\theta)x_4(t)/\boldsymbol{a}_E)_{\max} \tag{61}$$

$$\Delta Z_E(\theta) = \varepsilon^2\psi(\theta/\varepsilon)x_3(\theta)/(\boldsymbol{a}_E)_{\max} \tag{62}$$

Because of the delayed measurement $x_3(\theta + \Delta\theta_{\text{est}})$, the uncertain value of $x_3(\theta)$ is bounded by

$$[x_3(\theta)]_{\min} \le x_3(\theta) \le [x_3(\theta)]_{\max} \tag{63}$$

where the extreme values $[x_3(\theta)]_{\min}$ and $[x_3(\theta)]_{\max}$ can be computed by integrating (6) with $(\boldsymbol{a}^c)_E = -(\boldsymbol{a}_E)_{\max}$ and $(\boldsymbol{a}^c)_E = (a_E)_{\max}$ respectively:

$$[x_3(\theta)]_{\min} = x_3(\theta + \Delta\theta_{\text{est}})e^{-\Delta t_{\text{est}}/\tau_?} - (\boldsymbol{a}_E)_{\max}\left(1 - e^{-\Delta t_{\text{est}}/\tau_E}\right) \tag{64}$$

$$[x_3(\theta)]_{\max} = x_3(\theta + \Delta\theta_{\text{est}})e^{-\Delta t_{\text{est}}/\tau_?} + (\boldsymbol{a}_E)_{\max}\left(1 - e^{-\Delta t_{\text{est}}/\tau_E}\right) \tag{65}$$

The center of this "segment of uncertainty" is

$$[x_3(\theta)]^c = \{[x_3(\theta)]_{\max} + [x_3(\theta)]_{\min}\}/2 = x_3(\theta + \Delta\theta_{\text{est}})e^{-\Delta t_{\text{est}}/\tau_E} \tag{66}$$

As a consequence the new variable, replacing $Z(\theta)$, is defined as

$$Z^c(\theta) \triangleq Z^0(\theta) + \Delta Z^c_E(\theta) \tag{67}$$

where

$$\Delta Z^c_E(\theta) = \left[\varepsilon^2 \psi(\theta/\tau_E)\, x_3(\theta + \Delta\theta_{\text{est}}) e^{-\Delta t_{\text{est}}/\tau_E}\right] / (\boldsymbol{a}_E)_{\max} \tag{68}$$

Comparing Eqs. (59–62) with Eqs. (67) and (68), one obtains the relationship between the new state variable $Z^c(\theta)$ and the original one $Z(\theta)$:

$$Z^c(\theta) = Z(\theta) + \varepsilon^2 \psi(\theta/\varepsilon)\left[x_3(\theta + \Delta\theta_{\text{est}}) e^{-\Delta\theta_{\text{est}}/\varepsilon} - x_3(\theta)\right] / \boldsymbol{a}_E^{\max} \tag{69}$$

The derivative of $Z^c(\theta)$ with respect to θ is

$$\frac{\mathrm{d}Z^c}{\mathrm{d}\theta} = \frac{\mathrm{d}Z}{\mathrm{d}\theta} + \left(\varepsilon^2/\boldsymbol{a}_E^{\max}\right)\left\{\mathrm{d}\psi(\theta/\varepsilon)/\mathrm{d}\theta\left[x_3(\theta + \Delta\theta_{\text{est}}) e^{-\Delta\theta_{\text{est}}/\varepsilon} - x_3(\theta)\right]\right.$$
$$\left. + \psi(\theta/\varepsilon)\,\mathrm{d}\left[x_3(\theta + \Delta\theta_{\text{est}}) e^{-\Delta\theta_{\text{est}}/\varepsilon} - x_3(\theta)\right]/\mathrm{d}\theta\right\} \tag{70}$$

where

$$\mathrm{d}\psi(\theta/\varepsilon)/\mathrm{d}\theta = 1/\varepsilon\left(1 - e^{-\theta/\varepsilon}\right) \tag{71}$$

By integrating Eq. (6) between $(\theta + \Delta\theta_{\text{est}})$ and θ, using Eq. (8), one gets

$$\left[x_3(\theta + \Delta\theta_{\text{est}}) e^{-\Delta\theta_{\text{est}}/\varepsilon} - x_3(\theta)\right] = \left(\boldsymbol{a}_E^{\max}\right)/\varepsilon \int_{\theta+\Delta\theta_{\text{est}}}^{\theta} e^{(\theta-\sigma)/\varepsilon} \boldsymbol{v}(\sigma)\,\mathrm{d}\sigma \tag{72}$$

with $\sigma = (t_f - s)/\tau_P$. Consequently,

$$\mathrm{d}\left[x_3(\theta + \Delta\theta_{\text{est}}) e^{-\Delta\theta_{\text{est}}/\varepsilon} - x_3(\theta)\right]/\mathrm{d}\theta = \left(\boldsymbol{a}_E^{\max}\right)/\varepsilon^2 \left\{\varepsilon[\boldsymbol{v}(\theta) - e^{-\Delta\theta_{\text{est}}/\varepsilon} \boldsymbol{v}(\theta + \Delta\theta_{\text{est}})]\right.$$
$$\left. + \int_{\theta+\Delta\theta_{\text{est}}}^{\theta} e^{(\theta-\sigma)/\varepsilon} \boldsymbol{v}(\sigma)\,\mathrm{d}\sigma\right\} \tag{73}$$

Substituting Eqs. (20), (72), and (73), into Eq. (70), and setting $\rho = \sigma - \theta$ leads, after eliminating equal terms, to the expression

$$\frac{\mathrm{d}Z^c}{\mathrm{d}\theta} = \mu\psi(\theta)\,\boldsymbol{u}(\theta) - \varepsilon\psi(\theta/\varepsilon) e^{-\Delta\theta_{\text{est}}/\varepsilon} \boldsymbol{v}(\theta + \Delta\theta_{\text{est}})$$
$$+ (\theta/\varepsilon) \int_{\theta+\Delta\theta_{\text{est}}}^{\theta} e^{(\theta-\sigma)/\varepsilon} \boldsymbol{v}(\theta + \rho)\,\mathrm{d}\rho \tag{74}$$

Because the evader also knows Z^c, Eq. (74) represents the dynamics of a *perfect information game with delayed control*. By observing the definition of Z^c in Eq. (69), and remembering from Eq. (19) that $\psi(\alpha = 0) = 0$, the cost function of this game is identical to the original one in Eq. (22) with the same bounded normalized controls of Eqs. (8) and (9). The methodology leading to the solution of this game, detailed in a recent report[29] and a subsequent paper,[30] is out of the scope of this chapter. Here only the end results are repeated. The elaborate mathematical analysis[29] yields the optimal strategies as

$$\boldsymbol{u}^*(\theta) = \boldsymbol{v}^*(\theta) = \text{sign}\{Z^c(\theta)\}; \qquad Z^c(\theta) \neq 0 \tag{75}$$

reconfirming the validity of the intuitively derived guidance law.[26]

Substituting Eq. (75) into Eq. (74) and carrying out the integration leads to express the optimal game dynamics as

$$\frac{dZ^c}{d\theta} = \Gamma^c(\theta, \Delta\theta_{est})\,\mathrm{sign}\{Z^c(\theta)\} \tag{76}$$

where

$$\Gamma^c(\theta, \Delta\theta_{est}) = \left\{\mu\psi(\theta) - \varepsilon\psi(\theta/\varepsilon)e^{-\Delta\theta_{est}/\varepsilon} + \theta\left[e^{-\Delta\theta_{est}/\varepsilon} - 1\right]\right\} \tag{77}$$

similar to the form of Eq. (24), obtained for the solution of the perfect information games (such as DGL/0 and DGL/1). It means that the decomposition of the normalized game space (Z^c, θ) has the same structure as Fig. 2. Similarly, the coordinate of the "throat" θ_s^c is the nonvanishing solution $(\theta \neq 0)$ of

$$\Gamma^c(\theta, \Delta\theta_{est}) = 0 \tag{78}$$

and M_s^c, the value of the game in D_0 can be computed by integrating $\Gamma^c(\theta, \Delta\theta_{est})$ between $\theta = 0$ and $\theta = \theta_s^c$. By comparing Eqs. (76) and (77) to Eq. (26) one can directly observe that $\theta_s^c > \theta_s$ for all $\Delta\theta_{est} > 0$, and as a consequence $M_s^c > M_s$. It means that because of the estimation delay, the guaranteed miss distance *can never be zero*. The values of θ_s^c and M_s^c are plotted as the function of $(\Delta\theta_{est}/\varepsilon)$ in Figs. 20 and 21, respectively, for $\mu = 2.25$ and $\varepsilon = (0, 0.25, 0.5, 1.0)$.

C. Validation by Monte Carlo Simulations

The homing performance of the new guidance law (DGL/C) in comparison to DGL/0 and DGL/1 was tested by Monte Carlo simulations in an environment of

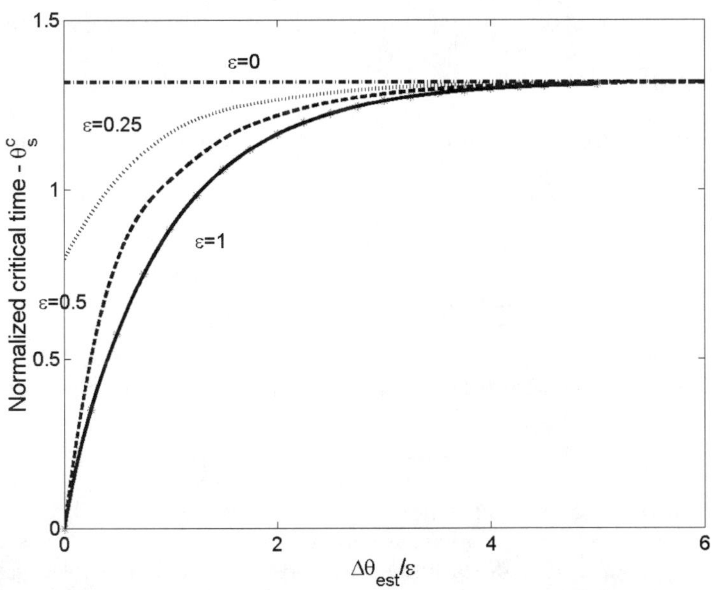

Fig. 20 Critical normalized time-to-go $\theta_s^c(\mu, \varepsilon)$ as a function of $(\Delta\theta_{est}/\varepsilon)$.

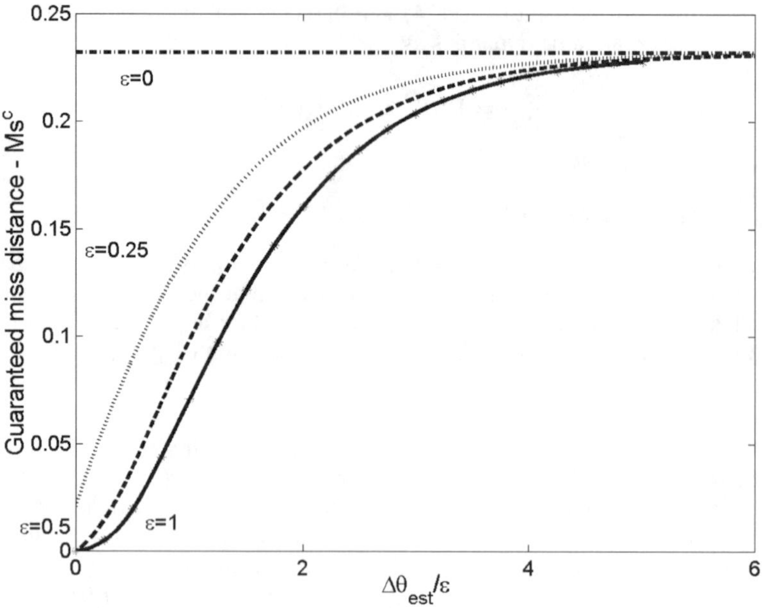

Fig. 21 Guaranteed normalized miss distance $M_s^c(\mu, \varepsilon)$ as a function of $(\Delta\theta_{\text{est}}/\varepsilon)$.

noise-corrupted measurements. The guidance law implementation requires an estimator. The well-known equations of an estimator can be found in the technical literature and therefore are not repeated here. The design of the estimator is based on the dynamic model of Eqs. (4–7). Because the tactical ballistic missile is *blind* with respect to the whereabouts of the interceptor, it must maneuver randomly. It is assumed (as often used in missile guidance analysis[15]) that the evader's maneuver is a stochastic process in the form of a random telegraph (RT) signal, characterized by a single parameter λ (the average frequency of the signal). For the estimator design, such a process is represented by white noise going through a first-order *shaping filter* with a time constant of $1/(2\lambda)$,[15] since both have the same autocorrelation function. It is assumed that the interceptor acquires measurements at a given frequency f. The measurement vector is

$$Y = \begin{bmatrix} 1 & 0 & 0 & 0 \\ 0 & 0 & 0 & 1 \end{bmatrix} \boldsymbol{x} + \begin{bmatrix} R & 0 \\ 0 & 1 \end{bmatrix} \begin{bmatrix} v_1 \\ v_2 \end{bmatrix} \tag{79}$$

where R is the accurately measured range, v_1 is the angular noise of the seeker, and v_2 is the measurement noise of the interceptor's own acceleration. The noise statistics are given by

$$v_i \sim WN\left(0, \sigma_i^2\right) \qquad i = 1, 2 \tag{80}$$

In simulating the implementation of the guidance laws DGL/0, DGL/1, and DGL/C, sets of 100 Monte Carlo runs with different noise samples were used. To allow comparison among the different cases, the same random number generator *seed* has been selected for each set of the 100 Monte Carlo runs. The simulation parameters are given in Table 4.

Table 4 Simulation parameters

Parameter	Description	Value	Remarks
$\boldsymbol{a}_E^{\max}$	Evader's maximal lateral acceleration	21.5 g	
$\boldsymbol{a}_P^{\max}$	Pursuer's maximal lateral acceleration	48.4 g	$\Rightarrow \mu = 2.25$
τ_E	Evader's auto-pilot time constant	0.2 s	
τ_P	Pursuer's auto-pilot time constant	0.2 s	$\Rightarrow \varepsilon = 1$
σ_1	Standard deviation of the angular noise	0.2 mrad	
σ_2	Standard deviation of the acceleration noise	0.1 g	
V_c	Closing velocity ($V_E + V_P$)	5.5 km/s	
R_0	Initial range	16.5 km	$\Rightarrow t_f = 3$ s
Δt	Discrete time step	0.001 s	
f	Measurement frequency	500 Hz	
λ	Assumed average RT frequency	1.5 1/s	

Because the maneuvers of the TBM are expected to be of a randomly switched bang-bang type, the worst maneuver timing (the one that creates the largest miss distance) has to be identified. The accumulated normalized miss distance distributions obtained by the bang-bang maneuvers for DGL/0 and DGL/1 are shown in Figs. 22 and 23, respectively. In Fig. 22 the guaranteed miss distance predicted by the perfect information game solution is also indicated. Note that for DGL/1 this guaranteed miss distance is zero. From these figures the timing of the worst-case maneuvers can also be identified as $\theta_{sw} = 7.5$ for DGL/0 and $\theta_{sw} = 2$ for DGL/1. These results are similar (although not identical) to those obtained with a different estimator and reported in a recent paper.[27]

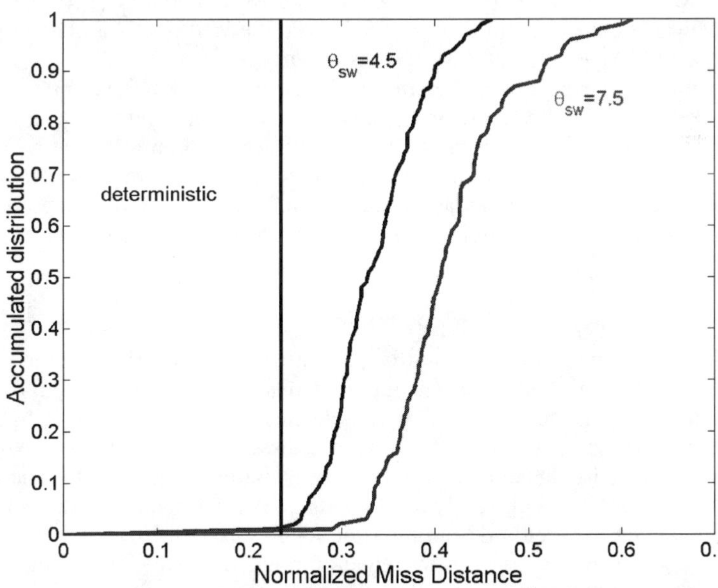

Fig. 22 Accumulated normalized miss distance distributions for DGL/0.

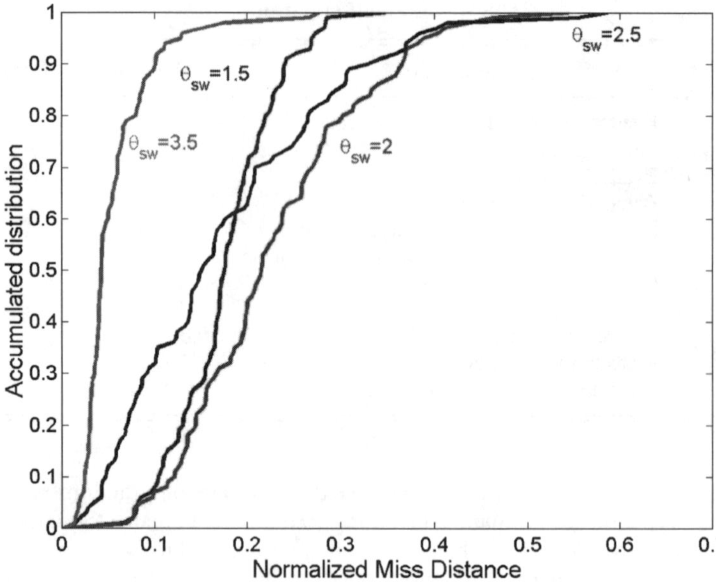

Fig. 23 Accumulated normalized miss distance distributions for DGL/1.

It turns out that the *worst* maneuver timing for DGL/C depends on the value of the assumed estimation delay to be compensated. This observation leads to perform a simultaneous min-max search for the *best* estimation delay and the *worst* timing of the evader maneuver. The accumulated normalized miss distance distribution obtained for the optimal pair (the best estimation delay being $\Delta\theta_{\text{est}} = 0.5$, while the worst evader maneuver timing is $\theta_{sw} = 7.5$) is shown in Fig. 24 and is compared with the worst-case results of the previous two figures.

The simulation results, presented in Fig. 24, clearly confirm the improved homing performance of DGL/C compared with the other guidance laws, as predicted by the deterministic analysis. The maximum miss distance (compared with DGL/1) is reduced to less than half and the entire distribution becomes more favorable. For example, given a normalized lethality radius of 0.2, DGL/C provides a probability of success of about 0.80, compared to a probability of 0.35 for DGL/1.

VII. Concluding Remarks

In this chapter the results of a multiyear investigation motivated by the lessons learned in the Persian Gulf War was reported. The challenging problem of intercepting highly maneuverable reentry vehicles, expected in the future, has been formulated and studied. Deterministic and stochastic analysis, as well as extensive simulations created an understanding of the complexities involved in the challenge. It was demonstrated that currently used guidance and estimation methods are unable to guarantee the required homing accuracy for a satisfactory defense against maneuvering future threats. The investigation pointed out the deficiencies of the currently used methods and outlined avenues of a new nonorthodox approach for guidance law design that represent a potential breakthrough. The elements of an

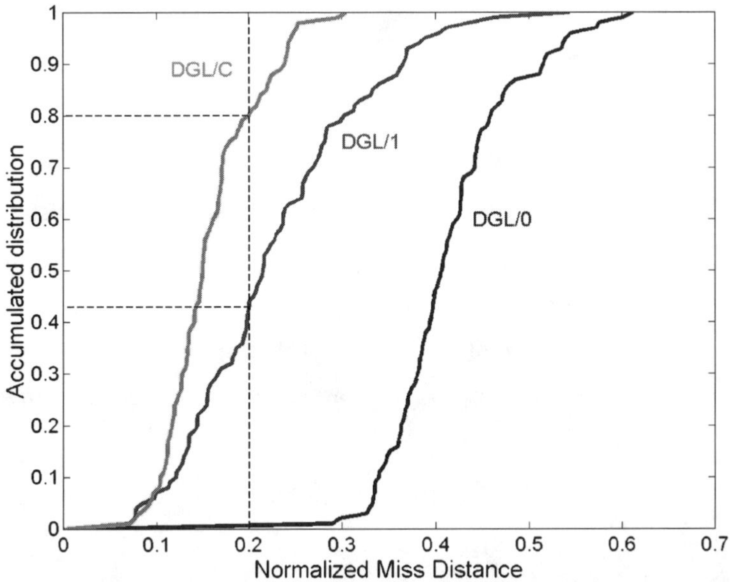

Fig. 24 Accumulated normalized miss distance distributions for DGL/C with the shortest estimation delay and the worst timing of evader maneuver.

innovative mind setting, such as the pursuit–evasion game formulation and abandoning the unjustified application of the certainty equivalence principle, project a hope that small miss distances can be achieved even in very stressing future TMD interception scenarios (where the maneuverability advantage of the interceptor is marginal).

The investigation summarized in this chapter strongly suggests for the designers of the next generation TMD systems to not only use an improved guidance law but also revise two basic design parameters: 1) interceptor end-game maneuverability has to be higher than it is considered in current designs assuming nonmaneuvering threats and 2) the feasibility of a hit-to-kill accuracy against future targets and the eventual need of a warhead have to be reconsidered.

Appendix: Linear Game Solution with Bounded Controls

Consider the class of linear pursuit–evasion games with the dynamics:

$$\frac{\mathrm{d}\boldsymbol{X}}{\mathrm{d}t} = \mathbf{A}(t)\boldsymbol{X} + \mathbf{B}(t)\boldsymbol{u} + \mathbf{C}(t)\boldsymbol{v}; \qquad \boldsymbol{X}(t_0) = \boldsymbol{X}_0$$

$$\boldsymbol{X} \in R^n; \qquad \boldsymbol{u} \in R^1; \qquad \boldsymbol{v} \in R^1 \tag{A1}$$

where $\mathbf{A}(t)$, $\mathbf{B}(t)$, and $\mathbf{C}(t)$ are matrices of appropriate dimensions and the controls are bounded

$$|\boldsymbol{u}| \leq 1; \qquad |\boldsymbol{v}| \leq 1 \tag{A2}$$

Let the cost function of the game be

$$J = |\boldsymbol{D}^T \boldsymbol{X}(t_f)| \tag{A3}$$

where $\boldsymbol{D}^T$ is a raw matrix of the form

$$\boldsymbol{D}^T = (1, 0, 0, 0, \ldots) \tag{A4}$$

and the final time t_f is given. This cost function is to be minimized by $\boldsymbol{u}$ and maximized by $\boldsymbol{v}$.

By using $\Phi(t_f, t)$, the transition matrix of the homogeneous system $\mathrm{d}\boldsymbol{X}/\mathrm{d}t = \mathbf{A}(t)\boldsymbol{X}$, the transformation of "terminal projection"

$$\boldsymbol{Z}(t) = \boldsymbol{D}^T \Phi(t_f, t)\boldsymbol{X}(t) \tag{A5}$$

allows reducing the vector equation (A1) to a scalar dynamic equation in reverse time

$$\frac{\mathrm{d}\boldsymbol{Z}}{\mathrm{d}t_{\mathrm{go}}} = -\{B(t_f, t)\boldsymbol{u} + C(t_f, t)\boldsymbol{v}\} \tag{A6}$$

where

$$B(t_f, t) = \boldsymbol{D}^T \Phi(t_f, t)\, \mathbf{B}(t) \le 0 \tag{A7}$$

and

$$C(t_f, t) = \boldsymbol{D}^T \Phi(t_f, t)\, \mathbf{C}(t) \ge 0 \tag{A8}$$

with the cost function

$$J = |\boldsymbol{Z}(t_f)| \tag{A9}$$

to be minimized by $\boldsymbol{u}$ and maximized by $\boldsymbol{v}$. The signs of $\mathbf{B}(t_f, t)$ and $\mathbf{C}(t_f, t)$ in (A7) and (A8) are the consequence of the pursuit–evasion game formulation.

The variational Hamiltonian of the game is

$$\boldsymbol{H} = \lambda_z[B(t_f, t)\boldsymbol{u} + C(t_f, t)\boldsymbol{v}] \tag{A10}$$

where λ_z is the costate variable, satisfying the adjoint equation

$$\lambda_z = -\frac{\partial \boldsymbol{H}}{\partial \boldsymbol{Z}} = 0 \tag{A11}$$

and the transversality condition

$$\lambda_z(t_f) = \left.\frac{\partial J}{\partial \boldsymbol{Z}}\right|_{t_f} = \mathrm{sign}\{\boldsymbol{Z}(t_f)\} \tag{A12}$$

It means that as long as $\lambda_z(t)$ is continuous

$$\lambda_z(t) = \mathrm{sign}\{\boldsymbol{Z}(t_f)\}; \qquad \boldsymbol{Z}(t_f) \neq 0 \tag{A13}$$

This allows determining the candidates for the optimal strategies as

$$\boldsymbol{u}^* = \arg\min \boldsymbol{H} = -\mathrm{sign}\{B(t_f, t)\boldsymbol{Z}(t_f)\} \tag{A14}$$

$$\boldsymbol{v}^* = \arg\max \boldsymbol{H} = \mathrm{sign}\{C(t_f, t)\boldsymbol{Z}(t_f)\} \tag{A15}$$

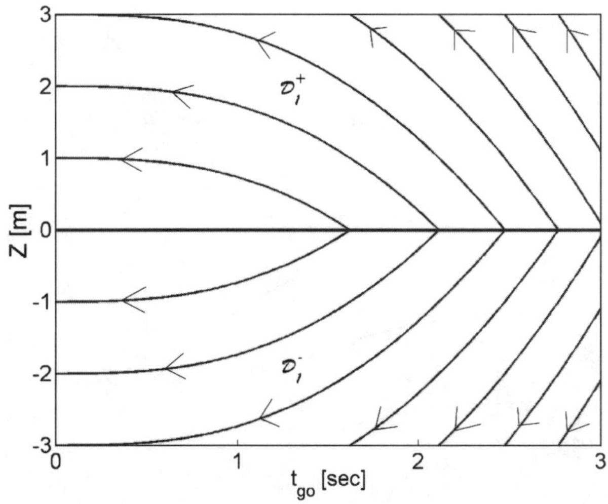

Fig. A1 Game space for case 1.

that lead, based on Eqs. (A7) and (A8), to

$$u^* = v^* = \text{sign}\{\mathbf{Z}(t_f)\}; \qquad \mathbf{Z}(t_f) \neq 0 \tag{A16}$$

Substituting Eq. (A16) into Eq. (A6) yields the optimized game dynamics

$$\frac{d\mathbf{Z}^*}{dt_{go}} = \mathbf{\Gamma}(t_f, t)\,\text{sign}\{\mathbf{Z}(t_f)\}; \qquad \mathbf{Z}(t_f) \neq 0 \tag{A17}$$

with

$$\mathbf{\Gamma}(t_f, t) = -[B(t_f, t) + C(t_f, t)] \tag{A18}$$

Candidate optimal trajectories are generated by integrating Eq. (A18) backward from any end condition $\mathbf{Z}(t_f)$. From the different cases that may occur, four are briefly discussed.

Case 1. If $\mathbf{\Gamma}(t_f, t) \geq 0$ for the entire interval $t_0 \leq t \leq t_f$, two families of monotonic optimal trajectories with can be generated, filling the entire game space (see Fig. A1). The two families intersect on the $\mathbf{Z} = 0$ axis, which serves as a *dispersal line* and dominated by the evader. In this case the optimal strategies can be expressed in a state feedback form

$$u^* = v^* = \text{sign}\{\mathbf{Z}(t)\}; \qquad \mathbf{Z}(t) \neq 0 \tag{A19}$$

and the value of the game is a function of the initial conditions.

$$J^*(\mathbf{Z}_0, t_0) = \left| \mathbf{Z}_0 + \text{sign}\,\mathbf{Z}_0 \int_{t_0}^{t_f} \mathbf{\Gamma}(t_f, t)\,dt \right| \tag{A20}$$

An example for such a case is the pursuit–evasion game with bounded control with ideal dynamics[31] and $\mu < 1$.

Case 2. If $\mathbf{\Gamma}(t_f, t) \leq 0$ for the entire interval $t_0 \leq t \leq t_f$, then the optimal trajectory pair generated from the point $\mathbf{Z}(t_f) = 0$ with different signs separates

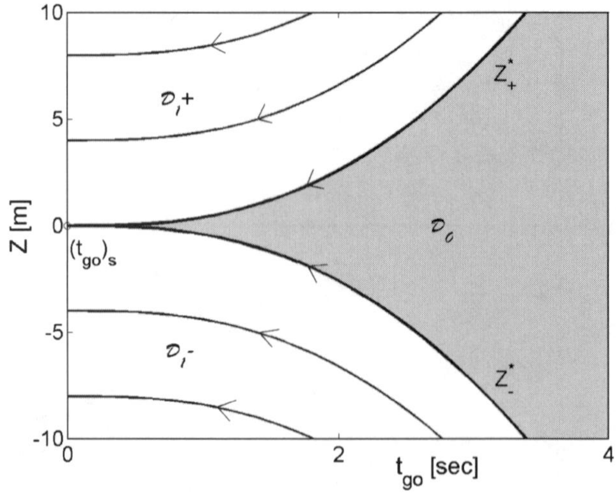

Fig. A2 Game space for case 2.

the game space into two regions of different solutions (see Fig. A2). Outside of these two optimal boundary trajectories, denoted respectively by $\mathbf{Z}^*_+$ and $\mathbf{Z}^*_-$, there is the region of *regular* trajectories denoted by D_1 where the solution is given by Eqs. (A19) and (A20). The boundary trajectories belong to D_1. Inside the other region, defined by

$$|\mathbf{Z}(t)| < \mathbf{Z}^*_+(t) \tag{A21}$$

and denoted by D_0, the optimal strategies are *arbitrary* and the value of the game is constant.

$$J^*_0(\mathbf{Z}_0, t_0) = 0 \tag{A22}$$

Inside this region $\lambda_z(t)$, which represents the gradient of the value function, is identically zero. Thus the game space is decomposed into three regions of different constant gradients $(+1, -1, 0)$ separated by the two semipermeable optimal boundary trajectories $(\mathbf{Z}^*)_+$ and $(\mathbf{Z}^*)_-$, which are the singular surfaces of the game. An example for such a case is the pursuit–evasion game with bounded control with ideal dynamics[31] and $\mu > 1$.

Case 3. If $\Gamma(t_f, t) = 0$ at $t = t_s \neq t_f$ and $\Gamma(t_f, t) > 0$ in the open interval $t_f > t > t_s$, while $\Gamma(t_f, t) < 0$ for $t_0 \leq t < t_s$, the optimal trajectories have a minimum at $t = t_s$. When an optimal trajectory, generated by backward integration, intersects the $\mathbf{Z} = 0$ axis, it ceases to be optimal because the change in sign$\{\mathbf{Z}(t)\}$. The two families of such trajectories define an evader-dominated dispersal line of the game. The boundary trajectories in this case, for which the decomposition of the game space is depicted in Fig. 2, in normalized form, are the pair of optimal trajectories that reach the $\mathbf{Z} = 0$ axis tangentially at $t = t_s$. The two regions of the different game solutions are

$$D_1 = \{(\mathbf{Z}, t) || \mathbf{Z}(t)| \geq \mathbf{Z}^*_+(t) \cup t_f \geq t \geq t_s\} \tag{A23}$$

$$D_0 = \{(\mathbf{Z}, t) || \mathbf{Z}(t)| < \mathbf{Z}^*_+(t) \cap t_0 \leq t < t_s\} \tag{A24}$$

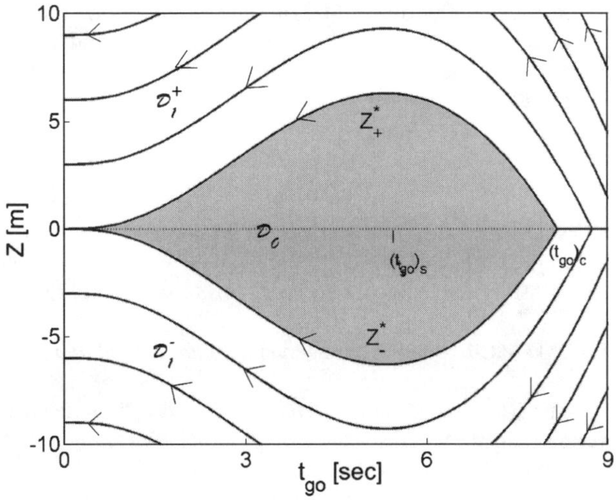

Fig. A3 Game space for case 4.

In D_1, Eqs. (A19) and (A20) provide the game solution. In D_0 the optimal strategies are arbitrary and the value of the game is constant:

$$J_0^*(\mathbf{Z}_0, t_0) = \int_{t_s}^{t_f} \Gamma(t_f, t)\,\mathrm{d}t \tag{A25}$$

The boundary trajectories and the dispersal line $\{\mathbf{Z}(t) = 0$ in the interval $t_f \geq t \geq t_s\}$, dominated by the evader, belong to D_1. An example is the game solved in Sec. II with $\mu > 1$ and $\mu\varepsilon < 1$.

Case 4. If $\Gamma(t_f, t_s) = 0$ and $\Gamma(t_f, t) < 0$ in the open interval $t_f > t > t_s$, while $\Gamma(t_f, t) > 0$ for $t_0 < t < t_s$, a different situation, depicted in Fig. A3, is created. The two optimal trajectories generated from the point $\mathbf{Z}(t_f) = 0$ with different signs intersect again on the $\mathbf{Z} = 0$ axis at $t = t_x < t_s$ (assuming $t_x > t_0$) and enclose the D_0 region. All other optimal trajectory pairs, terminating at different values of $|\mathbf{Z}(t_f)| \neq 0$, also intersect each other on the $\mathbf{Z} = 0$ axis at $t < t_x$ (if t_f is large enough) creating an evader-dominated dispersal line $\{\mathbf{Z}(t) = 0\}$ in the interval $t_0 \leq t \leq t_x$. Inside D_0 the optimal strategies are arbitrary and the value of the game is zero, as given by Eq. (A22). Everywhere else (in D_1) the solution is given by Eqs. (A19) and (A20). An example for such a case has not been yet encountered, but it can be generated for the game model of Section II with $\mu < 1$ and $\mu\varepsilon \geq 1$.

Remark. If the equation $\Gamma(t_f, t) = 0$ has more than one nonzero root, the structure of the solution will be slightly different depending on changing sign of $\Gamma(t_f, t)$ in the interval $t_0 \leq t \leq t_f$.

Acknowledgments

The multiyear investigation described in this chapter was partially supported by the U.S. Air Force Office of Scientific Research (AFOSR) Grant F49620-92-J-0527, AFOSR Contract F61708-97-C0004, and Ballistic Missile Defense

Organization Contract HQ0006-98-C-0014. The members of the research team involved in this effort, former doctoral students Y. Lipman and T. Shima, as well as research scientists M. Zarkh, A. Kepke, and V. Glizer, all deserve much credit for their significant contributions.

References

[1]Hughes, D., "Next Arrow Test this Summer after Scoring Direct Hit," *Aviation Week and Space Technology,* 24 March 1997.

[2]Philips, H. E., "PAC-3 Missile Seeker Succeed," *Aviation Week and Space Technology,* 22 March 1999.

[3]Wall, R., "THAAD At Crossroads After Intercept," *Aviation Week and Space Technology,* 9 Aug. 1999.

[4]Axelrod, A., Tahan, D., and Shinar, J., "High Endo-atmospheric Interception of Randomly Maneuvering Ballistic Missiles, *Proceedings of the 40th Israel Annual Conference on Aerospace Sciences,* Feb. 2000, pp. 211–218.

[5]Zarchan, P., "*Tactical and Strategic Missile Guidance,*" Progress in Astronautics and Aeronautics, Vol. 124, AIAA, Washington DC, 1990.

[6]Basar, T., and Olsder, G. J., "*Dynamic Noncooperative Game Theory*" Series of Mathematics in Science and Engineering, Vol. 160, Academic, London, 1982.

[7]Isaacs, R. "*Differential Games,*" Wiley, New York, 1965.

[8]Anderson, G. M., "Comparison of Optimal Control and Differential Game Intercept Missile Guidance Laws," *Journal of Guidance and Control,* Vol. 4, No. 2, 1981, pp. 109–115.

[9]Shinar, J., "On New Concepts Effecting Guidance Law Synthesis of Future Interceptor Missiles," *Proceedings of the AIAA Guidance, Navigation, and Control Conference,* CP 89-3589, AIAA, Washington, DC, Aug. 1989.

[10]Shinar, J., "Solution Techniques for Realistic Pursuit-Evasion Games" *Advances in Control and Dynamic Systems,* edited by C. T. Leondes, Vol. 17, Academic, New York, 1981, pp. 63–124.

[11]Gutman, S., "On Optimal Guidance for Homing Missiles," *Journal of Guidance and Control,* Vol. 3, No. 4, 1979, pp. 296–300.

[12]Lipman, Y., and Shinar, J., "A Linear Pursuit-Evasion Game with State Constraint of a Highly Maneuverable Evader," *New Trends in Dynamic Games and Applications,* Annals of the International Society of Dynamic Games, Vol. 3, edited by G. J. Olsder, Birkhäuser, Boston, 1995, pp. 143–164.

[13]Lipman, Y., and Shinar, J., "Mixed Strategy Guidance in Future Ship Defense," *Journal of Guidance, Control, and Dynamics,* Vol. 19, No. 2, 1996, pp. 334–339.

[14]Lipman, Y., Shinar, J., and Oshman, Y., "A Stochastic Analysis of the Interception of Maneuvering Anti-Surface Missiles," *Journal of Guidance, Control, and Dynamics,* Vol. 20, No. 4. 1997, pp. 707–714.

[15]Fitzgerald, R. J., and Zarchan, P., "Shaping Filters for Randomly Initiated Target Maneuvers," *Proceedings of the AIAA Guidance and Control Conference,* AIAA, New York, Aug. 1978, pp. 424–430.

[16]Shinar, J., and Zarkh, M., "Interception of Maneuvering Tactical Ballistic Missiles in the Atmosphere," *Proceedings of the 19th ICAS Congress* (Anaheim, CA), Sept. 1994, pp. 1354–1363.

[17]Garber, V., "Optimum Intercept Law for Accelerating Targets," *AIAA Journal,* Vol. 6, No. 11, 1968, pp. 2196–2198.

[18]Cottrell, R. G., "Optimal Intercept Guidance for Short Range Tactical Missiles," *AIAA Journal,* Vol. 9, No. 7, 1971, pp. 1414–1415.

[19]Shinar, J., and Zarkh, M., "The Guidance Challenge in Ballistic Missile Defense Scenarios against Maneuvering Threats," Technion Aerospace Engineering Rept. 777, Haifa, June 1996.

[20]Shinar, J., Shima, T., and Kebke, A., "Evaluation of Guidance Laws for the Interception of Highly Maneuvering Targets—Comparison to Linear Analysis," TAE Rept. 808, Nov. 1997.

[21]Shinar, J., Shima, T., and Kebke, A., "On the Validity of Linearized Analysis in the Interception of Reentry Vehicles," *Proceedings of the AIAA Guidance, Navigation, and Control Conference,* CP98-4303, Reston, VA, Aug. 1998.

[22]Shinar, J., and Shima, T. "A Game Theoretical Interceptor Guidance Law for Ballistic Missile Defense," *Proceedings of the 35th IEEE Conference on Decision and Control,* Inst. of Electrical and Electronics Engineers, New York, Dec. 1996, pp. 2780–2785.

[23]Shinar, J., "Requirement for a New Guidance Law Against Maneuvering Tactical Ballistic Missiles" 6th Annual AIAA/BMDO Technology Conf., San Diego, CA, Aug. 1997.

[24]Shima, T., and Shinar, J., "On the Extension of Linear Pursuit-Evasion Game Model Applied for Interception Analysis," *Proceedings of the 39th Israeli Annual Aerospace Conference,* Feb. 1999, pp. 142–152.

[25]Witsenhausen, H. S., "Separation of Estimation and Control for Discrete Time Systems," *Proceedings of the IEEE,* Vol. 59, No. 11, Nov. 1971, pp. 1557–1566.

[26]Shinar, J., and Shima, T., "A New Application of Bernhard's Certainty Equivalence Principle," *Proceedings of the 8th International Symposium on Dynamic Games and Applications,* Maastricht, The Netherlands, July 1998.

[27]Shinar, J., and Shima, T., "Robust Missile Guidance Law against Highly Maneuvering Targets," *Proceedings of the 7th IEEE Mediterranean Conference on Control & Automation,* CP-218, Haifa, Israel, June 1999.

[28]Petrosjan, L. A., "*Differential Games of Pursuit,*" Series on Optimization, Vol. 2, World Scientific Publ. Singapore, 1993, Chap. 6, pp. 169–177.

[29]Shinar, J., and Glizer, V., "Complete Solution of a Delayed Information Linear Pursuit-Evasion Game with Bounded Controls," Technion Aerospace Engineering Rept. 841, Haifa, Nov. 1999.

[30]Shinar, J., and Glizer, V. Y., "Solution of a Delayed Information Linear Pursuit-Evasion Game with Bounded Controls," *International Game Theory Review,* Vol. 1, No. 3–4, 1999, pp. 197–218.

[31]Gutman, S., and Leitmann, G., "Optimal Strategies in the Neighborhood of a Collision Course," *AIAA Journal,* Vol. 14, No. 9, 1976, pp. 1210–1212.

V. Measures of System Effectiveness and Risk Management

Chapter 14

Analytical Methods, Measures of Effectiveness, and Simulations

Dror Cohen,* Ronia Lapid,† and Ayala Gur ‡
WALES Ltd., Ramat-Gan, Israel

I. Introduction

THE present chapter is devoted to analytical methods and simulations employed in the development and analysis of TMD systems performance. Let us stress, at the outset, that it is not the authors' intent to provide an in-depth presentation of all known and familiar operations research techniques used in weapon systems development. Such a thorough treatment merits a book unto itself, and may not be of interest to prospective readers of this volume.

The goal we have set for ourselves is to highlight several techniques and issues that are either unique to theater missile defense (TMD) systems or in which problems and trends that may be relevant to future weapon systems developments are first brought to the surface through TMD analysis.

Indeed, it is the view of the authors that TMD, which was the last major development in weapon systems in the twentieth century (together with information warfare), highlights certain trends and problems that will characterize the future development environment of weapon systems, and hence is a good framework in which to discuss the required analytical methods and computerized tools.

Two main issues will be discussed in this chapter. The first deals with the question of what are the important measures that characterize TMD system performance—the so-called measures of effectiveness (MOE). In dealing with this issue we will identify several MOE specific to TMD. We will also attempt to establish a generalized view of the role of MOE based on the experience gained in their development for TMD, and to highlight some methods and ideas, which may be useful for other systems as well. The second issue discussed is the use of simulations and computerized tools for TMD systems analysis. We shall attempt

Copyright © 2000 by the American Institute of Aeronautics and Astronautics, Inc. All rights reserved.

*President. Member AIAA.

†Executive Vice President. Member AIAA.

‡Senior Systems Analyst. Member AIAA.

to highlight some unique applications and analytical resolution of issues that arose in the study of antitactical ballistic missile (ATBM) systems, and point to possible generalizations for other applications in the future.

The goal of this chapter is, therefore, not to teach the reader specific approaches and implementations, but rather to clarify the logic and thought processes that brought about the resolution of specific issues, so that the reader may apply them to his or her problems, which may be different from our own. This chapter should be read in that spirit.

II. Measures of Effectiveness

A. General

Measures of effectiveness (MOE) are those quantities, typically achieved through various methods of data gathering (actual weapon system test, simulation run, analytic calculation, etc.), that are used for evaluating the performance of a specific element/weapon system/architecture in achieving a defined goal. MOE may be used to compare alternative defense architectures, deployment options, defensive strategies, firing doctrines, etc., and may also be used for determining optimal development goals.

Because this definition is broad almost to the extent of being useless, an attempt should be made to classify performance qualities into narrower groups, containing quantities that have some common denominator, making it easier to identify useable MOE. Such a classification will be attempted in the current section.

B. Classification of MOE

MOE may be classified in a variety of ways. The classification described here involves grouping at three levels, as follows.

1) MOE of level one: Basic quantitative "one on one" performance parameters. These include parameters such as weapon probability of kill [against a specific tactical ballistic missile (TBM) under specific engagement conditions], radar detection range, footprint of a certain weapon system (against a specific threat), etc. MOE of level one (sometimes referred to as MOP—measures of performance) are often used by engineers and scientists engaged in developing parts of the weapon system, or as building blocks for higher level MOE.

2) MOE of level two: Quantities that measure weapon system/architecture performance against a specific (many-on-many) attack scenario. Level two MOE are developed from level one MOE and the threat scenario chosen. The connection between levels one and two MOE is not immediate, but is affected by the decisions of the battle manager (e.g., deployment, rule of engagement). An example of a MOE of level two is the leakage rate (see further discussion to follow). MOE of level two are the ones most generally used in weapon system/architecture analysis and comparison.

3) MOE of level three: Quantities that measure attributes of the defense system performance, which are independent of the attack scenario (i.e., are inherent in the system itself) or an aggregate of MOE (level one or two) over an entire range of scenarios. Examples of such qualities are the system's robustness, flexibility, etc. These weapon system qualities, sometimes referred to as MOM (measures of merit), are usually not considered as part of the MOE spectrum, because they are

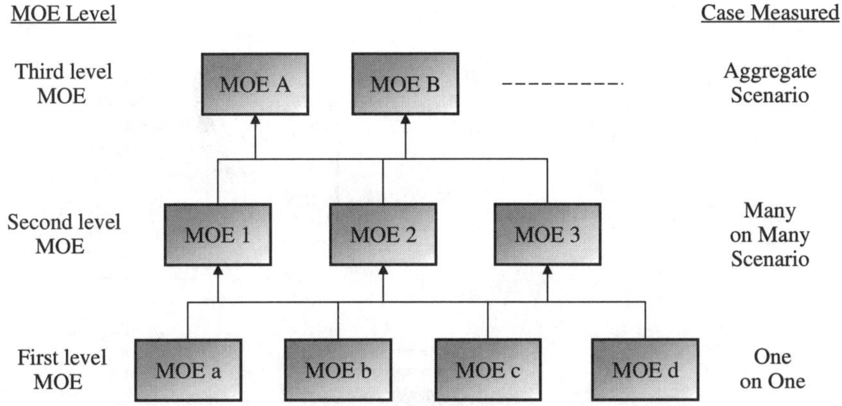

Fig. 1 General hierarchy of MOE.

thought to be nonquantifiable. In this chapter, we shall attempt to show that, at least for some of these qualities, this assumption is inaccurate.

Figure 1 illustrates the general hierarchy of MOE.

C. Level-One MOE as Building Blocks for Level Two

The level-one MOE are concerned with element or subsystem performance against a single threat. As such, they are useful in engineering and development applications, as demonstrated in other parts of this book. The focus of the present chapter is on the use of analytic methods and tools in the study and development of architectures, rather than subsystems. Our interest in level-one MOE stems, therefore, from their role in determining the architecture performance against a full-attack scenario. That is, their integration to level-two MOE.

Level-one MOE are not linked directly to the level-two MOE. Rather, they are linked through the set of operational decisions of the commanders and operators of the overall defense architecture. For example, a particular weapon system's probability of kill P_k against a particular TBM (level-one MOE) may be high, but if the architecture planner chooses to deploy, or use the system in such a way that its performance would be degraded, then this quality (the high P_k) will not be realized. In that case, to achieve a low leakage or leakage rate (level-two MOE), one would have to depend on the performance of a different defense component.

Figure 2 illustrates the connections between several level-one MOE, the operational decisions and threat scenarios, and the level-two MOE. For example, enemy doctrine affects the time line of specific events in the defender's architecture, because it affects the time line of the attack, and thus the sequence of events in the sky to which the architecture is expected to respond. The same MOE (time line) is also affected by the defender's rules of engagement (ROE), which dictate, for example, interception altitudes. Figure 2 is illustrative and does not in any way attempt to include all the level-one or level-two MOE.

Understanding the mechanisms governing these interconnections is essential for effective planning and operation of a defense architecture.

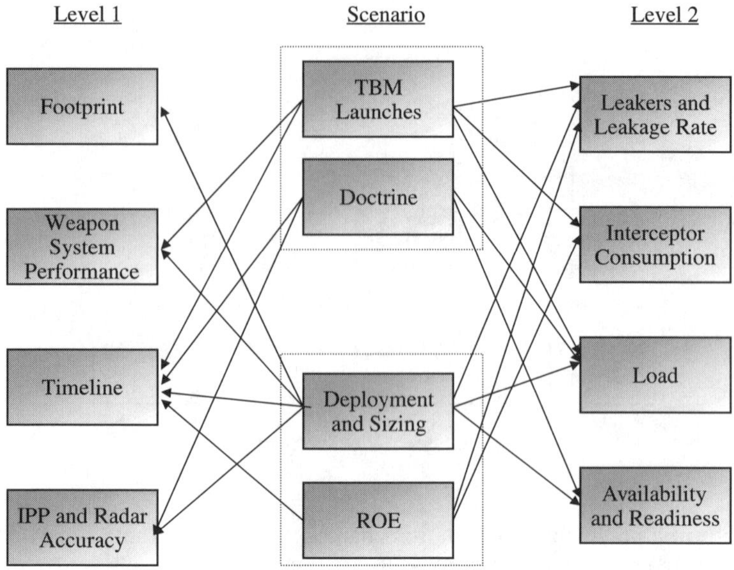

Fig. 2 Connections between MOE and operational decisions.

D. Level-Two MOE

The level-two MOE represent aspects of the performance of the architecture against a specific threat scenario. Level-two MOE are interconnected in various ways. Figure 3 illustrates these connections using several (obviously not all) level-two MOE.

Typically, the connection between level-two MOE is one of direct cause and effect. For example, radar load problems encountered during the attack may cause certain TBMs to pass undetected, thus increasing the leakers (and the leakage rate).

Even from this partial figure, it can be seen that the level-two MOE contain a certain hierarchy of their own, in the sense that some of them represent "causes" most of the time, whereas others represent "effects." This distinction is important. Level-two MOE are the ones most often used in architecture analysis. Because, most of the time, budget and timing constraints limit the resources devoted to analysis, analysts seek to concentrate on as few measures as possible. Obviously,

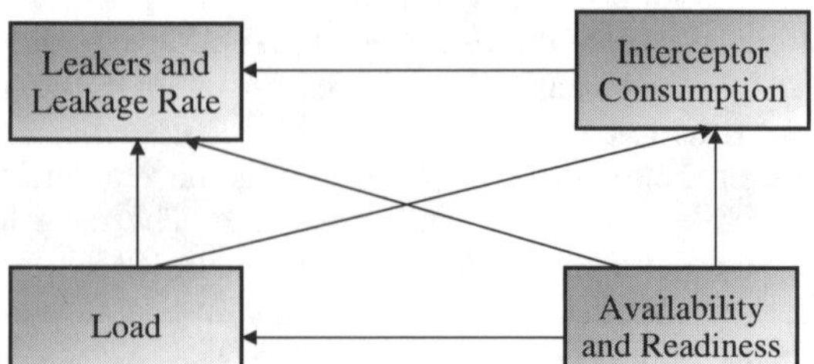

Fig. 3 Connections between level-two MOE.

it is most beneficial to concentrate on the MOE representing "effects," because in this way more characteristics are included in the measured, if not fully analyzed, set.

It is possible to show that, for level-two MOE, in the final analysis there are only two main "effects"—interceptor consumption and leakers (or leakage rate). There is no rigorous mathematical proof of the preceding assertion, but the reader is invited to try his hand at identifying any level-two MOE that does not lead to one of these two. For example, the availability of the defense system to engage a TBM threat may be expressed in terms of the resources available at a given moment. This may in turn result in poor/no defense plans, or lack of resources due to load, both directly affecting number of leakers and interceptor consumption.

It is possible, therefore, to express the commutative effects of level-two MOE by only two measures: leakers (leakage rate) and interceptor consumption. These two MOE are the subject of the next section.

E. "Natural" MOE—Leakage Rate and Interceptor Consumption

Our first step will be to define several basic terms and quantities. If we assume a simple defense architecture made of one weapon system defending one attacked asset, we may define the following basic parameters: 1) attack size N is the number of TBMs that attack the defended asset (DA), 2) leakers L is the number of TBMs (out of N) that hit the DA, 3) interceptor consumption IC is the number of interceptors fired during the attack, and 4) kills – K is the number of TBMs (out of N) that are killed by interceptors.

Using these basic values, it is possible to calculate the following parameters. Leakage rate:

$$\mathrm{LR} = \frac{L}{N} \tag{1}$$

Interceptor consumption rate:

$$\mathrm{ICR} = \frac{IC}{N} \tag{2}$$

Effective interceptor consumption [(a variant of Eq. (2)]:

$$\mathrm{EIC} = \frac{IC}{K} \tag{3}$$

When the situation is made more complex by adding more weapon systems and DAs, the following variants are seen, in addition to the basic definitions:

1) L, or LR, per DA (or group of DAs).

2) IC, ICR, or EIC per weapon system per DA.

3) Weighing of interceptors according to "interceptor cost." Interceptor cost represents the value attributed to an interceptor type under given circumstances (not necessarily directly reflecting its price).

4) LR or L per DA, weighed according to the DA value (importance, vulnerability).

5) Any of the above, for a given subperiod of the attack scenario.

In any of the preceding variations, these MOE express a very "natural" view of the TMD war. A defense architecture is deployed to kill TBMs, and if possible, to do so efficiently (i.e., using the least interceptors). Therefore, its success may be measured in terms of how well it achieves these two goals.

The difference between the quantitative and the "rate" versions (e.g., between L and LR) implies knowledge of the attack scenario (in this case, the total number of attacking TBMs). Obviously, the leakers L by themselves are of limited utility to the analyst if the entire attack scenario is not known (four leakers out of four attacking TBMs is one result, four out of four hundred is a totally different matter). The LR does not assume a knowledge of the scenario (a 4% LR means the same thing under any attack scenario: out of any 100 attacking TBMs, four are expected to leak). On the other hand, the defense commander does not care that the LR is, say, 10%. All he cares about is whether 1 or 10 TBMs hit the ground in his DA. This causes a situation in which the LR level considered acceptable by a decision maker/commander varies with the scenario. This makes the LR a difficult tool to use for comparison of architectures across a range of attack scenarios, though very important as a basic analysis parameter.

The same logic applies to interceptor consumption. The defense planner tries to minimize the rate of consumption of interceptors per TBM whereas the commander is interested in the numbers of interceptors remaining for future battles.

An important point that should be clarified is that, while the L (LR) and IC (ICR) are the two most commonly used MOE to measure architecture performance, they are not independent. In the simplest case of a single-system architecture, having full coverage and an unlimited number of interceptors, and with a ROE in which one interceptor is allocated per TBM, the relationship between IC and L is given by the interceptor P_k. Because in this case the expected number of leakers is

$$L = (1 - P_k)IC \tag{4}$$

F. Combining the "Natural" MOE—The Baseline System Effectiveness Approach

As has been stated, leakers and interceptor consumption are the most often used level-two MOE when analyzing architecture performance. Furthermore, these two measures "contain" all of the information needed to compare architectures although, naturally, it is sometimes necessary to turn to less all-encompassing level-two MOE to reveal information which is "hidden" within these two measures. Finally, as explained in the previous section, these two MOE are linked.

The idea behind the baseline system effectiveness (BSE) MOE is to construct a single measure, which combines all of the knowledge contained in level-two MOE about architecture performance against a given threat scenario. The need for such a measure arises for two reasons: First, to reach a simple and easily understandable comparison between two architectures, and second, To supply a single number, representing the results of level-two analysis, when constructing higher level MOE.

Based on the considerations outlined in the preceding sections, it is clear that the BSE should consist of a combination of L (LR) and IC (ICR). For the purpose of the present chapter, we shall use the L and IC as basic values, although a similar analysis can be performed using LR and ICR (mixing rates with actual values is, however, not advisable).

It is possible to define a L–IC plane, as presented in Fig. 4. The performance of a particular architecture against a specific threat scenario can be mapped as a single point on this "plane." The BSE is defined as the "norm" of the point on

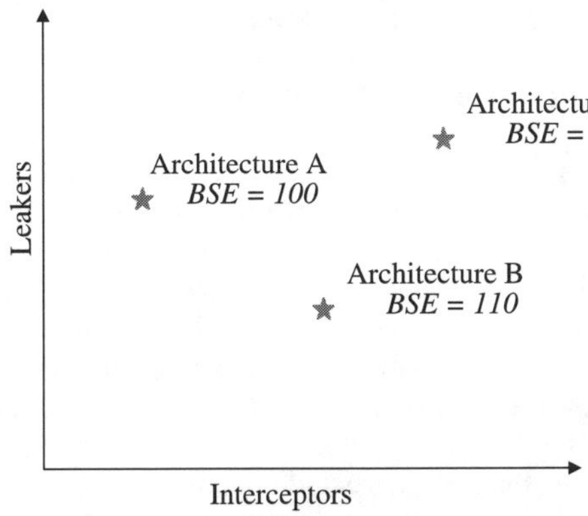

Fig. 4 BSE defined on the *L–IC* plane.

the plane. Because an increase in either one of the parameters (*IC*, *L*) indicates that the architecture performance is less effective, a smaller BSE value indicates a better architecture.

In general the norm between two partially dependent values such as L and IC includes the values themselves and a correlation factor. Therefore, the BSE is defined as

$$\text{BSE} = \sqrt{L^2 + IC^2 - 2rL \cdot IC} \tag{5}$$

where r is the correlation factor between L and IC.

Mathematically, this equation is true only if r is constant in all points of the *L–IC* plane. The relationship between IC and L is the effective P_k [Eq. (3)], and r represents this P_k. It is determined according to the actual P_k of the defense system throughout the battlespace on all the threats, the ROE used and the number of interceptors available. It is clear that r is not constant in the entire *L–IC* plane because, for large attacks relative to the number of interceptors, leakers will be caused by lack of interceptors as well as system performance limitations. As a result, the BSE is not actually a norm in the *L–IC* plane. However, it will be shown that the sensitivity of the BSE at a specific *L–IC* point, to changes in the value of r, is low. Also, the change in r with L and IC (given a specific architecture) is gradual and slow, and so for all practical purposes r may be viewed as a constant within any relevant section of the plane.

Equation (5) represents a basic version of the BSE. However, one more factor may be included, and that is the architecture planner's, or decision-maker's, preference between L and IC. If we designate this preference factor α, Eq. (5) becomes

$$\text{BSE} = \sqrt{(\alpha L)^2 + \left(\frac{1}{\alpha} IC\right)^2 - 2rL \cdot IC} \tag{6}$$

which is the final version of the BSE.

The value α represents the preference of the decision makers as to whether or not to save interceptors for later attacks at the cost of a less effective defense against the present attack, α may be deduced from the decision-maker's stated priorities and previous decisions. For a specific scenario, these decisions are seen in the defense levels and ROEs that are defined. The preference defined by α may change during any given scenario (through real-time decisions). However, because we are defining a measure to distinguish between architectures on a range of threat scenarios, we may safely claim that this comparison should be made based on the decision-maker's preferences at the outset of the war, disregarding subsequent changes.

A few observations need to be made regarding this formula: 1) When there are a number of different interceptor types in an architecture, the *IC* is the sum of the number of interceptors used of each type normalized by the relative value of each type. If one type of interceptor is twice as valuable as another, its weight in the *IC* value will be twice as high. Value should be determined according to various parameters including purchase cost, availability, and effectiveness 2) r is a negative number between 0 and -1. $r = -1$ when the architecture P_k is 1. 3) $\alpha \in (0, 1]$ (i.e., α can take any value between zero and one, except zero). 4) Clearly, low BSE is good (i.e., better architecture performance). 5) The equation is not universal. Once the range of threats (scenarios) is defined, r is determined by the architecture. Different architectures may have different values of r.

Equation (6) is useless unless we define α and r in some meaningful way. For a given application (seeking an architecture to defend a specific country/region against a specified range of threat scenarios) r may be found by testing several candidate architectures against a representative subset of the threat scenarios in a battlefield simulation. The r value is the average P_k over all tested cases. Figures 5 and 6 show an analysis of r and α for a number of architectures (different numbers of interceptors) over a range of attack sizes. Using such graphs it is possible to choose the relevant r and α values for comparing architectures.

We will now analyze the sensitivity of the BSE to the specific values of r and α. From Figs. 5 and 6, representative values of r and α were chosen ($r = -0.6$, $\alpha = 2$). Figure 7 shows the equi-BSE lines for this case. To test sensitivity, the impact

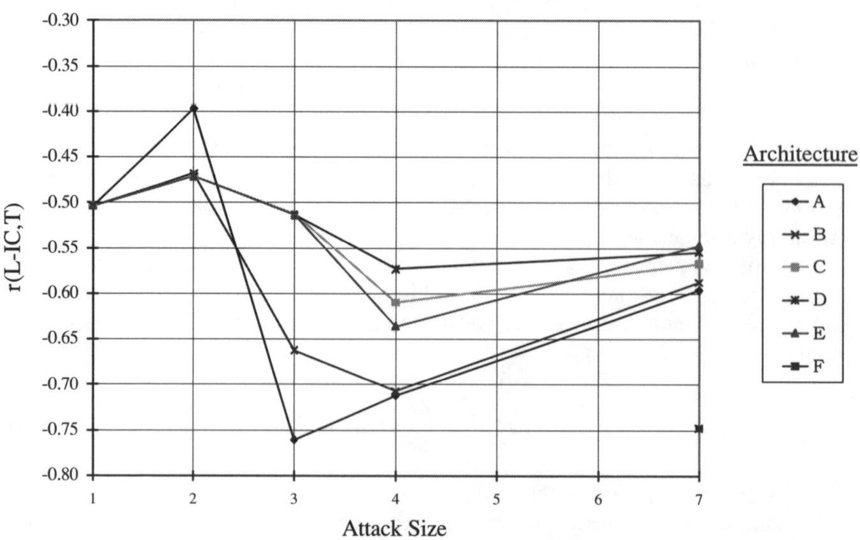

Fig. 5 Calibration for different architectures: *r*.

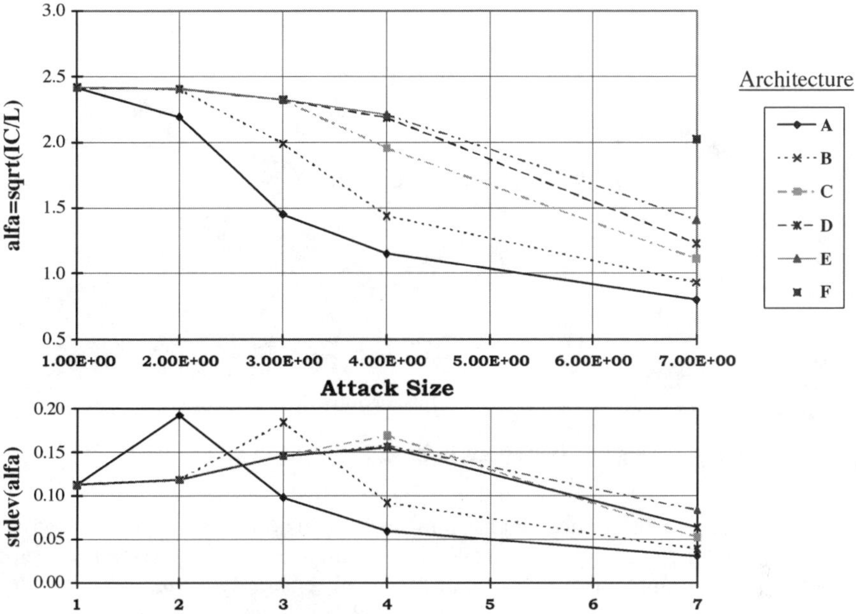

Fig. 6 Calibration for different architectures: α.

on the BSE if r or α were varied, was calculated. The possible values of r are between -0.8 and -0.4, which is a deviation of ± 0.2 relative to the chosen value. Figure 8 shows the maximal error in BSE caused by a deviation of 0.25 in r. As expected, little sensitivity can be seen.

The range of possible values for α is 1 to 2.5 (from Fig. 6). We repeat the same calculation testing $\Delta\alpha = 1$. This is presented in Fig. 9. We see a much greater sensitivity than in the case of r.

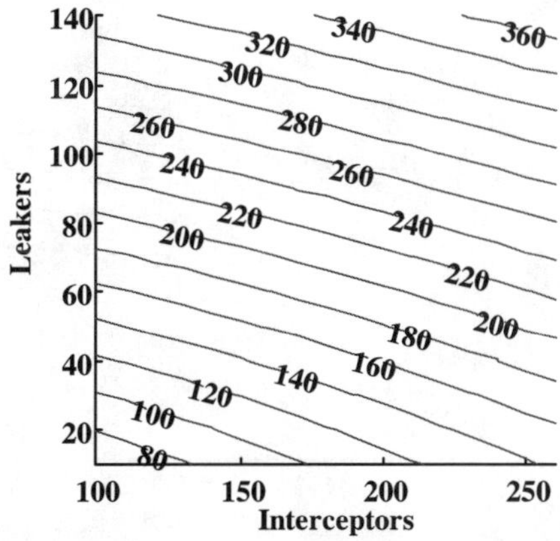

Fig. 7 Equi–BSE lines.

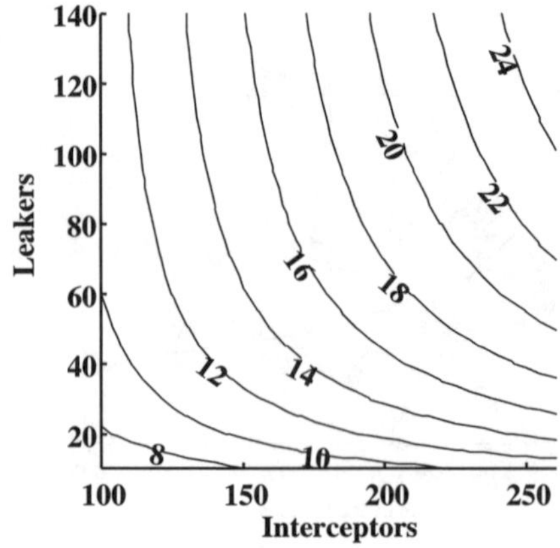

Fig. 8 Deviations in BSE, $r = -0.6 \pm 0.25$.

It therefore may be deduced that as long as the decision-maker's preferences (α) are fixed (and they usually are) the BSE is a useful tool for comparison between a wide range of architectures (because of the small sensitivity to r).

G. MOE of Level Three

MOE of level three are quantifications of general qualities of the architecture. They should reflect either architecture performance over a large set of attack scenarios or architecture potential performance (i.e., independent of the scenario). Third-level MOE, being quantifications of abstract terms, are difficult to define and implement, but are important for gaining a clearer understanding of the mechanisms governing the architecture performance and thus also architecture design. In the current section, two such MOE will be presented in some detail as examples. These MOE (robustness and flexibility) were developed and used in architecture

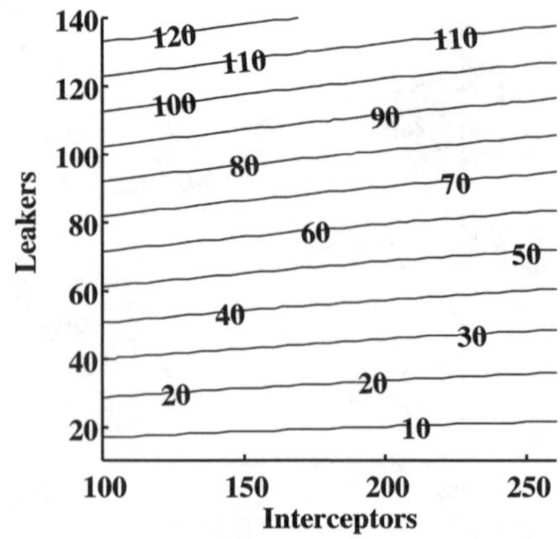

Fig. 9 Deviations in BSE, $\alpha = 2 \pm 1$.

studies conducted in Israel. However, it should be noted that they are not the only possible MOE of level three, and some other possible MOE will be mentioned subsequently.

We believe that the processes used in defining the two example MOE described next will be general enough to serve as a reference for further work on this topic.

H. Example 1—Architecture Robustness

A defense architecture is developed for a set of performance parameters, which represent its standard operational domain. The domain includes the set of threats that the architecture was planned against, the standard expected values of the defense system's level-one MOE, and external parameters (i.e., environment). An architecture is considered valid from the point of view of architecture developers, if it achieves the operational goals set by decision makers within the operational domain.

1. Robustness: Threshold Performance

The robustness of a defense architecture is defined as its ability to withstand changes in its operational domain without suffering a severe degradation of performance. To clarify this definition, let us look at Fig. 10. The figure shows the change in BSE value of two architectures both designed to withstand an attack size of up to *M* attacking missiles (the figure is notional and does not represent results for any particular architecture).

We indicate as BSE_t the highest BSE value that the decision makers are willing to tolerate, i.e., it represents the operational requirement. Clearly, both architectures in this figure are valid, because they achieve the required performance over the defined operating domain (up to *M* attacking missiles). However, when we exceed

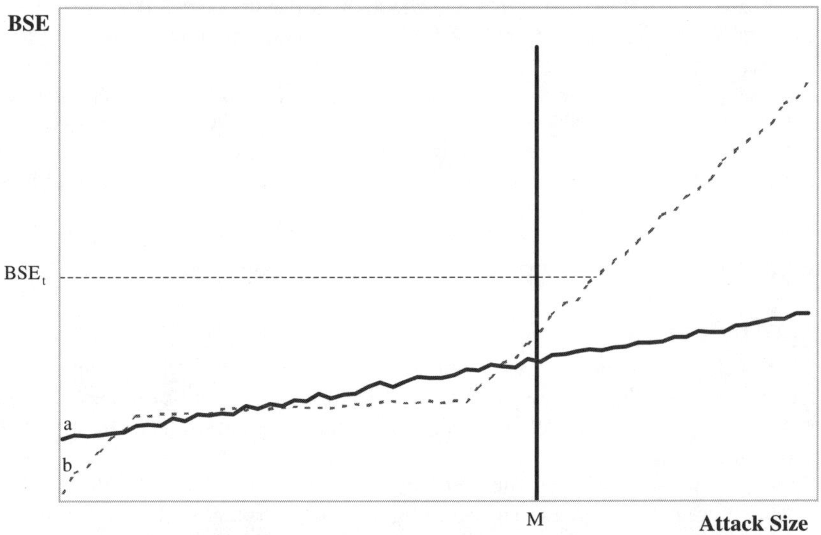

Fig. 10 Architecture BSE as a function of attack size.

the expected number of attacking missiles, architecture a continues to function adequately, whereas b experiences a rapid deterioration in its performance. We say that architecture a is more robust than architecture b, with respect to attack size.

The robustness MOE is based on decision-maker–defined threshold requirements of the defense effectiveness expressed in terms of BSE, LR, or any other suitable measure. When an architecture ceases to be able to achieve the designated threshold performance, we say the architecture fails. The MOE is based on the ratio between the number of events (or parameter values) tested and the number of events in which the architecture failed.

$$\text{Robustness } (A) = \frac{\sum_{\text{all events}} P_{\text{event}} \cdot I_{\text{fail}}}{\sum_{\text{all events}} P_{\text{event}}} \tag{7}$$

where

A = the tested architecture
P_{event} = the probability of event occurrence (parameter value)
I_{fail} = 0 if the architecture does not fail in this event and 1 if the architecture fails in this event

From the equation it is clear that a lower value for the robustness MOE indicates a more robust architecture. Figure 11 presents the robustness as a function of two different concurrent parameters. Though the peak performance is identical for both architectures, A has a higher effectiveness over a wider range of parameters. Therefore, according to the measure, architecture A is more robust than architecture B.

To actually implement the robustness measure, two questions have to be answered: 1) How to define the probability of each event or parameter value. This needs to take into account the likelihood of unexpected events. 2) How to prioritize between failure events caused by different parameters.

For the Israeli architecture study, we chose the following answers: 1) Define, for each parameter, a set of "nominal" values. Then create groups of events based on discretization of the distance of the parameters value chosen from the "nominal" range (i.e., define 1α events, 2α events, etc.). 2) Because the failure event is defined discreetly, do not prioritize between parameters but rather between the categories, i.e., an architecture that fails in a 1α event (no matter by which parameter the problem was caused) is less robust than an architecture that only fails in 2α events.

The resulting "realization" of the robustness idea is termed the risk measure and is described in the chapter dealing with architecture assessment.

2. *Robustness: Performance Stability*

The basic robustness concept admits other realizations than the one just described. For example, it is possible to identify the failure point of the architecture not as an unacceptable level of performance but as a significant change in the performance.

In Fig. 12 we present the same two architectures as in Fig. 10. Our definition of the robustness MOE implies that the point at which architecture b fails for the first time is the point designated P_f. The corresponding point for architecture a is not seen in the figure (it may occur at an attack size greater than shown in the figure).

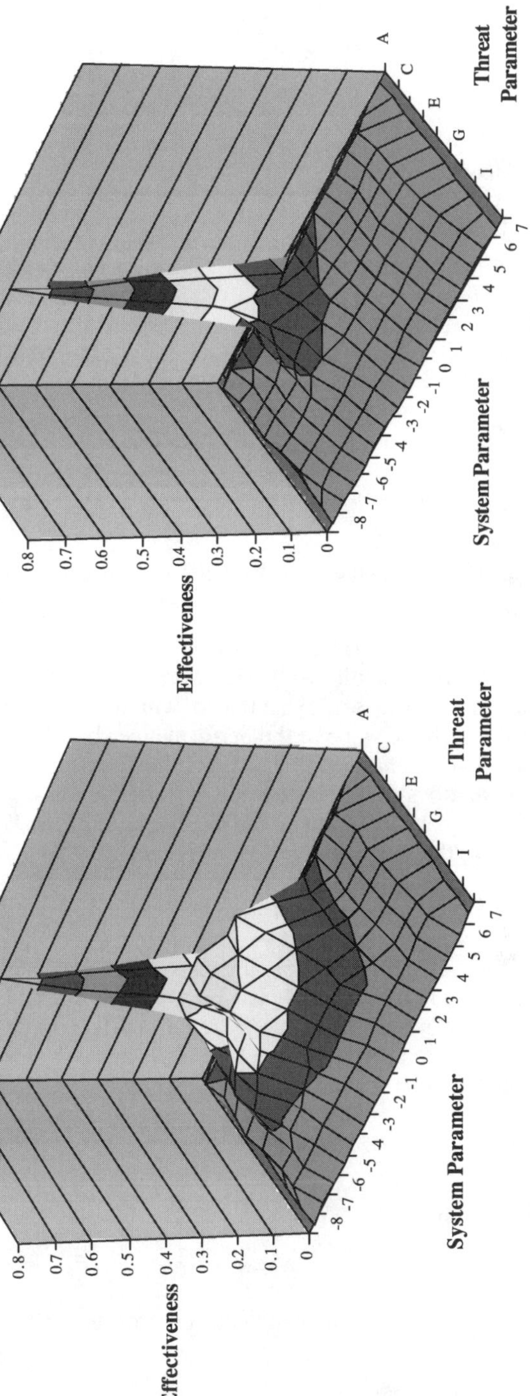

Fig. 11 Multiparameter robustness.

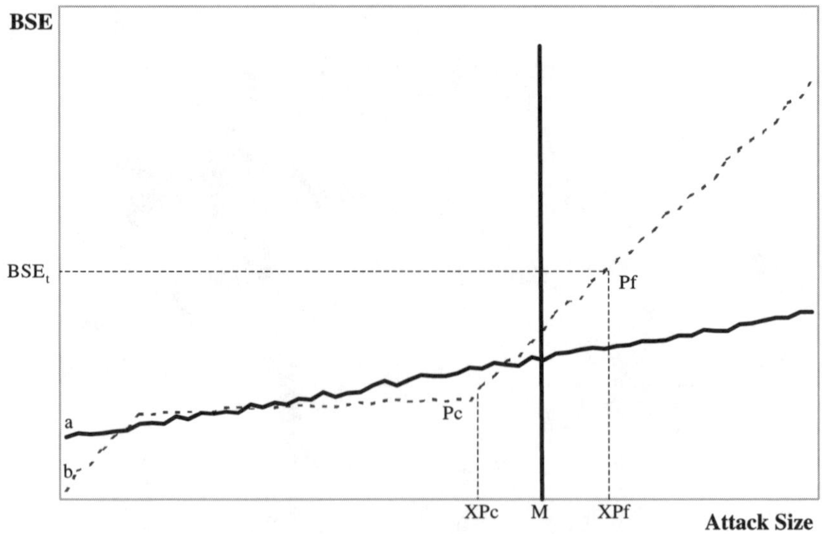

Fig. 12 Robustness using performance degradation.

The definition is based on the performance threshold that is an external number, not related to the architecture itself. However, two elements in the figure clearly define architecture b to be less robust than a, which are inherent to the architecture: 1) the point at which the slope of the performance changes and 2) the slope of the line following that point (steep line = less robustness).

An alternative robustness measure may be based on these values. To define such a measure, let us mark the point of the change in slope as Pc (point of collapse), its location along the X (parameters) axis is marked XPc. Our first problem will be to locate Pc among the points in the graph, because, as Fig. 12 shows, the graph representing architecture performance is a blurred picture, and not a uniform function of the parameter changed.

Let us assume that n points (parameter values) were tested. Without loss of generality, we may assume that X_1 is a point below X_{pc} and X_n is a point above. Take any point X_i between the two extreme points, and define M_1 as the slope of the linear regression line between X_1 and X_i and M_2 as the slope of the linear regression line between X_i and X_n.

Then,

$$X_{pc} = X_i \mid \max(M_2 - M_1) \tag{8}$$

The angle of the line after Pc is

$$\alpha = \tan^{-1}(M_2) \tag{9}$$

If we designate the probability of occurrence of the given point X_{pc} as P_{xpc}, we may define

$$\text{Robustness } (A) = \frac{1}{P_{xpc} \cdot \sin\alpha} \tag{10}$$

As before, this is a measure of the likelihood of an architecture to behave at less than the desired level. This measure includes the severity of the collapse as well as its likelihood. Other versions are also possible, for example, by inserting into the calculation the difference between *Pc* and *Pf*.

In all of its various forms, we feel that the robustness measure allows evaluation of an important quality, relevant for the analysis of defense architectures. The particular implementation chosen will depend on analyst preference and on external factors, such as the level of available simulations and tools and the types of data supplied.

I. Example 2—System Flexibility

The second MOE of level three that we are presenting is system flexibility. System flexibility is the ability of the system to adapt to changes in its operational domain, by actively changing its performance parameters or mode of operation. Unlike robustness, which measures to what degree the system (or architecture) can maintain a desired level of performance under changes in its operating environment, without any modifications, Flexibility measures the system's capability of change, in response to unforeseen developments.

In defining a system flexibility MOE, one must be aware of the fact that the "unknown-unknowns" cannot be predicted before the battle. Thus, the full range of circumstances that must be accommodated through change cannot be known in advance. In fact, even when an event occurs, it may not be possible to understand immediately exactly what has happened, and only its effect on defense system performance may be observed. Thus, the analysis of flexibility should be performed at the system level, independent of the scenario.

Two more observations should be made before we define an MOE for flexibility. First, because a TMD system must operate during a battle that may extend over only several days, it is very desirable to be able to implement a change that improves the defense system performance as quickly as possible. Therefore, time must be factored into the MOE definition. In our analyses, we chose to deal with the timing issue by introducing a threshold value, that is, system flexibility measures the change that can be made to the system within a threshold time T_t.

Second, to change the system to improve its performance, one must understand why a change is necessary, and to identify the change that is required. This sequence of events may be described as follows:

$$\text{Flexibility Requirement} = T_{\text{fault-recognition}} + T_{\text{change-identification}} + T_{\text{change}} < T_t \quad (11)$$

where $T_{\text{fault-recognition}}$ is the time it takes the system to identify the fact that a fault has occurred, $T_{\text{change-identification}}$ is the time required to analyze the failure and identify the required change, and T_{change} is the time taken by the actual changing process.

Clearly, the requirement set forth in Eq. (11) implies the existence of an efficient near-real-time debrief system. Such systems are discussed in the chapter dealing with the defense process.

To measure system flexibility, we must first define a few terms. For the analysis of flexibility we look at a defense architecture from the point of view of the defense process, rather than from the point of view of a set of linked systems and their individual attributes. These definitions may be different from those used in other analyses.

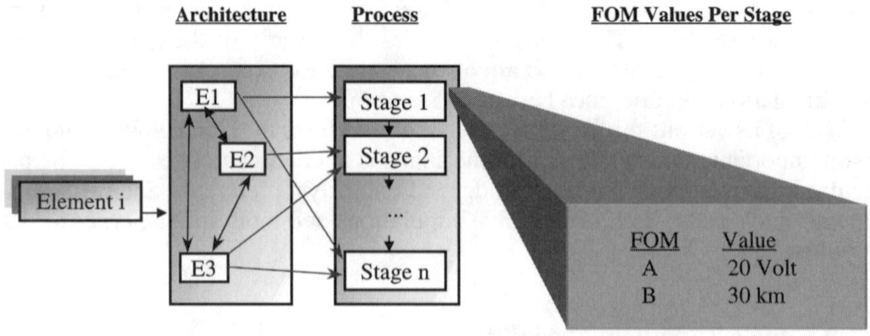

Fig. 13 Architecture, process, and FOM values.

An architecture is defined as a linked set of systems that perform an integrated function. The flexibility is analyzed in accordance with the process and subprocesses involved. A process is defined as a series of steps that can be measured by a particular figure of merit (FOM)—a FOM is usually a level-one MOE. For example, a FOM for the detection of a TBM is the detection range (average); another possible FOM for the same process is the detection probability. Note that for the analysis of flexibility, it is immaterial whether one or more sensors perform the detection. The value of the FOM is what matters. Figure 13 presents the general concept. Each architecture element participates in a number of stages of the process. At each stage, the element has required values (or range of values) and an actual value for the various performance parameters.

The analysis of flexibility now becomes an analysis of the FOM. If we analyze the entire defense process and come up with a series of FOM that are not scenario dependent, and represent the important subprocesses, it is possible define the flexibility of each FOM as the maximum change capability given a feasible change in the relevant elements. The system flexibility is limited by the FOM that can be changed the least:

$$\text{Flexibility}\ (A) = \min\{\max[\text{change}\ (f)]\}_{f=\text{FOM1},}^{\text{FOM}_n} \tag{12}$$

To use Eq. (12) we must 1) identify the scenario-independent FOM for each subprocess of the architecture; 2) find the feasible changes in the defense system that affects the FOM; and 3) find the maximal change possible in each FOM.

The analysis leading to the achievement of the these goals will be specific to the type of systems that compose the architecture analyzed. We shall give one example of such an analysis.

In Fig. 14, the process of engaging a TBM by a fragmentation warhead interceptor is analyzed. The leading FOM for this process is the system battlespace. This FOM is analyzed, identifying two nonscenario dependent FOM and the system elements that can affect them: fragment velocity and total impact energy.

To determine the impact of changes in element values on the FOM it is necessary to test variations of the values. Table 1 was generated using a fusing simulation and relevant intercept parameters. It provides representative results for the amount of change possible in each element and its effect on the FOM.

The table shows, for each parameter of the interception end-game, how much a change in its value from the nominal value required will affect each of the various FOM identified. For example, a decrease of 10% in the fusing time (fusing

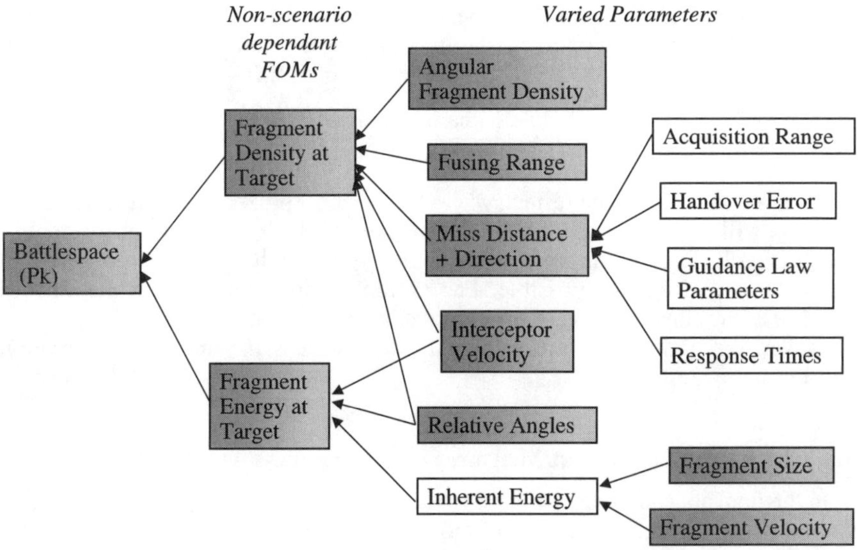

Fig. 14 Battlespace breakdown to FOM (fragmentation warhead).

earlier by 10% relative to the required fusing time) causes a change of 37% in the fragments density at the required impact point.

There are two ways of looking at Table 1. First, find the maximum change in FOM available and return to Eq. (11) to calculate architecture flexibility. In some cases, depending on the FOM, any positive change is clearly beneficial. In other cases it is the absolute size of the change that is relevant. Second, identify the

Table 1 Representative results—FOM change as function of parameter change

Parameter	Change, %	Fragment density change, %	Total energy change, %	Maximum energy change, %
Velocity	−10	2	−6	−8
	10	20	27	6
	20	7	11	8
	30	11	15	28
Angle	−10	0	−26	−26
	10	24	57	25
	25	0	57	57
	35	−5	58	67
Fusing time	−20	50	57	4
	−10	37	39	0
	10	−28	−29	−1
	20	−56	−56	−8
MD	−10	−7	−6	−3
Distribution	+10	15	18	3
	+20	1	5	−10

system element in which it is most beneficial to invest for increasing architecture flexibility. Typically, this will be the one that achieves the minimum change in parameter value that gives the maximum change in FOM:

$$\min \frac{\%\text{ change parameter}}{\%\text{ change FOM}} \tag{13}$$

Because, in general, the tested system has been optimized for performance, the changes will come at some cost (performance-wise). It is important to identify these as well. Definitions for system flexibility other than the one presented in Eq. (11) are, of course, possible. For example prioritizing among the various FOM to allow consideration of the complexity and/or cost of the added capability. However, the underlying principles will remain the same under any definition chosen.

J. Closing the Loop: Cost/Measures of Effectiveness Analysis

In the final analysis, a decision maker has to choose one course of action among several possibilities. It is the task of the analyst to supply the decision maker with tools to assist in arriving at his or her decision. Most of the time, the mechanism employed in arriving at final decisions is cost-effectiveness (cost/MOE) analysis. The cost of an architecture can be defined in a number of ways. Each definition is appropriate depending on the question being asked.

The BSE MOE that was previously discussed in this chapter includes the *cost of consumed elements* (interceptors). This is appropriate when comparing different methods of employing a given architecture (deployments, ROE) or comparing architectures with similar elements in which the purchase cost is not a main consideration. In principle, the BSE approach can be expanded to include any type of consumed entity. However, when comparing the merits of one architecture vs another, or when deciding on the sizing (the number of purchased elements) of a given architecture, the other elements of cost come into play, including the development cost and purchasing cost.

When considering purchase cost we have to take into account both the cost per element and the number of elements purchased. Let us look first at the number of purchased elements. For a fixed threat using any relevant effectiveness measure, the resulting graph of system effectiveness vs acquisition cost will appear as the one seen in Fig. 15. The graph is asymptotic, which means that above a certain number of elements, the contribution of any additional element becomes marginal. The effectiveness measured cannot be significantly improved with more of the same, considering the reference threat. It is important to note that in reality it is not possible to calculate the asymptotic effectiveness of each element of the defense architecture separately. For example, let us look at launchers and interceptors. If you buy too many interceptors, there will not be enough launchers to launch them at the given scenario time, and their incremental effect will be nullified. However, taken in combination, the effect of Fig. 15 will be clearly seen and the most cost effective mixture of elements can be identified.

We next consider the cost per element of an architecture. In suitably developed architectures there is a relationship between the cost of an element and its performance; usually a more expensive element will perform better. Figure 16 compares two architectures, one that is more expensive (B) to purchase relative

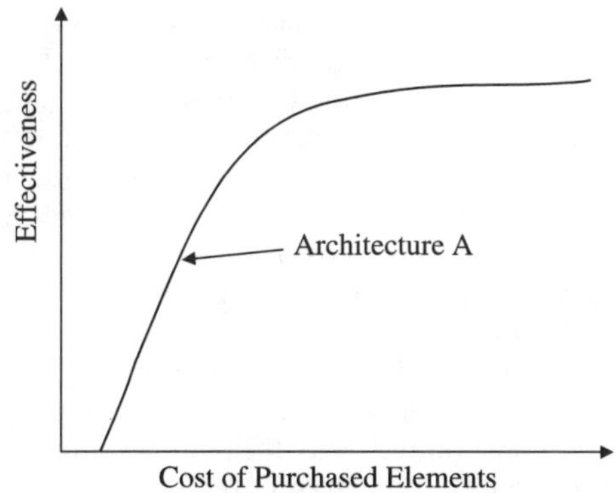

Fig. 15 Notional cost-effectiveness phenomena.

to the other (A). The values to which the architectures go asymptotically will be different (the more expensive architecture will ultimately provide better performance), however it is not clear, whether for a desired effectiveness level it is necessary to buy more quantities of one architecture, or fewer quantities of a more expensive architecture.

It should be mentioned that the picture depicted in Fig. 16 also occurs when we look at purchased elements vs other MOE (such as robustness) that do not directly measure architecture performance. However, the exact shape of the graph will be different.

The full cost of the architecture includes, along with the purchase cost, the non-recurring development costs. These costs are important to consider when determining which architecture option to buy or how to further develop the architecture. Basically, two approaches exist to compare architectures when the full cost is taken into account:

1) Integrating the development costs of each architecture into the previously described purchase cost by setting the initial cost of each architecture according to the non-recurring costs. In this case it is possible to compare different cost and effectiveness levels of the same architectures.

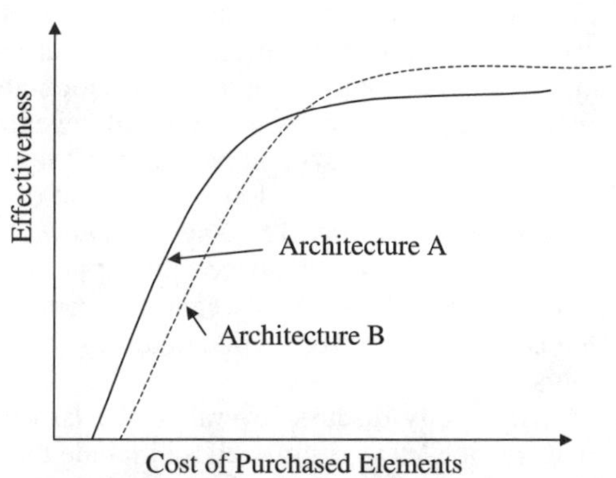

Fig. 16 Notional cost-effectiveness phenomena—comparison.

2) In many cases it is difficult to calculate a continuous cost effectiveness function for an architecture. In this case it is possible to define several cost categories and the different architectures are defined at various cost categories. The defined architectures cost level is determined according to all the development required and all the elements to be purchased. The comparison between architectures is performed only for those belonging to the same cost category.

The analysis of cost-effectiveness (cost/MOE) closes the loop and allows intelligent comparison of development/procurement options.

The MOE presented in this chapter are only a partial set of the qualities of TMD architectures that can, and should, be considered during development, procurement, and use. In the process of working on defense architecture development, we found that the need for more complex and difficult measures (typically, level-three measures) increases as the development progresses. As deployment of these systems nears, the need will arise to study complex qualities, which may be paramount for the correct utilization of the systems, either in their originally intended role, or in possible secondary roles. Some qualities of TMD architectures that should be considered for MOE development are deterrence value, diversity (i.e., the possibility of dealing with non-TBM threats, such as cruise missiles), interoperability quality (i.e., the degree to which an architecture is capable of interoperability with friendly systems), and combat readiness.

The field of MOE for TMD systems (beyond the most commonly used leakage rate) remains largely an uncharted territory, never before treated in a carefully laid out, systematic approach. This is true for other systems as well. We hope that this chapter will constitute an initial step to fill this gap. It is certain that a great deal more work needs to be done before a fully systematic theory of MOE can be created.

III. Computerized Models and Simulations

Computerized models and simulations of various levels are today an essential part of any weapon system development process. The use of computerized tools starts with checking the basic idea for the new weapon system in battlefield models, to assess its possible contribution, and continues throughout the development process as engineering models, system level representations, and battlefield level tools are used by the developers and analysts. Even after development is completed, widespread use is made of computerized simulators and trainers, to facilitate operational crews' learning and to provide experience in operating the system.

It is not the authors' intent to provide general information about computerized tools and their usage. Rather, our goal is to highlight several aspects of TMD weapon system development and deployment, which merit somewhat unorthodox and innovative use of computerized tools. Let us stress, at the outset, that these aspects are not limited to TMD systems. TMD systems are one of the first major systems for the new millenium to enter the development phase, and thus allow us a look at the new problems and dilemmas of weapon system development for the future battlefield. In this context, it is worthwhile to discuss the role of simulations and computerized tools.

In this section we will briefly discuss several of the issues that have special importance in the analysis of TMD systems. These include the ways to handle an uncertain, ever changing threat, the use of simulations in preparing for interoperability between weapon systems, the importance of analysis of near-real-time decision-making effects on battle results, and the role of simulators and trainers in maintaining system readiness against a rarely appearing (low likelihood) threat. A brief discussion on the future of simulations as interoperable entities, using DIS/HLA protocols, will be presented at the end this chapter.

A. Dealing with an Ever-Changing Threat

1. Threat Characteristics

One aspect of TMD systems that is important to stress is that they are, by nature, responding to, rather than initiating, systems. In this sense they are akin to surface-to-air missiles (SAMs). However, the much larger operating envelope (at least of upper-tier systems), and the short time frame available for response, create a unique response requirement from the system. The TMD system has to handle a situation in which the threat generation occurs far away, and the enemy has almost complete freedom in choosing the timing and characteristics of the attack (launch locations, salvo size, and distribution) as well as a wide latitude in determining the characteristics of the threat itself (payload, trajectories). This is particularly true when discussing isolated operations by terror organizations, or attacks mounted as part of a conflict in which the country attacked by TBMs is not a participant (as happened to Israel during the 1991 Persian Gulf War). The TMD system must therefore be able to respond to an unknown, uncontrolled threat. Moreover, because the TMD systems development processes are widely reported in the mass media, including technical details, the system has to be prepared, from the start, to deal with responsive threat, i.e., the means employed by the enemy to counter the effect of the defensive system. The rate at which various responsive threats can be developed and the specific development options that will be chosen by the enemy are unknown to the defense planner. However, it may be possible to define a maximum capability based on existing technologies and enemy engineering and economic capabilities.

The preceding discussion leads us to conclude that in analyzing a defense system's performance, it is important to take into account the numerous dimensions of the threat. This goes against the usual practice of defining a few highly detailed reference attack scenarios and using them throughout the development and evaluation process.

There are several techniques for dealing with such threats. One technique was already discussed, when dealing with the robustness MOE. Returning to Fig. 9, and the related discussion, we can look at the robustness MOE as a way of systematically analyzing excursions from the nominal threat scenarios. In this way, it is possible to analyze both single and multiparameter excursions. Another method, discussed later in this chapter, is to introduce the "enemy" into the simulated environment, i.e., conducting two-sided wargames. This approach, while very beneficial from an analytic point of view, is too cumbersome and costly to be used for a systematic evaluation of various parameter excursions. Rather, it should be used for in-depth analysis of specific, interesting cases.

2. Statistical Threat Model

Another approach, and one that has been successfully utilized in Israeli studies, is that of creating a statistical representation of the threat. The main idea behind this approach is to create a computerized tool that will automatically generate *reasonable* attack scenarios. The term "reasonable" is taken to mean scenarios that will be considered plausible from the point of view of an intelligence specialist. This, in turn, means that not only all of the parameters of an attack fall between well defined boundaries but also that the combination of all parameters makes sense from an intelligence point of view. A simple example will serve to clarify this point. Suppose that the random threat generation model draws n missiles as the enemy's initial stock. Then, although it is possible to draw $m > n$ launchers as initial stock, that will not be a reasonable scenario.

In the model actually designed, some numbers are drawn randomly using distributions defined by intelligence experts, whereas some others are derived from a database whose point of entrance is determined by the random draws. For example, in our particular realization, the number of available missiles and launchers in certain enemy countries is fixed by an intelligence assessment. The number out of those that participate in a given attack is drawn, based on the probability of participation by each enemy country and possible combinations of participants, that were provided by intelligence assessment.

Statistical threat modeling allows the generation of many reasonable attack scenarios that can be used in the analysis. In our realization, the statistical threat model has been linked to a battlefield simulation and used to study the performance of a given architecture. Notional results of this analysis are presented in Fig. 17.

The figure presents the number of leakers suffered by the architecture under different attack scenarios, arranged by one particular parameter of the attack (in this case, attack size). Each point on the graph represents the result of one or more scenarios. The analysis was performed on 1000 scenarios generated by the statistical threat model. The parameters that were varied between the scenarios include attack size, attack timing, and attack distribution (launch and impact points). It can be seen from the graph that there is a general trend in the behavior of the defense system—as the attack size increases the number of leakers increases. For

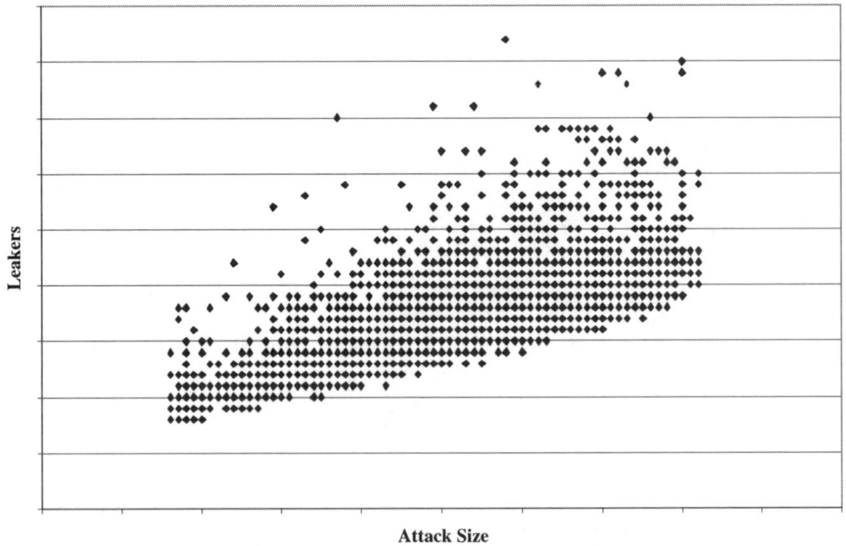

Fig. 17 Example of the use of a statistical threat model.

any attack size there are cases when the resulting number of leakers is higher than for other cases. This is caused by attack parameters other than attack size (e.g., distribution of TBMs between the targets).

Looking at Fig. 17 and the data used to generate the graph, the many possible uses and the amount of information revealed by the use of a statistical threat model become apparent. One possible use is to test for the number of events in which the architecture fails to achieve a certain threshold performance (as is defined in the robustness MOE). Another use might be to identify the points in which a particular combination of parameters causes a severe deterioration in performance (the "spikes" in the figure) and to analyze them in depth.

The issue of systematically describing a many faceted and rapidly changing threat is something that should be dealt with by developers of weapon systems for the future battlefield, both in TMD as in other areas. The approaches suggested here might serve as a starting point for such a treatment.

B. Computerized Tools in Interoperability Analysis

1. Interoperability Problem

The TMD weapon system is characterized as being, in itself, a "system of systems," that is a set of systems (radar, battle management center, interceptors) that work together to perform a specific mission (for example active defense against a TBM threat in the reentry phase). The TMD architecture is characterized from the outset as being a "family of systems," that is, a group of weapon systems, each of which performs a specific defensive mission that contributes to the same overall goal. In our case, the goal is TMD and the missions include passive defense, active defense in boost, midcourse, and reentry phases, as well as counter force. This characterization implies more than mere semantics. Most other defense systems either interact by mutual noninterference (i.e., predefined division of areas of responsibility) or mutual assistance against a set of threats. The level of data-sharing is at most a common battlefield picture. TMD systems are planned for *continuance* of the defense effort against a single threat (i.e., upper and lower tier interception of the same target) and are meant to share (in one method or another) all of the relevant interception information.

This very tight interoperability between weapon systems, both in time and in mission, needs special handling if performed within a single defense force, but especially in a situation of coalition warfare. This situation, in which a defense architecture that has a single mission comprises a number of separate systems, linked by data and/or vocal connections, and sometimes employing a dual command structure, calls for very elaborate definition of intersystem links, and for continuous training. Situations involving coalition warfare bring into the "family of systems" problems related to different command structures and rules, different understanding of the activity going on in the battlefield, and even language barriers. All of this in a system that has to collaborate in an interception process lasting at most only several minutes and sometimes only a few seconds.

2. Interoperability Study Tools

The appropriate use of simulations and computerized tools can significantly contribute to dealing with these issues. The most important of these are human-in-the-loop (HIL) simulations. Our experience in this field is based on running the Israeli test bed (ITB)* in a number of experiments, both with and without coalition (U.S.) partners. The use of a test bed with extensive HIL capabilities to conduct interoperability exercises enables analysis of the aforementioned interoperability issues and an evaluation of various possible solutions. These include coordination assistance tools, threat information sharing (TIS) techniques, roles of operators of the different weapon systems, etc. Any simulators used for this purpose should include adequately accurate representations of all the weapon systems involved, including the HIL capability.

This type of operation can either be carried out through the use of a single, highly complex, simulation, or by connecting a number of specific system simulations through distributed integration simulations/high level architecture (DIS/HLA) (see later section). Working on interoperability in HIL simulations requires several unique analysis techniques, because all of the verbal communication between the systems and all the decision-making processes occur outside of the simulators. For example, in an exercise with human participation the reasons for the failure to intercept a TBM include, in addition to architecture effects (resources, P_k, etc.), the potential impact of the human participants. Leakers can result from wrong coordination, command decision, or faulty operation. It is almost impossible to determine these types of causes using recordings of the simulation because only the performed actions are recorded and not the reasons for the actions. Recording the voice coordination channels provides some assistance for this analysis. However the need to synchronize between the voice and data files and the difficulty in efficiently analyzing the voice channels makes this task virtually beyond the capabilities of a reasonably sized analysis team.

3. *Use of Observers*

An alternative method, developed and used during numerous ITB experiments, involves the employment of trained observers, sitting at key points in each weapon system operating post, monitoring the coordination process while it occurs, including the generation of real-time reports. In this way the coordination between the decision process and the actual events is immediately provided, enabling the analysis of the impact of human intervention on the battle performance. A typical setting of such an experiment is depicted in Fig. 18.

In this case the coordination between two different weapon systems is tested. The command structure of each weapon system battle management center (BMC) includes a commander, various intermediate functions including assistant commanders, work managers and specialized officers, and finally coordinators. The lowest level trained is the execution and coordination level where the actual launch and hold fire commands are performed. There are two different communication links between the two systems. A data link is used to automatically transfer data for the creation of a unified sky-picture. A voice link is used for coordination. The commanders generate policy decisions and guidelines based on the battle picture. These are transferred to the coordinators via the various intermediate functions. The task of the coordinators is to execute the defense based on commander guidelines. This includes coordinating the defense with additional weapon systems if necessary.

The location of the observers is determined according to the analysis goals and is one of the important parameters to be determined during the planning of the

*The ITB is a product of Tadiran Electronic Systems, Ltd., Israel, and is jointly developed and operated by the U.S. and Israeli governments.

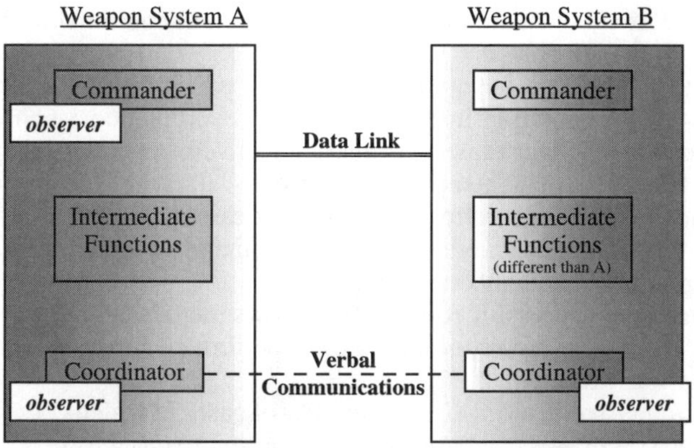

Fig. 18 Typical interoperability experiment setup.

simulation runs. Because the purpose of the analysis (in this example) involves the impact of the commander's guidelines and the coordination on the defense performance, observers are placed at the commander and coordinator levels only.

The observers record the exchange of verbal coordination between the coordinators on each track together with appropriate battle-picture data (track numbers, time, and events). These observers later form a part of the analysis team and can, based on comparison of their notes, direct the focus of the team to specific events, thus avoiding the need for elaborate search among piles of recordings and computer reports. The participants in each experiment are also interviewed about their perception of what transpired immediately after the run, to analyze their situational awareness and gain insight into the possible methods of improving performance. Typically, participants are trained military personnel.*

4. *Interoperability Measures*

In analyzing interoperability, particular emphasis is placed on the measurement of quantities that are significant in determining the effectiveness of the coordination process. The purpose of the coordination process is to generate an appropriate defense plan for each TBM. The appropriate defense plan is not fixed throughout the battle, but changes according to command-level decision making. The commander's decisions are based on battle development parameters including damage actually suffered during the combat, remaining inventory of weapons per ATBM system, intelligence information, etc.

The measures for coordination efficiency should therefore be based on the number of cases (attacking TBM) for which it succeeded/failed in bringing about the desired defense plan. Such measures include the following.

1) Coordination errors are the number of cases where the coordination resulted in a defense plan that was contradictory to the prevailing policy at this point in the run.

2) Timing problems are the number of cases in which the coordination worked correctly, but time line problems prevented carrying out the resulting defense plan

---

*For the development of a large part of this methodology, we are indebted to Dr. Colin Kessel, of PAMAM, Ltd.

(the existence of an adequate timeline for interception coordination is of utmost importance).

3) Operating errors are the number of cases in which the human operator performed the wrong operation in spite of correct coordination (such as pressing the wrong button). This parameter is also indicative of operator inexperience or inappropriate HCI (human–computer interface).

4) Double interceptions reflect the number of cases in which as a result of incorrect coordination or no coordination, more than one weapon system incorrectly launched against the same incoming TBM.

5) Percentage of successful coordination shows the percent of cases (out of all the required cases) in which coordination was performed correctly and the correct defense plan was executed.

It is important to remember that the number of cases in which coordination was required is not set in advance but changes according to changes in defense policy and therefore should be monitored by the observers during the run.

To reach relevant conclusions in these analyses, it is necessary to perform a number of runs with different operators and with different scenarios. In most cases the results are reported as averages over all of the runs performed.

5. Subjective Workload Analysis Tool

Figure 19 depicts another important analysis tool employed in interoperability analysis in the Israeli test bed, the subjective workload analysis tool (SWAT). The SWAT is a measure of the level of workload a particular operator felt during the run. At the end of each run, the participants' reply to a specially designed questionnaire that includes questions about perceived workload and perceived degradation of performance. The SWAT number is arrived at according to the participants' answers. By comparing the SWAT of different command configurations as reported by different subjects performing different functions, it is possible to determine which configuration places the least stress on the operators and what functions

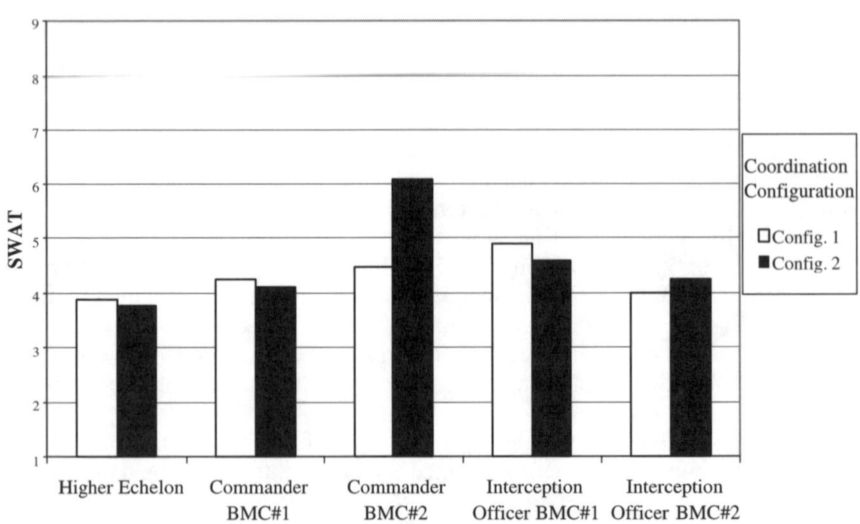

Fig. 19 SWAT example.

need special tools or modified configurations. The final results of a HIL experiment include a combination of the quantitative performance results, observers, reports and the SWAT.

The methodology presented above has been extensively used in interoperability exercises, yielding insights into the proper ways to deal with this complex issue. The types of issues that have been analyzed with this methodology include BMC structure, coordination methodologies, the benefit of various computerized coordination tools and the flow of information within the command structure.

C. Training for Rare Occurrence Threats

TMD systems, once they are deployed, will face a very difficult problem, which is not unique to them, but in this case is manifested in its most severe form. The problem is that it is almost impossible to realistically train the operators of such systems in the performance of their combat tasks. In fact, it is impossible to perform such training systematically at regular intervals.

A number of reasons for this problem may be cited: The enormous cost of the consumed assets (interceptors) during live firing, the lack of "targets of opportunity," and the relative rarity of actual combat conditions (all of these as opposed to, for example, SAM systems). In the first stages of deployment, it will be possible for operational crews to participate in weapon system development tests, but even these are rare, require a unit to drop its alert level including redeployment, and will become rarer as development ends and deployment progresses. All of the aforementioned considerations are even more prominent for the exercising of a full architecture (including interoperable systems).

Simulations, in particular those that include HIL, will form a part of the effort to solve this problem. The requirements from simulations to perform these tasks need to be identified and developed as early as possible.

The major role that wide scope simulations (other than the simulators that are part of the weapon systems themselves) can play in training exercises is that of emulating the other defense systems deployed in the battlefield. Thus, a given unit can train with other (emulated) units of its own architecture, without materially degrading the entire defense architecture's alert level. Alternatively, a unit can train with friendly forces simulatively deployed on the battlefield. To be able to effectively emulate peer weapon systems for actual weapon system coordination, it is necessary to guarantee a uniform "truth" picture using something like the DIS/HLA protocol. In addition, the actual communication system and protocol used by the two systems must be available to the simulations. A simulation used in such an exercise must have all of these capabilities to be valid as a training tool.

Another aspect of using simulations as training aids is the need for a highly qualified team of simulation operators able to support the activities of both the real and the simulated weapon systems. Aspects of communication across long distances (to avoid physically moving various units), remote displays, etc., have also to be taken into account.

D. Impact of High-Level Decision Making

The TBM–ATBM war, fought mostly by remote forces, is strongly affected by decisions made at higher echelons regarding force deployment, ROE, and defense policy. The effect of these high-level decisions on battle results is more easily traceable in a conflict fought mainly by machines than by individual human combatants. This will be true of many of the battles to come in the 21st century, the TMD war being the first example.

Analysis teams working on defense architecture development should not overlook this major influence on the effectiveness of the defense architectures. Both TBM and ATBM systems are agile in terms of the ability to change battle plans quickly, sometimes even in the midst of a single attack, and the effect of such changes should be analyzed. Also, changes in battle plan and operational objectives carried out during the war have an impact on the resulting performance of the weapon systems. Neglecting to include these factors in the simulations and analyses may cause erroneous conclusions. For example, choosing between either launching large numbers of interceptors against early salvos or conserving interceptors for later stages of the conflict can affect the measured effectiveness of the architecture.

Obviously, there are several dimensions to the problem: timewise (real-time decisions vs non-real-time), attacker vs defender decisions, the perception of the enemy's doctrines and plans, the ability to make decisions based on available (rather than "God's eye view") information, etc.

Several approaches to this problem have been tried, each yielding some benefits to the analysis process. No single method that provides all of the answers has been identified. We shall now list the most beneficial approaches and discuss each one of them in brief. However, it should be pointed out that none of them offers a complete solution.

1) Rely on running a large amount of scenarios generated by a statistical tool (as already discussed). Choose the most severe cases (the "spikes" in Fig. 17) and analyze what caused the architecture failure. Determine if decision-maker actions (deployment, ROE) could improve the results. In this approach, the analysis focuses on possible defender responses, whereas the attacker is looked at as "arbitrary." On one hand, this brings to the surface unforeseen situations. On the other hand, the logic that guides the attacker's decisions is not explained and the probability of the occurrence of any such decision or action by the enemy is not addressed. Obviously, this form of analysis can only deal with non-real-time decisions.

2) Include a higher echelon element in HIL simulations (e.g., add a higher echelon unit to the structure depicted in Fig. 18). In this way, the high-level real-time decisions of the defending side may be effectively analyzed. This method is effective only if actual higher echelon personnel (high ranking officers) participate in the training and simulations. This approach has been proven to be very productive to test the defense architecture, but as in the previous method it is problematic if testing of the impact of decision making of the attacker is desired. It is also costly because of the complexity of tools required and numbers and types of manpower required.

3) Insert into an automatic simulation a model to change policy decisions based on clearly defined criteria. This method allows for some flexibility in representing the battle and its results. It also allows treatment of attacker responses, and is relatively inexpensive to implement. However, responses are limited to a few, well-defined situations, and the simulation will make predictable decisions, based on only a small fraction of the data available at each phase of the battle. Otherwise, the

Table 2 Benefits/drawbacks of alternative approaches

Method	Benefits	Drawbacks
Statistical threat	Can test many options Can identify problematic situations Limited expense	No responses to events Limited "sense" to the events
Higher echelon	Can change defender policy in response to events Participation of higher-ranked individuals in study	Participation of "expensive" personnel No attacker decision making complex to perform
Automatic decision making	Can change policies of both sides	Limited, predefined choices
War game	Can change policies of both sides using actual decision makers	Participation of "expensive" personnel Complex to perform

required databases and algorithms become too complex to be manageable within a reasonable amount of time and resources.

4) Use of a two-sided war game. This approach entails the creation of an independent attacker, defender, and management teams. The management team generates a situation and provides the attacker and defender sides with relevant parameters. Each of the two sides makes decisions at regular intervals based on management-provided results and events. The decisions of each side are then fed into a battlefield simulation that generates the battle results. The management team, in accordance with the collection devices available to each side, filters the results of the simulation. This is, obviously, the most complete approach, but it is the most expensive to implement, because of the large manpower requirements, and allows the analysis of only a few, not necessarily representative, scenarios.

None of the approaches just described is definitive, and any analysis should include a combination of methods to enable a wide understanding of the TMD problem. Table 2 summarizes the benefits and drawbacks of the methods described.

E. Simulations as "Systems"—DIS/HLA

The previous sections have discussed a number of important issues in the TMD environment that need to be analyzed using advanced simulations and methods. In many cases, the problems analyzed include a number of weapon systems. It is extremely difficult to create and maintain individual simulations that contain adequate models for all weapon systems operating in a given theater (both own and allied) including HIL, and also include all of the connections between the systems. The limitations result both from the required complexity of such a tool as well as the required level of understanding of all participating defense systems.

There are complete simulations for single weapon systems that are developed for analysis and training. The idea of a protocol that will allow simulations to work together to create a joint representation of a fuller battlefield, seems therefore to be a step in the right direction. It remains to be seen whether this alone will suffice, or whether other measures need to be taken.

For the benefit of readers unfamiliar with the terminology, we shall provide a very simplistic definition of the main terms involved. DIS is a standard communication protocol that allows real-time simulations to maintain a uniform simulated environment, by sending and receiving protocol data units (PDUs). PDUs represent entities (identity, location, status), events (e.g., interceptor launch) and decisions (e.g., hit/miss). By implementing DIS in a set of simulations it is possible to have one simulation provide the threat, another provide TMD systems and yet another provide airbreathing targets.

The HLA is the next phase after DIS in simulation connectivity. It allows also connection of non-real-time tools. In Israel, there is limited experience in using DIS, particularly for large-scale exercises, and so the remarks made here are based on an overview of DIS without considering details and variations of its use. However, a few remarks still seem in order.

1) Work on interoperability between weapon systems requires development of new coordination tools (software) and procedures in all systems that are to interoperate. If a single simulation is used as the main study tool, it is relatively simple to develop the new software and include it in the simulation for testing before implementation decisions are made. If different simulations are used for different systems, the proposed software needs to be implemented in all of these systems, and therefore it must be developed several times (for each system) resulting in increased testing cost.

2) The way most simulation developers cope with the need to communicate with other simulations is by creating HLA "federations" with particular simulations. Other simulations wishing to participate in exercises need to abide by the rules of the earlier defined federation or create a new ad-hoc federation, which involves further work on the communication between the tools. More standardization is required for this trend to become the common practice in simulation development.

Simulations and computerized tools will have a much larger role in development and deployment of weapon systems in the near future. The DIS/HLA approach to connecting simulations is a very significant step on the way to achieve the future goals, some of which were outlined here. We hope that this chapter assisted at least in pointing out some of the issues that should be handled and the ways to approach them.

Chapter 15

Theater Missile Defense Systems Readiness and Training

Karel Pick* and Joseph Zack†
WALES Ltd., Ramat-Gan, Israel

I. Introduction

ANTITHEATER ballistic missile (ATBM) systems, like many military systems, face the problem of having to operate successfully on very short notice after being dormant for long periods of time. Moreover, one of the most important uses of theater ballistic missile defense (TBMD) would be in countering a first strike/surprise attack during the opening stages of a war. Under these circumstances, a long warning time will not be available, and the system may be called upon to act literally within minutes from the first received warning. This implies that once fielded, an ATBM system must maintain a very high level of operational readiness even after years of peacetime. However, there are factors peculiar to ATBM systems that make it difficult to achieve and maintain the readiness level necessary under the aforementioned circumstances.

The most obvious factor, and the hardest to overcome, is the difficulty in training the ATBM units under "real-life" conditions. Most of the time, the ATBM radar will not detect any target. Even if it can be made to detect and track various other targets such as aircraft, this will not correctly simulate the operation of the system against TBMs, because of the large differences in target behavior, mostly trajectory and velocity. Training by exercising the system against TBM-like targets (including firing of interceptors) is limited by the high cost of such practice and by safety considerations. If the interceptors' stock is limited, the training may be reduced to the use of simulators with little actual hands-on experience with the real system. This means that the operation of the defense system as a whole, from radar to battle management and control (BMC) to launcher to interceptor, is very difficult to test. The problems facing the independent operation of the ATBM weapon system are intensified when interoperability with other systems or with allies is considered.

Copyright © 2000 by the American Institute of Aeronautics and Astronautics, Inc. All rights reserved.

*Systems Analyst.

†Senior System Engineer for Advanced Weapons and Technologies. Member AIAA.

The need to train and test the various systems together is usually recognized, but is complex to achieve.

In the following sections several topics affecting the training and readiness issues will be defined and explained: 1) definitions, 2) the impact of a maintenance policy on system readiness and performance, and 3) the impact of human factors on system readiness and performance.

It should be emphasized that while many of these problems are common to all military systems, in the case of the ATBM they are exacerbated by the special demands of ballistic missile warfare: short time constants and the high price of one-shot hardware.

II. Definitions

System readiness is the capability of a defense system to perform its functions when and where required. System readiness is quantitatively composed of the probability to intercept the first TBM attack and the interception effectiveness over the entire attack.

Reliability is the probability that the system will perform as specified at a given time, assessed by mean time between failure (MTBF) hours.

Availability is the probability of performing as specified, during certain time periods, assessed with the help of MTBF, mean time to repair (MTTR) and mean time to test (MTT).

Maintainability is a characteristic of design and installation, expressed as the probability that an item will be retained in, or restored to, a specified condition within a given period of time, when the maintenance is performed in accordance with prescribed procedures and resources (Federal Standards FS-1037C and MIL-STD-188).

Maintenance levels are level O—operational level, level I—intermediate level, and level D—depot/production level.

Testability of a (sub) system is the extent or percentage of circuits or components tested at a certain level during a specific test type.

III. Impact of Maintenance Policy on System Readiness and Performance

It is generally assumed that any periodic maintenance regime, performed at its different alert levels, may be optimized in such a manner that the maintained system is simultaneously at an appropriate technical condition and maximum operational availability. This assumption is a close analogy to the ones applied to other complex weapon system units such as interceptor aircraft squadrons. System availability requirements may be used for the optimization, when the requirement for its maximum availability implies a certain well-defined rate of preventive maintenance actions.

The goal of an optimized maintenance policy is to perform all maintenance and other necessary actions to achieve certain readiness and availability within a given set of constraints (technical and operational). This policy includes testing of certain portions (subsystems) of the system at the O, I, and D maintenance levels.

These maintenance levels are (or should be) consistent with system alert levels in the sense that during the highest alert level (fielded and erected, when we are talking about missiles) the system will be at level O maintenance level with certain

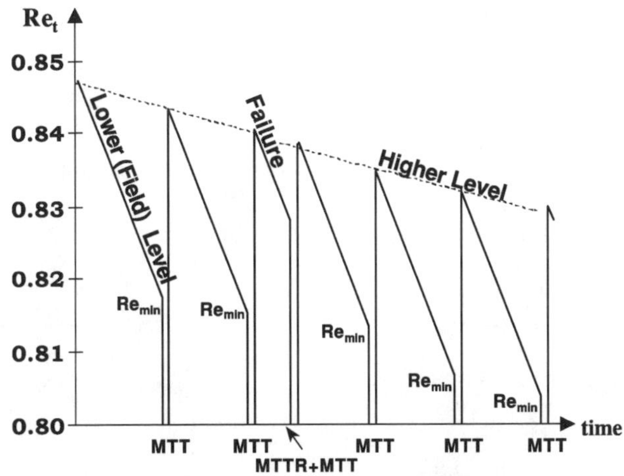

Fig. 1 Typical behavior of reliability in a system that operates periodically: Re_t is reliability as a function of time and Re_{min} is the reliability level before testing (higher than a predefined value).

built-in-test capabilities verifying the system's serviceability. When dormant or at the home base, maintenance levels I or D are applied.

The system's life cycle principles are assumed to be as follows: Immediately after being tested, a subsystem has certain reliability, which is a function of its testability. The reliability of a subsystem decreases exponentially with time (except for certain devices, such as pyrotechnics, which have a fixed reliability, constant with time, of less than one). It is also assumed that at the depot level the system is fully tested, and at the end of the test its reliability is close to one. Typical periodic life-cycle reliability behavior for such a system is displayed in Fig. 1.

The graph in the figure shows a number of system-on runs, separated by MTT time periods. If each system run lasts the same time, then the Re_{min} value decreases with time, where Re_{min} is the reliability level before testing. Note that after a "failure" occurs, the system undergoes repair action and test, both lasting an average MTTR and MTT time period. After a certain number of system runs the system is fully tested at the depot level, and its initial reliability is close to one.

The availability of the system depends on certain system parameters and on the arbitrary decision of how many times during the life cycle the system is stopped (for MTT hours), maintained, and tested. The system's availability may be maximized by the selection of an appropriate number of maintenance actions that yield maximal value of the area under the reliability curve as displayed in Fig. 1. The availability of the system is evaluated as follows.

The system performance expectation $E(T)$ is defined as the expected (average) period of time of actual system operation (statistically evaluated) during a given time period T, the major cycle. This leads to the definition of the system availability A as the average system probability to perform a mission during the given time period T, i.e.,

$$A = \frac{E(T)}{T}$$

This definition introduces the integral

$$A = \frac{1}{T}\int_0^T Re(t)\,\mathrm{d}t$$

where the geometrical meaning is the magnitude of the area under the $Re(t)$ line for $t \in [0, T]$ [$Re(t)$ is the reliability as a function of time and Re_0 is the initial reliability at the beginning of the T].

This formula is developed by means of the minor time intervals, $[t_i, t_{i+1}]$, into

$$A = \frac{Re_0 c}{T}\sum_{i=1}^{n-1}\int_i^{i+1-\mathrm{MTT}} \exp\left[-\frac{t}{\mathrm{MTBF}} + \frac{t_i}{\mathrm{MTBF}_T}\right]\mathrm{d}t$$

Where c is the repair scaling factor,

$$c = 1 - \frac{\mathrm{MTTR}}{\mathrm{MTBF}}$$

Then, implementing the definite integration, one arrives at the following expression:

$$A = \frac{Re_0}{T}\cdot c\cdot \mathrm{MTBF}\cdot\left\{1-\exp\left[-\left(\frac{T}{n}-\mathrm{MTT}\right)\frac{1}{\mathrm{MTBF}}\right]\right\}\sum_{i=1}^{n-1}\exp\left(-\frac{iT}{n\mathrm{MTBF}_N}\right)$$

MTBF_N denotes MTBF of the nontested components (circuits), MTBF_T refers to the tested part of the system. The following expression correlates among MTBF_N, MTBF_T, and the overall system MTBF:

$$\frac{1}{\mathrm{MTBF}} = \frac{1}{\mathrm{MTBF}_N} + \frac{1}{\mathrm{MTBF}_T}$$

As was already mentioned, the availability depends on the number of maintenance actions during the related time period. Figure 2 shows this behavior. It should be mentioned that the choice of the maximum availability is not necessarily the best one. It can be seen from Fig. 2 that with a much smaller number of maintenance actions, the availability is still close to the maximum one.

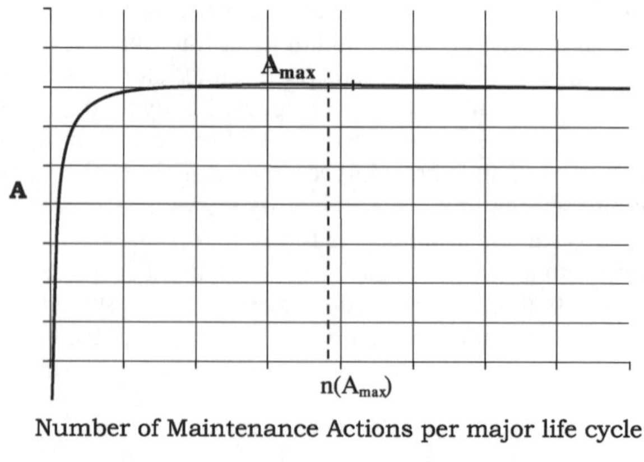

Fig. 2 System availability as a function of the number of maintenance actions.

There exist a certain number of maintenance actions for which the availability is maximal. The maximum point depends of course on the values of MTT, MTTR, and MTBF. These values depend both on technical system characteristics as well as personnel performance. Untrained or tired technicians make mistakes or, even if they don't, the tests and repairs take longer. This issue is discussed in the next section.

IV. Impact of Human Factors on System Readiness and Performance

Human factors may affect the readiness of the ATBM system through a series of mutually interrelated processes.

A. Deployment and Maintenance

The deployment and maintenance process comprises home base preparations, deployment and setup preparations, and infield routine and emergency maintenance actions.

B. Planning the Engagement and the Interception Process

In each process the possible performance degradation of the system due to the condition and skill of the human operators is quantitatively related to specific availability-model's parameters. The intervention of the human operator in defense system actions influences the timing of key processes and the defense plans (see Chapter 7) produced by the system. The impact on system effectiveness is expressed by means of the number of consumed interceptors and the number of leaking TBMs because of wrong decisions or subnominal performance of the technical team. Table 1 presents the effect of technical personnel on system readiness.

The expected impact of the technical personnel abilities is incorporated in the system readiness in the following way: We assume that the system is at its highest alert level and it is continuously controlled by automatic built-in-test (BIT). It is convenient to estimate the minimum reliability (worst case) during a T time period, which includes MTT and MTTR as illustrated in Fig. 3.

Table 1 Technical personnel capabilities effect on system readiness

Mission stage	Task	Possible effect	Affecting
Preparations for leaving home base	Opening and packaging Preliminary testing Preparations for transportation	Mechanical damage Wrong test procedure Lengthy time	Time required to change to higher level
Maintenance in the field	Periodic maintenance Repair maintenance	Mechanical damage Wrong procedure Lengthy time	MTBF MTTR
Maintenance during emergency	Periodic maintenance Repair maintenance Support of mission	Mechanical damage Wrong procedure Lengthy time	MTBF MTTR

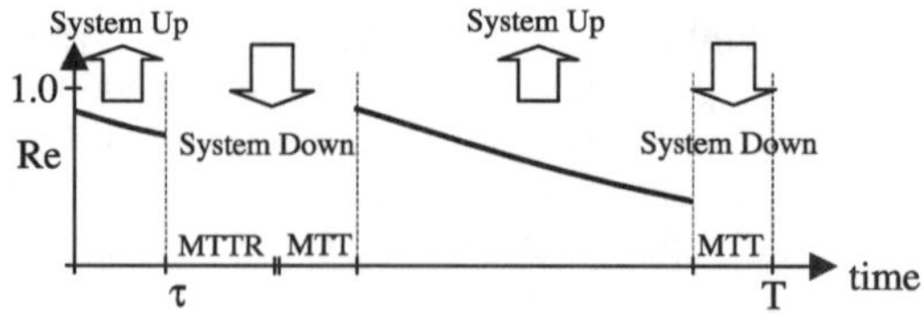

Fig. 3 Model for reliability assessment.

The system's probability to succeed in a mission is based on the hardware reliability and on the reliability of the personnel. The minimum possible reliability, $Re_{\min}(T)$ during T time period including MTT and possible MTTR + MTT (in case of failure, which happens at time instant τ) is given by the following expression:

$$Re_{\min}(T) = \frac{Re_0}{T} \min_{\tau \in (0, T-\text{MTT})} \left\{ \int_0^{\tau} \exp\left(-\frac{t}{\text{MTBF}}\right) \mathrm{d}t + \int_{\tau+\text{MTT}+\text{MTTR}}^{T-\text{MTT}} \exp\left(-\frac{t}{\text{MTBF}}\right) \mathrm{d}t \right\}$$

In the preceding expression the min operator seeks the least reliability in the whole time period T, between two consecutive maintenance tests (one week, one month, etc.), which was determined by the optimized availability process and must be higher than a predefined value.

The changes in timing and in the quality of the various parameters arise from the training level that affects MTT and MTTR. Fatigue and battle load affect the technical personnel performance as well. To illustrate this effect, three performance (and training) levels were assumed for technical personnel: good, intermediate, acceptable (lowest). We assumed that MTBF = 700 h for a particular system, and that it is fully tested once a week. Table 2 presents the system's availability for each technical personnel performance level.

A clear degradation in $Re_{\min}$ is seen when going from "good" to "acceptable" operator quality, demonstrating that human effect on readiness may be significant. $Re_{\min}$, being a measure of the system's readiness, also affects the number of required spares, as follows: if n_N denotes the number of spares of a certain subsystem, then, based on simple probability considerations, the number of required

Table 2 System availability and minimum possible reliability as a function of technical personnel skill level

Technical personnel skill level	MTT, h	MTTR, h	System availability	$Re_{\min}$
Good	1	2	0.86	0.97
Intermediate	2	4	0.85	0.95
Acceptable	4	8	0.84	0.90

spares for this subsystem, n_{spares}, is assessed by the following expression:

$$n_{\text{spares}} \geq (1 - Re_{\min}) \cdot n\_N,$$

where $Re_{\min}$ is the minimum allowable reliability for that subsystem.

To carry out successfully either a simple or a complex activity, a certain level of skill is required. Such skill level, however, is a function of time and training through an initial training course, advanced courses, and periodic refresher courses. Three types of skills are defined, mainly, in reference to the BMC framework of operational actions: psychomotor, procedural, and cognitive. The cognitive skill family may be further divided into two subtypes: skills dealing with situational awareness and skills concerning the quality and speed of decision making.

The following are some examples of such skills as they are manifested in the operational work of BMC operators.

1) Opening of the defense plan and choosing the appropriate action, both relying on procedural skills.

2) Choosing one of the items from the defense plan menu, an action that depends mainly on psychomotor skills.

3) Because of high battle load, disregarding important defense system parameters such as footprints of particular interceptors, inventories etc.

4) Based on good decision-making practices, taking reasonable decisions such as holding fire toward certain incoming TBMs because of a shortage of resources.

The skill levels have typical behavior, which may be summarized by the following statements.

1) Skill level decreases with time.

2) With appropriate training it is possible to regain or even improve the original level of the skills.

3) Repetitive training time is (much) shorter.

4) As longer time intervals elapse between training and operational activity, so is the time required for skill acquisition

5) Procedural skills require longer retraining time then psychomotor skills.

6) Psychomotor skills are easier to learn than other (cognitive).

Further on, and with accordance with appropriate general principles, it is possible to sketch a typical refresher curve. Such curves are given in Fig. 4. It should be noted that Fig. 4 presents a typical graph that does not represent results of any specific system, but rather gives a general idea of the skill behavior.

To construct a human readiness model tailored to reflect the actual parameters of a TMD system, it is necessary to calibrate the theoretical curves just presented, using actual values obtained from system training, courses, or exercises. Defense-system simulators may be used for this purpose, where a number of operators may be trained and tested several times in a periodic fashion. This seems to be a simple plan but it includes a number of very difficult issues, which have to be resolved. Firstly, key activities, which have to be measured, should be identified, and it is to be ascertained that these activities are the ones that mostly affect system performance. Secondly, measures of effectiveness (MOE) must be defined for each activity. These MOE must accurately represent the trainees' capability to perform the measured task. They should also be indicative of the impact that adequate (or inadequate) performance of this task will have on the overall system. The impact

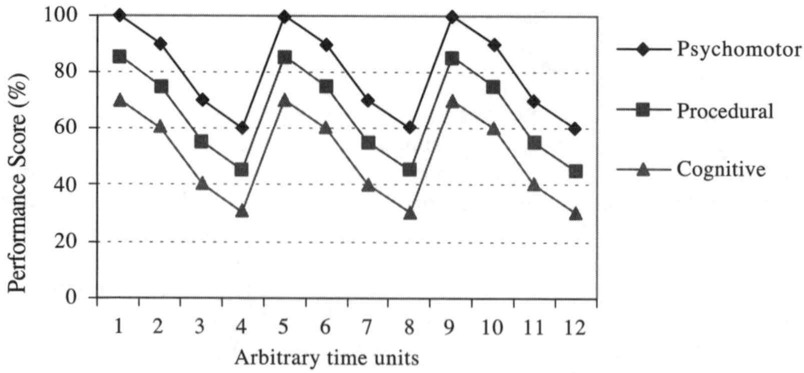

Fig. 4 Typical time behavior of three types of skills.

of the battle load and fatigue on the human performance must also be adjoined to all above human readiness dependencies on the training regime.

V. Overall System Readiness

Finally, the human readiness and the defense system equipment's technical condition should be combined to assess the overall system readiness. The overall system readiness expression may consist of a series of conditional probabilities derived from the readiness and reliability measures already described.

A. Derivation of the System-Readiness Expression Model

The impact of the human factor on the system performance (and vice versa) is quite complex, and their mutual relations are as follows:

1) Under normal conditions, the defense system equipment is expected to perform its functions almost automatically.

2) If the threat exceeds the nominal threshold or if to some extent the equipment fails to perform, then on occasion the human operator is capable of restoring the system's performance to acceptable levels.

3) In any event the operator's readiness level will determine the possible success of such action.

4) There are such events during which the defense system performs successfully its actions even in case of operational–personnel error.

5) Subnominal human readiness may cause overall system failure even if the system's equipment performs nominally.

B. Concept of Conditional Probability

The concept of conditional probability is used when combining human performance with equipment performance. In this context three types of events are defined:

1) System's equipment (such as BMC and radars) performance S is determined by the reliability threshold – $Re_{\min}$.

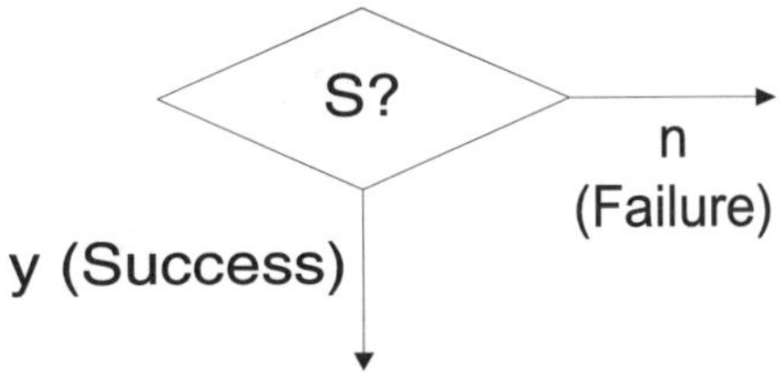

2) Operational personnel activity H reflects how the BMC personnel react to the displayed information. The human operator may succeed in choosing the correct action or may fail.

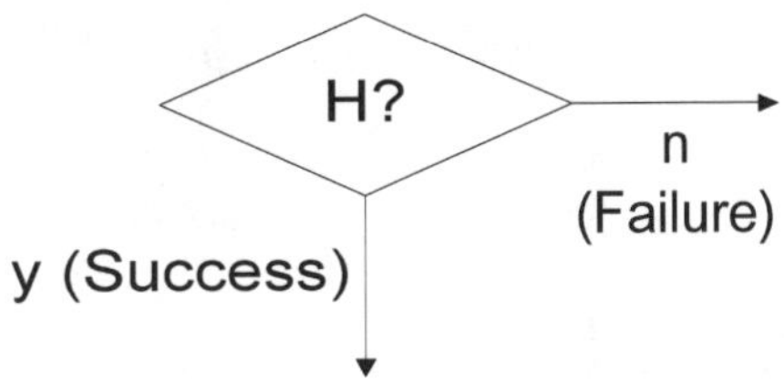

3) Interceptor launch I_{xx}, which may occur or not (when required) with certain probability. It should be noted that an interceptor that was not launched may be a success if that was the right decision. I_{xx} is the probability to correct action of the interceptor depending on the success or failure of S and H. For example: $I_{S\bar{H}}$ is the probability that the interceptor will perform properly when the system performs properly, but the personnel failed.

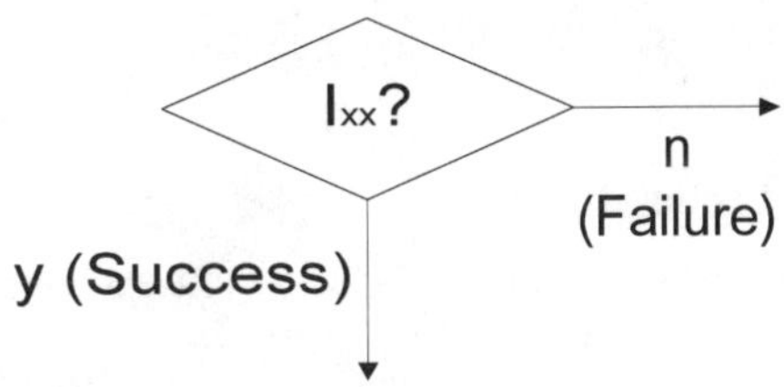

C. Conditional Probability Theory

As was already stated, the overall system readiness is a function of the equipment's threshold (minimum) reliability and the minimum value of the human skill. The exact expression, a convolution of the individual processes, is assessed by means of the conditional probability theory.

D. Battle Management Center Process

The BMC process, consisting of the three events, is integrated in the following chart.

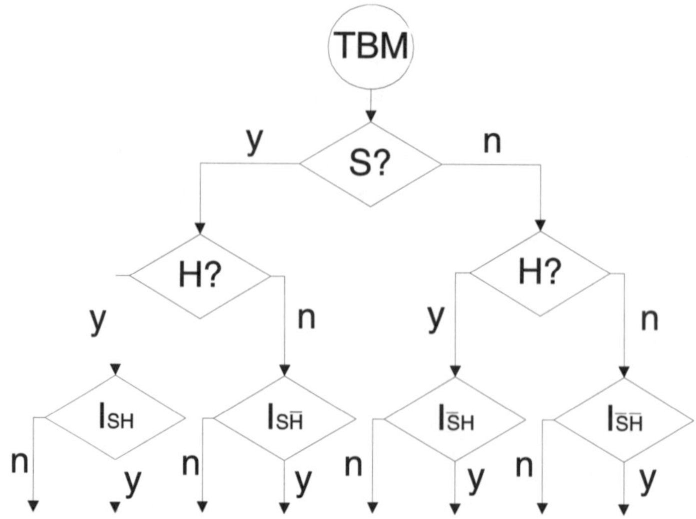

$P(I_{SH})$ $P(I_{S\bar{H}})$ $P(I_{\bar{S}H})$ $P(I_{\overline{SH}})$

Four event paths conclude with positive results, i.e., successful operation of an interceptor. The resulting overall probability, the system readiness *SR*, is a sum of these event paths:

$$SR = P(I_{SH}) + P(I_{S\bar{H}}) + P(I_{\bar{S}H}) + P(I_{\overline{SH}})$$

It is obvious that $P(I_{\overline{SH}})$ (probability of proper performance while both the system and the personnel failed) is negligible, so the system readiness is

$$SR = P(I_{\mathrm{SH}}) + P(I_{\mathrm{S\bar{H}}}) + P(I_{\mathrm{\bar{S}H}})$$

E. Calculation of Probabilities

The calculation of the probabilities is specific to a specific weapon system, and the application to such a system is left to the reader.

VI. Conclusions

The equipment reliability and the human factors issues were discussed with reference to the readiness of TMD systems. To arrive at the overall high-level effectiveness of the defense system and to make the system efficient to the largest possible extent, human activities and the system's procedures must be "properly tuned." This means that maintenance actions and human training actions must follow adequate cycles, which depend on the system's reliability, availability, and maintainability factors and on human factor characteristics, which were outlined in this chapter. Furthermore, this "tuning" must be based on equipment–human interactive relations.

Chapter 16

Development Program Risk Management: Principles and a Case Study

Joseph Z. Ben-Asher,* Joseph Zack,† and Moshe Prinz‡
WALES Ltd., Ramat-Gan, Israel

I. Introduction

THE design of a theater missile defense (TMD) system, being a system-of-systems, poses a great challenge to the system engineer. The challenge rises not only from the technical complexity but also stems from the managerial point of view. The chief architect has to put together a coalition of independent systems with predesigned additional objectives, to operate coherently in a TMD system.

A risk in a system development process is a measure of the uncertainty to comply with a specified requirement. A risk may be technical, programmatic, related to cost, or a schedule risk. Fig. 1 presents typical relations among the risk categories.

Risk management is the set of activities aimed to handle the development risks by tracking, mitigating, or avoiding them, if necessary. The following three preliminary remarks apply to most development programs:

1) There are always risks involved in development processes. The only way to avoid risk entirely is by developing systems using existing technologies, well within the performance envelope of these technologies, and with large funds and flexible schedules. However, a system, either commercial or military, developed along these guidelines will seldom be competitive, either commercially or in the ultimate test on the battlefield.

2) Risk management, although an important and integral part of the development process, is *not* identical to the development process. Major parts of the system can be developed with no risks attached. Nevertheless their development should be managed and controlled as well. The natural tendency to focus the attention to risks, and frequently, to shape the entire development process around them, is a common mistake that may turn nonrisky activities into risk-driving ones in terms of cost and schedule.

Copyright © 2000 by the American Institute of Aeronautics and Astronautics, Inc. All rights reserved.

*Special Consultant; also Associate Professor, Aerospace Engineering, Technion—Israel Institute of Technology. Senior Member AIAA.

†Senior System Engineer for Advanced Weapons and Technologies. Member AIAA.

‡Project Manager; currently with Rafael. Member AIAA.

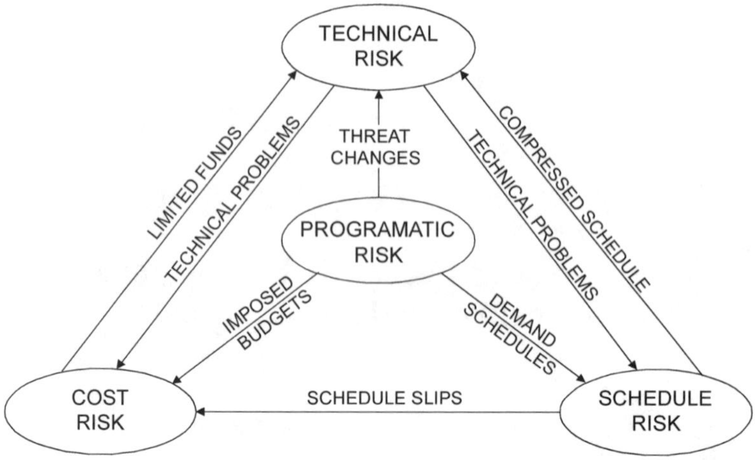

Fig. 1 Main risk components (reprinted with permission of INCOSE).[1]

3) Unfortunately not every risk can be handled by the developers. Programmatic risks, like a change in the threat characteristics in a TMD system development process or a competitive new product in a commercial environment, are typically driven by external causes over which the developer has no real control. One should recognize when this is the case and pursue only the relevant activity, namely, keep close track of all the external developments that may unexpectedly affect a program, possibly culminate in endangering it altogether.

The TMD development process is an excellent example of these processes in action. To start with, because of the basic technical challenges, these programs have to "push the technological envelope" so to speak in a most aggressive manner, and furthermore, necessitate choosing the best technical solution from myriad promising but untried ones.

Secondly, because of the very active nature of ballistic missile technology proliferation, the antiballistic missile (ABM) community has to keep being aware of these developments so as not to be caught short by an unanticipated new technical or strategic development.

Finally, because this field is emotionally volatile and internationally highly charged, the political decision-making atmosphere is unstable. This affects fund allocation. Unfortunately, this is a field of long-term programs, which need stability and steady funding to proceed successfully. Furthermore, in democratic regimes, changes of administration often bring about changes in perceptions and priorities. Expensive risk-fraught defense programs are often the victims of such changes, unless solidly justified strategically and technologically. Risk management thus has a special meaning in the field of TBM defense.

This chapter is organized as follows. In the next section the risk management activities will be described in general terms. In Sec. III various ways of evaluating risk will be discussed and compared. Section IV presents a case study of a risk mitigation phase in a recent development effort, and Sec. V provides concluding remarks.

II. Risk Management Principles*

There are five major steps involved in the risk management process: planning, identification, assessment, analysis and handling.

A. Planning

The aim of the planning process is to define how the risks are to be managed in a program, what procedures will be applied, and who will be responsible for this process.

B. Identification

In the identification step all possible risks are recognized, classified, and listed. To this end, the technical specifications should be taken one by one. A compliance table should be constructed. Requirements that are straightforwardly complied with are not considered as risks. All other requirements, quantitative as well as qualitative, should appear in the operational and technical risks list.

The statement-of-work should be considered next. Time tables should be reviewed and critical paths should be identified. These critical paths, and those paths that are nearly critical, should be carefully reviewed, based on previous experience and expert advice, and if appropriate (i.e., when uncertainty is involved) should appear in the schedule risk list.

Cost estimates should be reviewed along similar lines. Life-cycle cost estimates should be made including all program phases from the preliminary design to the operational use and system disposal. Whenever uncertainty is involved, implying a possible cost excess, a cost-related risk is identified and listed.

Finally, programmatic risks should be considered. Possible future changes in needs, policies, fund allocations, etc., should be identified, and their effects on the program development should be recognized.

C. Assessment

The risk assessment step introduces quantitative and qualitative measures to assess and prioritize the program risks. To this end, two factors are considered. First, the likelihood of the risk, namely the probability of its occurrence, is estimated. Second, the consequences of the risk occurrence, in terms of excessive cost, reduced budgets, reduced performance, etc., are evaluated. Based on these two factors the risk is classified as low, medium, or high. The assessment methods will be detailed in Sec. III.

D. Analysis

The objective of the risk analysis step is to determine, based on the risk nature and classification, the appropriate way to handle the risk. Typically low risks are handled by monitoring only, whereas medium or high risks require specific risk

*This section is based in part on principles summarized in Ref. 1.

mitigation activities or, when possible, risk avoidance (e.g., alternative solutions, changes in the requirements, etc.).

E. Handling

The risk handling constitutes the final risk management step. There may be a designated risk-mitigation phase in the program (as in the example to come), or it may be part of the development program. In the later case, it is important that the risks be tracked, monitored, and/or mitigated as separate identified entities, with well-defined responsibilities and procedures to avoid the danger of hidden or ignored risks.

III. Risk Assessment Methods

As described earlier, risk assessment involves two factors: The probability of its occurrence and the consequences of its materialization. The risk factor determination, required for the risk prioritization and the consequent handling, mixes these two influencing factors.

A. Probability of Risk Occurrence

The probability of the risk occurrence is determined by three factors.[1,2]

1) Maturity factor: A factor reflecting the likelihood of risks caused by exploring new technologies.

2) Complexity factor: A factor reflecting the likelihood of risks caused by the intricacy of the developed system.

3) Dependency factor: A factor reflecting the likelihood of risks caused by dependencies on facility, associate contractors, etc.

In Ref. 2 a risk level (0.1 to 0.9) is defined to each factor, according to its intensity. For example, the complexity factor is varied from a simple design (0.1), through minor (0.3), moderate (0.5), significant (0.7), and extremely complex (0.9) designs. The definitions of the risk levels for the probability of risk occurrence are defined in Table 1, based on Ref. 2.

After evaluating the risk components, the average probability of occurrence can be calculated. The averages can be calculated by using weighting factor for each component.

B. Consequences of Risk Occurrence

The consequences of the risk occurrence are determined by three factors (see Ref. 2): 1) performance factor, a factor reflecting the performance degradation, 2) cost factor, a factor reflecting the cost increase, and 3) schedule factor, a factor reflecting the schedule delay. A risk level (0.1 to 0.9) is allocated to each factor, according to its impact.

The performance factor is considered to be the performance that can be achieved (subject to the risk occurrence), without additional cost and time investments. The cost and schedule factors are estimated to be the additional investments needed to achieve the original spec goals. The consequent levels of the risk occurrence are defined in Table 2. Here again, the average consequences can be calculated by

Table 1 Probability rating of risk

Probability, P	Maturity factor	Complexity factor	Dependency factor
Low (0.1)	Similar design exists	Design is simple or straightforward; trivial interactions between components	No dependency on external resources
Low/Medium (0.3)	Different from an existing design by several well-proven aspects	Level of complexity has grown; some nonelementary interactions between components	Some dependency of the program on external resources that are available
Medium (0.5)	Different from an existing design by several technically feasible aspects	Level of complexity is moderate; integration of the components is a nontrivial issue that requires special attention	Strong dependency of the program on external resources that are available
Medium/High (0.7)	Conceptually new design, based on existing technology	Level of complexity is high; integration of the components is complex and some tradeoffs are necessary	Some dependency of the program on external resources that need to be developed
High (0.9)	Conceptually new design, based on new (state-of-art) technology	Level of complexity is extremely high; integration of the components is a major development effort	Strong dependency of the program on external resources that need to be developed

using weighting factors for each component, based on the accumulated experience in the relevant fields.

C. Risk Factor Calculation

To calculate the risk factor, several alternatives have been proposed in the literature. The most straightforward approach is given in Ref. 3:

$$RF = P \times C \tag{1}$$

where

RF = risk factor
P = average probability of risk occurrence
C = average consequences of the risk occurrence

There are two drawbacks of this approach. The first is equal weighting of probability and consequences. For example, a probability of 0.9 with consequences

Table 2 Consequences of risk

Consequence level, C	Performance factor	Cost factor	Schedule factor
Low (0.1)	No reduction in technical performance; Some inconveniences or nonoperational impact	Risk does not affect the overall budget; reallocation of budgets in the program	Risk does not affect the overall schedule; some changes in activities milestones
Low/Medium (0.3)	Minimal or small reduction in technical performance	Minor increase in the overall cost	Minor slippage in the critical path of the overall schedule
Medium (0.5)	Some reduction in technical performance; degradation of the secondary mission	Small increase in the overall cost	Small slippage in the critical path of the overall schedule
Medium/High (0.7)	Degradation of technical performance; mission success is questionable	Significant increase in the overall cost	Significant slippage in the critical path of the overall schedule
High (0.9)	Significant degradation of technical performance that would result in mission failure	Critical increase in the overall cost (order of magnitude of the original budget)	Large slippage in the program schedule; program continuity is questionable

of 0.1 (high probability with negligible consequences) yields the same risk factor (0.09) as a probability of 0.1 with consequences of 0.9 (low probability with very high consequences). This is counterintuitive. To emphasize this inadequacy, it can be compared with an insurance policy. Insurance is always available for severe consequences with low probability (earthquake, car total loss, etc.), but not vice versa.

The second drawback is that a minor probability (0.3) with minor consequences (0.3) yields the same risk factor (0.09) as a low probability (0.1) with severe consequences (0.9).

Another approach is given in Ref. 2. The risk factor is calculated as follows:

$$RF = P + C - P \times C \tag{2}$$

This expression resolves the second discrepancy, because now

$$\begin{array}{lll} P = 0.3 & C = 0.3 & RF = 0.51 \\ P = 0.1 & C = 0.9 & RF = 0.91 \end{array}$$

and so severe consequences with low probability of occurrence weigh more than moderate consequences with moderate likelihood. However, because of the symmetry between C and P in Eq. (2), the first drawback has not been resolved.

To give higher weight to the consequences one can use another expression:

$$RF = \beta_1 \times P + \beta_2 \times C, \qquad \beta_1 < \beta_2 \tag{3}$$

For example let $\beta_1 = 0.3$ and $\beta_2 = 0.7$, than we obtain

$$\begin{array}{lll} P = 0.3 & C = 0.3 & RF = 0.30 \\ P = 0.9 & C = 0.1 & RF = 0.34 \\ P = 0.1 & C = 0.9 & RF = 0.66 \end{array}$$

Based on practical experience, this approach seems to classify and rank the risks better than the previous methods, and therefore is the one advocated by the present authors.

Remark: Because expression (3) is empirical, it does not cover extreme cases like $P = 0$ or $C = 0$, but these cases are of no interest to us since they do not represent any risk.

To verbally classify the risks as low, medium, or high, we need to define thresholds for the various risk factor ranges. Following Ref. 1, and based on practical experience with technical experts, we advocate classifying $\{0 < \mathrm{RF} < 0.4\}$ as a low-risk range, $\{0.4 < \mathrm{RF} < 0.7\}$ as a medium-risk range, and $\{0.7 < \mathrm{RF} < 1.0\}$ as a high-risk range.

Another approach is proposed by Ref. 1. This approach replaces the single-valued expressions (1–3) with the Table 3. This table produces similar results to our empirical expression [Eq. (3) with $\beta_1 = 0.3$ and $\beta_2 = 0.7$ with the already defined thresholds].

IV. Case Study—IBIS (Israeli Boost-Phase Interception System)

Whereas the previous discussion of risk management may apply to many technical developments, we chose to illustrate the practical side of this concept with an example from the TMD field.

Table 3 Risk factor calculation[1]

Consequences	Frequent (High) $0.7 < P < 1$	Probable (Medium) $0.4 < P < 0.7$	Improbable (Low) $0 < P < 0.4$	Impossible $P = 0$
Catastrophic 1.0-0.9	0.9 (High)	0.7	0.4	0.0
Critical 0.8-0.7	0.8	(Medium) 0.6	0.3	0.0
Marginal 0.6-0.4	0.6	0.4	0.2 (Low)	0.0
Negligible 0.3-0.0	0.3	0.2	0.1	0.0 (None)

A. System Description

A boost-phase interception mission has been studied under a joint American–Israeli effort during the past decade. The concept is based on patrolling constellations of unmanned air vehicles (UAVs) equipped with high-speed interceptors and with infrared search and track systems (IRSTs) that fly over suspected launch areas during crisis times. Launched TBMs are detected and identified by the IRSTs and missiles with the appropriate interception envelopes are launched to hit the TBM before the end-of-boost.

The concept is based on four basic elements: 1) a fleet of UAVs, 2) search and track systems, 3) high-speed interceptors, and 4) battle management, command, control, and communication (BMC^3).

The principle of independence is mandatory in establishing the concept-of-operation. A constellation of UAVs should be able to perform the mission without ground intervention, employing their onboard BMC^3. Moreover, each UAV should be able to perform its mission with no help from the others. For the sake of independence, each UAV is equipped with search and track systems, with the high-speed interceptors, and with a BMC^3 system.

Collaboration among UAVs, however, results in higher measures of effectiveness beyond the simple effect of power multiplication. The merits of collaboration are achieved by several factors.

1) Targets are shared under the common effort, thus avoiding multiple kills.

2) Backups are provided by other members, thus interceptors can be launched from one UAV against a target acquired by another.

3) Intraconstellation BMC^3 (IBMC) with identical algorithms, in each UAV guarantees adequate threat response without ground intervention.

4) The constellation provides multiple redundancy for communication links, both within the constellation and with the ground stations.

5) Target position is dramatically improved by sharing information both in accuracy and in timing (critical for BPI).

Although the mission can be performed autonomously, the ground-based human operator may intervene at any time, changing loitering patterns, rules-of-engagement, or any other mission parameters, including mission abort and return-to-base.

Table 4 Risk factors

Risk no.	*P*	*C*	RF	
A1	0.62	0.77	0.73	High
A2	0.17	0.43	0.35	Low
A3	0.37	0.57	0.51	Medium
A4	0.33	0.50	0.45	Medium
A5	0.57	0.30	0.38	Low
B1	0.57	0.50	0.52	Medium
C1	0.90	0.57	0.67	Medium
D1	0.56	0.60	0.59	Medium
D2	0.78	0.7	0.72	High
D3	0.46	0.60	0.56	Medium
D4	0.57	0.37	0.43	Medium

Work sharing between the human operator and the autonomous BMC^3 is determined following the philosophy of maximal autonomy with minimal necessary human intervention. Thus human control is sacrificed for the sake of efficiency.

The human operator acts mainly through a ground-positioned central battle management and control (CBMC). The main functions of the CBMC are mission planning, mission management and monitoring, coordinating with headquarters and air-traffic control, and debriefing ad training. Additionally, automatic landing and takeoff functions are monitored by a ground control center (GCC) with the responsibility over the UAVs in the airbase and its neighborhood. Figure 2 depicts the BPI system architecture.

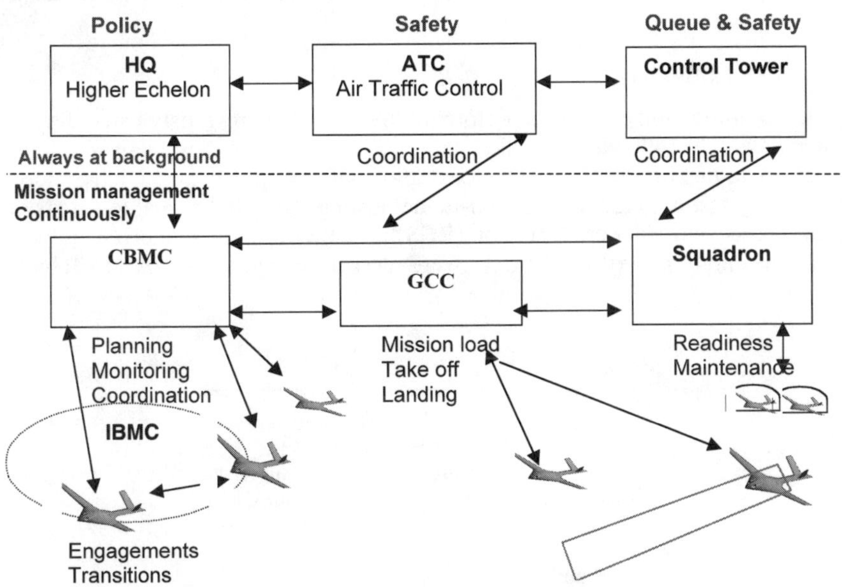

Fig. 2 BPI system architecture.

Table 5 Risk factors

Risk no.	*P*	*C*	RF	
A1	0.46	0.53	0.51	Medium
A2	0.17	0.43	0.35	Low
A3	0.17	0.57	0.45	Medium
A4	0.2	0.47	0.39	Low
A5	0.17	0.30	0.26	Low
B1	0.37	0.52	0.48	Medium
C1	0.63	0.3	0.4	Low
D1	0.28	0.43	0.39	Low
D2	0.22	0.60	0.49	Medium
D3	0.46	0.57	0.54	Medium
D4	0.17	0.30	0.26	Low

B. Risk Assessment

IBIS may be decomposed into four main elements: A, B, C, and D. For each element, one or more risks has been identified by a group of experts. Table 4 contains the estimated figures for the probability of risk occurrence P, the consequence of risk occurrence C, and the resulting the risk factor RF, for the various risks, as estimated by experts to be the case before the risk mitigation effort (risk no. A1 is the first risk associated with element A, A2 is the second, etc.).

As already mentioned, RF was evaluated by

$$RF = 0.7 \times C + 0.3 \times P \tag{4}$$

and the thresholds are $RF > 0.4$ for medium risks and $RF > 0.7$ for high risks.

C. Risk Mitigation

A risk mitigation effort was performed to handle the previously listed development risks. The following were the main risk handling activities: analysis, simulations (including Monte-Carlo), demonstration with computerized model, prototype laboratory testing, high-speed wind-tunnel testing, hot wind-tunnel testing, static rocket tests, and radar cross section (RCS) measurements on models.

At the end of this effort, the risks were reestimated as summarized in Table 5.

Table 6 Summary of risks

	Risk quantity	
Risk level	Start of risk mitigation	End of risk mitigation
High	2	0
Medium	7	5
Low	2	6

D. Results and Conclusions

The results of the risk mitigation program show reduction of the IBIS program risk level, as summarized in Table 6. Notice that no major risk ("high") that can endanger the project was left. The goals of risk mitigation effort have been obtained, and the program can be continued toward more advanced stages.

V. Conclusions

The core of risk management is the risk assessment activity. It is this assessment that determines the risk-handling activities throughout the program. To determine the risk level and to prioritize the risks, one should separately assess the risks' likelihood and the risks' consequences, and then combine them into a single risk factor. The weights should reflect the fact that consequences are emphasized over probabilities of risk occurrence. TMD systems are risk-fraught by nature, hence an appropriate risk management is an indispensable part in their development programs. The case study of IBIS provides a good example to this approach as manifested during its risk mitigation phase.

References

[1]INCOSE, *Systems Engineering Handbook*, Release 1, San Francisco, Jan. 1998.

[2]Blanchard, B. S., and Fabricky, W. J., *Systems Engineering and Analysis* third ed., Prentice Hall, Englewood Cliffs, NJ, 1998.

[3]*Systems Engineering*, NASA Electronic Industries Association EIA/IS-632, Washington DC, 1994.

VI. A Look to the Future

Chapter 17

Future Trends in Offense and Defense

Azriel Lorber* and Ben-Zion Naveh†
WALES Ltd., Ramat-Gan, Israel

I. Introduction

SINCE the inception of the Strategic Defense Initiative (SDI) program, a considerable amount of work has been done in the field of ballistic missile defense by several countries. In fact several systems are at the time of this publication operational or at the stage of an initial operational capability. These include the U.S. PAC-2, the Israeli Arrow weapon system and the Russian S-300 (in its several configurations). Furthermore, several additional U.S. systems are at advanced stages of actual interception testing.

It is safe to assume that the advances in the United States and Israel stem from their recognition of the meaning of the threat and its potential evolution, and from being in the past on the receiving end of ballistic missile salvos. Also, being technologically developed they possess the know-how to develop suitable defense systems.

Surprisingly, in several developed countries, seemingly little consideration is given to the likelihood or necessity of actual deployment of ballistic missile defense (BMD) systems. In these countries the problem is not technological but essentially one of perception.

Both the military and political decision makers view armed forces either as purely conventional ground, air, and naval forces, or see them in terms of massive retaliatory systems, possibly even weapons of mass destruction (WMD): chemical, biological, and nuclear. Conventionally armed ballistic missiles, being neither fish nor fowl are, for the time being at least, almost ignored. The problem of the ballistic missile threat is exacerbated by three other factors. The first is proliferation. Before its demise, the Soviet Union sold or gave away to many countries (mostly in the Third World) considerable quantities of simple, single-stage, liquid-fuel, guided missiles. This was enough to start many of the recipient countries on the path of copying, improving, and manufacturing. As these skills grew so did the

Copyright © 2000 by the American Institute of Aeronautics and Astronautics, Inc. All rights reserved.

*Senior Consultant. Senior Member AIAA.
†Special Consultant and Chief Systems Architect. Member AIAA.

sophistication of the final product, including a change to solid-fuel motors, improved guidance and generally better overall design.

Here enters the second factor. Technology, by its very nature, is in a constant state of flux, continually improving its products. The same of course is true of military technology. Furthermore, much of this technology can be obtained from open sources (and we will just mention the Internet), bought on the open market (from a different version of mercenaries), or studied by almost anybody in the engineering departments at many reputable universities.

Furthermore, in many countries the acquisition of highly sophisticated weapon systems is not always dictated by what appear to us as rational strategic reasons, and it is often carried out on the whim of the current ruler.

The end result of all this is that most of the advanced military technology developed by the industrialized countries sooner or later may find its way into the arsenals of less developed, often irresponsible, rogue, states. (This subject was extensively treated in the past. See for example Refs. 1 and 2.) We consider this process to be an inevitable one in the long run.

When we talk about future trends in the field of military technology, it is somewhat naive to predict the development or fielding of particular technologies or systems. At best we can talk about broad paths, essentially scientific disciplines, and see what potential direction weapon systems might take within that pathway. Furthermore, any forecast we present, hazy as it might be, will be influenced in the future by three additional factors: 1) further development of current technologies, 2) the emergence of unexpected novel technologies, and 3) the reaction of decision makers to the preceding two factors (which we take for granted) and to the global political situation.

From past experience, of one thing we can be sure. If something has a potential as a weapon sooner rather than later it will become one. Thus, in the present chapter we will not go into improvements in particular technologies and will assume that the future will see steady improvements in all of them.

Two additional points. First, it is generally agreed that for myriad reasons all efforts should be made to avoid military confrontations. However, once one is unavoidable it is better to be properly prepared. In fact, just being properly prepared may avert war: *Si Vis Pacem, Para Bellum.* Second, it is obvious that there is no percentage in discussing future trends in defensive weapon systems without describing the threat they are supposed to defend against. The mechanism of threat assessment was described in a previous chapter, and in this chapter the currently perceived trends in the evolution of threat and defense will be described jointly.

II. Some Thoughts About the Future Battlefield

A. Battlefield Use of Ballistic Missiles and the Problem of Accuracy

We will begin by stating that we will not go into the technicalities of achieving higher accuracy. There are many excellent texts on the subject and it will be hard to improve on them here. We will deal with the effect of better accuracy on the usage of ballistic missiles and later with the effect that better accuracy in offensive systems will have on the defense.

Both from the point of view of the strategist and the tactician, ballistic missiles possess several advantages that can be easily exploited. For one, ballistic missiles prove the old truism about the ideal weapon system: "The work of geniuses to be operated by morons." While not really morons, missile operators need not be equal to pilots or even aircraft ground crews, and literally and figuratively they can achieve a lot of "bang" for many fewer bucks. Secondly, at longer than tube-artillery ranges, a ballistic missile's time of flight to any chosen target is extremely short, compared with aircraft or even cruise missiles. This makes them an almost ideal surprise weapon, to be used extensively at the opening stages of a war.

However, the accuracy of many of the present guidance systems of such missiles as the SCUDS and their derivatives leaves much to be desired. It is obviously sufficient if the missile is used as a terror weapon, against population centers in the hands of an unscrupulous warlord, but it is not always suitable as a frontline weapon, except against large concentrations of troops or materiel.

These factors point to the first future major improvement in offensive missile capabilities. Achieving improved accuracy, or in today's parlance, a smaller CEP (circular error probability—the radius of a circle into which 50% of the weapons will fall—serves as a measure of weapon efficiency). If, and when, such improvements will be achieved, they will convert the ballistic missile into a true battlefield weapon capable of hitting small, high-value targets. While this will necessitate much-improved means for target acquisition, the solutions to this part of the problem are in a process of constant improvement because of the requirements of the conventional battlefield. Improved accuracy will enable ballistic missiles to be used as a precision bombardment tool against chosen infrastructure targets, with the expenditure of relatively few resources and without endangering pilots.

Better accuracy will enable smaller (and lighter), more specialized warheads and the attendant gains in range or reduction of overall system weight. In turn, a reduction in weight will make missile systems more mobile, either easier to disperse locally or to be quickly sent as support to a far away ally. While possible improvements in more energetic fuels or novel concepts in motor design will contribute also to lighter missile systems, it is our estimate that these fields have reached, or are about to reach, their technological plateau, and in the foreseeable future their contribution to missile technology will be small. It should be emphasized that the technological level, in all disciplines, of many of the potential aggressors is far from this plateau (mostly defined by the industrialized nations), and they do have yet much leeway to improve their products.

B. Threat of the Accurate Cruise Missile

Up to now, when discussing long-range offensive weapons, the reference points for these discussions were manned attack aircraft and ballistic missiles, the advantages and disadvantages of which were widely discussed in the literature.[3] However the proliferation of sea-to-sea weapons and of reconnaissance unmanned air vehicles (UAVs) and the growing sophistication and availability of long-range navigation systems (global positioning system, for example) are opening the door to conversion of either (or of aircraft) to long-range, unmanned, land-attack systems, in other words cruise missiles. Although in theory conventional air defenses should be able to handle this threat their low, often terrain-masked flight profiles, may present a thorny problem that will require novel thinking and expensive solutions.

C. Warhead Developments

Although a warhead is usually perceived as a hunk of explosive, packaged in a cast iron envelope, the race to achieve better performance for a given investment in money or weight brought about major improvements in this field. None of the developments we will discuss here were used in an actual conflict but most of them were proved on test ranges and can now be found in active arsenals. Basically these new developments consist of three types: bomblets (submunitions), nuclear, biological, and chemical (NBC) warheads, and various forms of penetration aids.

The first of these, the bomblets, were designed to improve the distribution of explosives over the target. While used extensively in aerial bombs and missiles and in the warheads of rocket artillery, as of now no record exists of their use in guided ballistic missiles. This technology has several advantages from the point of view of the ballistic missile user. Individual bomblets are too small to be intercepted by the current antitactical ballistic missiles (ATBMs). Consequently, although (because of the flight environment) paying a huge penalty in weight and accuracy, bomblets dispersing warheads can release their loads early in flight and thus be practically immune to terminal-phase interception. The potential advent of the use of chemical warfare agents makes bomblets almost the configuration of choice, because of problems of agent dispersion from a unitary warhead, which are not insurmountable but degrade efficiency.

Without splitting hairs, in many respects biological agents and their weaponization problems are similar to those of chemical agents. Nuclear warheads on the other hand are inherently large so that, even if employed in a multiple independently targetable reentry vehicle warhead, they are still large enough to be individually detected and intercepted.

Before proceeding to the question of the credibility of NBC usage, we will mention penetration aids. Although not strictly weapons they are usually part of the warhead design and include various Electro-optical decoys, reflectors, and active radio frequency energy generators, designed to confuse the various sensors of the interception system.

D. Potential Use of Weapons of Mass Destruction

The question now turns to the possibility of use of WMD warheads in a future conflict. Chemical antipersonnel weapons were extensively used in World War I by all combatants and since then by many countries. There are huge stocks of various chemical agents and many weapon configurations, including ballistic missiles to employ them, and production of both goes on unabated. In view of the current lenient attitude of the world community to the use of these weapons, it is only a question of time before once again means and intent come together.

One of the proposed solutions to this problem is the concept of deterrence. While admittedly deterrence kept the world's peace (at least in the nuclear arena) for more than 40 years, the situation now developing is inherently different and unstable. For one, some of the new possessors of WMD can be classified as rogue states. This in turn leads to the question of relative values and gains from warfighting, which may be totally alien to the Western (democratic) way of thinking. Furthermore, no amount of condemnation or retaliation will help the initial victims.

So without going again into the pros and cons of the missile defense debate it is obvious that there is a difference in the level of the technological challenge when attempting to counter a conventional threat or a WMD armed weapon. This in essence influences the investment of resources and the question of tradeoffs between various forms of defense and deterrence. This of course is the domain of national security policy and we will not go in that direction here.

So what are the presumed technological directions these defenses will take?

III. Future Trends in Missile Defense

A. Introduction

There are several broad areas where meaningful contributions can be made to antiballistic missile warfare. These are 1) detection and early warning, 2) ballistic missile kill systems including boost-phase interception (BPI) and launcher destruction, 3) improving the self-defense of antimissile systems, 4) increasing mobility, and 5) battle management and interoperability.

B. Future Developments in Detection and Surveillance Systems

In view of the success of satellites in the detection of missile launchings during the 1991 Persian Gulf War, it is certain that this technology will be further expanded into several new areas, as follows.

1) Specialized microsatellites with quick launch capability. With some technological development such satellites might have the capability to detect prelaunch activities. These two attributes, quick launch and improved technology, will answer the problem of satellite vulnerability to hostile action and will enable better surveillance of suspected areas during times of tension.

2) Increased observation efforts of "nonfriendly" missile system production, launches, testing, and exercises. This will be done by means of satellites and other collection means. Even more important will be pooling this data between more of the concerned nations.

C. Ballistic Missile Kill Systems

Without doubt this is technologically the most challenging area, but also the one with the potential for the largest dividends, because, to a large extent, successful developments in this field may compensate for shortcomings in early detection and even for mediocre battle management and control of the defenses.

Destruction of theater ballistic missiles (TBMs) is based today almost solely on antimissile missiles of various kinds. Additional work (for future applications) is being performed on high-energy laser beams (the airborne laser, ABL) and in the past some effort was put into the development of a hypervelocity gun system as a local, last-ditch defense.

Some work was also performed on concepts involving UAVs or even manned aircraft that will haunt suspected TBM launch areas and destroy them at their moment of greatest vulnerability, during the boost phase. (In fact, the ABL just mentioned belongs to this category.) An added bonus (or a consolation prize, as the case might be) is the potential for destroying the launcher itself and its support equipment, even after the launch of the missile itself.

While the BPI systems are relatively simple technologically (this is in essence an air-to-air attack against a highly radiating target), its global realization is fraught with geographical and (consequently) political difficulties. The ABL, because of its weapon's considerably longer range, is more suited for this mission, but on the other hand its price tag is somewhat daunting. It has, however, better chances to come to fruition because of the potential spinoffs from this technology and the other uses to which such a system can be put, in addition to fighting missiles.

The growing proliferation of TBMs, both in terms of the number of states having them and the variety and numbers of missiles in the hands of potential aggressors, may lead to the danger of saturation and overwhelming of any single layer or multilayered defense system. Performance of the individual defensive missile systems will have little bearing on this problem because it will be one of sky-picture, debris, and fratricide. To solve this, the volume of the battlespace will have to be increased, possibly by an order of magnitude, to enable longer engagement times. This means an increase of its altitude or along the flight path of the incoming threat. However, because times of ascent to such altitudes and distances will be excessive, it seems certain that because of necessity, the idea of space-based defenses (high-energy, kinetic, or explosive) will be resurrected.

While not strictly a part of the "kill mechanism," one additional attribute of the ATBM will probably be improved to a considerable degree, to enable a successful "kill." This is the capability to discriminate between the warhead and its attendant decoys or other masking systems. It should be pointed out that this capability is quite distinct from the technology of detecting the incoming missile itself. Suffice it to say here that both the technology of the hardware and the various algorithms for performing this task are really still in an embryonic stage and can be vastly improved.

D. Improving the Self-Defense of Antimissile Systems

Because TBMs are going to grow in importance in any future military confrontation or large-scale terrorist attack, the aggressor will be well aware of the important role of the ATBM defense systems and their potential to undo his schemes. The steadily increasing number of available weapons will enable any aggressor to direct a heavy attack against the defense systems themselves (in a form of a latter day Pearl Harbor). If successful, the target country will be stripped of the means to defend its population and infrastructure, and the military's offensive and retaliatory components might be compromised to an irreversible degree.

While ATBM assets can be ringed by enough defensive missiles, to protect them against any such conceivable attack, in many respects this is a wasteful approach. A shorter range (and smaller footprint), less expensive weapon might be a better answer. We will not presume to predict whether this will be a hypervelocity gun or some updated version of a laser weapon or any other concept. However, it is self evident that the ATBM assets will need considerably better and less costly self-defense, and some solution is bound to be introduced.

E. Increasing Mobility

While today's battlefields are far from static, the ones of the future will be characterized by even more mobility and the so-called sparse battlefield. As already mentioned, increasing real-time target acquisition capability and increasing accuracy of offensive missiles will make them dangerous to high-value targets, and even to small mobile formations.

In principle this can be solved in two ways. One of them is to make any missile defense system have such a wide footprint that it can cover any conceivable area of military operations from a few chosen locations within the boundaries of the country. Without going too deeply into technical issues, it seems that such an approach will be terribly wasteful, have inherent problems of battle management, and probably will be impossible to implement against short-range weapons that will be the biggest menace against the targets to be defended.

One of the truisms of mobile warfare is that all parts of the force have to have similar mobility, otherwise the force is reduced to the rate of movement of the slowest component. To provide defense for mobile operations will require ATBM systems with similar movement capability, meaning high-speed movement on the ground, extremely short travel-to-deployment times and possibly even some capability to be air lifted by tactical transport. While the technical problems of this approach can be argued, at least for the present, we are certain that the requirements of the future battlefield will bring about this evolution.

F. Battle Management and Interoperability

Although in this book three different chapters were devoted to these two topics, in many respects they are two sides of the same coin. Battle management strives to integrate the different components of the defense system, the sensors, the decision making, and the weapons into a single coherent entity. Interoperability tries to integrate different weapon systems into a synergistic force. Interoperability may stem from attempted cooperation between different systems of the same military or from cooperation between different countries' armed forces.

Technical compatibility between systems (communication protocols, computer programs, and even the shape of electrical plugs) should not be considered simple when discussing interoperability. But the real problems in such instances are those of intracommunications among the personnel involved, of all ranks, starting with language barriers and nuances of language, and ending with questions of national pride, different war goals, and different priorities.

As ATBM systems mature and are widely exported, the use of similar systems will bring more technical cooperation. Of necessity, this will lead to mutual exercises between recipient countries with the major contributors of the hardware and software, or, if politically acceptable, with armed forces with more experience in ATBM operations. Such exercises and cooperation will contribute immensely to all concerned because it will allow cross-fertilization of ideas and improved technology and procedures.

IV. Conclusions

The aforementioned enumerated advances in the capabilities of both ballistic missiles and ATBM defense systems will evolve from two major sources. In general these technologies will be driven by real or perceived threats to national security and the conclusion that improved weapons (of either type, as needed) can solve the problem. It is obvious that in western countries the present emphasis is on defensive systems, from the National Missile Defense in the United States to the Israeli Arrow. Furthermore, all of these defensive systems are based on novel and evolving technologies. From the anti-missile-missiles to high-power lasers, both ground-based and airborne. It should be borne in mind, though, that for the time being defensive systems carry a considerably larger price tag, and so necessities will be tempered by the availability of resources.

For obvious reasons, most of the Third World is concerned more with offensive systems. However, because of their inferior scientific and technological infrastructure, these countries are more interested in mastering existing technologies available to the superpowers. It should be remembered though that in most of the regions of interest in this respect, even the introduction of old technologies constitutes a step function in local capabilities, and in many cases is the first step on the way to creating an indigenous industry of sophisticated weapons. With the application of sufficient resources this may lead to almost anywhere.

References

[1]Lorber, A., "TBM Proliferation Control—Fact or Fiction," AIAA 4th Multinational Conference on Theater Defense Technologies and Applications, Washington, DC, March 1991.

[2]Rubin, U., and Levite, E., "Missile Saturation and Missile Defense," AIAA 13th Multinational Conference on Theater Missile Defense, June 2000.

[3]Lorber, A., "The Missile Threat Against Israel" "*Ballistic Missiles, The Threat and the Response*," edited by A. Stav, Brassey's, London, 1999.

Chapter 18

Concluding Remarks

Alik Hermetz*
WALES Ltd., Ramat-Gan, Israel

I. Introduction

THIS book marks an important milestone in the ongoing development effort of active defense against ballistic missiles. This notion, that incoming missiles can be actively shot down, originated in fact in the navies when the vulnerability of ships to guided (sea-to-sea) missiles was first realized. It slowly percolated into the thinking about the defense of other valuable targets and culminated in the initial research efforts of the Strategic Defense Initiative. Trouble was that shooting down (by whatever means) the extremely fast reentering warhead of a ballistic missile bordered, for a long time, on science fiction. Bringing a defensive missile to the vicinity of an attacking warhead was described as "hitting a bullet with a bullet." Actually the problem was even harder to solve. A typical bullet, after all, moves only at about Mach 2.5. An incoming warhead moves at Mach 6 and more, and although the problem was initially broached at the end of World War II, it was obvious to all (and remained so for many years) that the technology was not yet mature enough to tackle this task. Some later solutions to this problem depended on nuclear weapons to knock out incoming missiles. However, because of the realization that the cure was not much better than the disease and the evolution of political intercourse between the two blocks these efforts too essentially died out.

The ever-increasing proliferation of tactical ballistic missiles finally brought things to a head in 1991. Although ballistic missiles were used before, it was in local wars in the Third World, and none of the industrialized nations really worried about that. However, the 1991 Persian Gulf War (Desert Storm) changed all of that. Scores of SCUD missiles (and their Al-Hussein derivatives) were fired against population centers in Israel, causing some casualties, and against Saudi cities, causing there numerous casualties to U.S. personnel. However, the Patriot air defense missiles, hastily pressed into antimissile service, failed to intercept them. This failure exposed many basic problems in the technical design and furthermore in the overall system thinking about ballistic missile interception. Being a totally

---

Copyright © 2000 by the American Institute of Aeronautics and Astronautics, Inc. All rights reserved.

*President and Program Manager, Israeli System Architecture and Integration. Member AIAA.

new field, most of these problems were never before properly addressed, even on the theoretical level.

II. Technological Considerations

It turned out that ballistic missile interception is considerably more complicated than originally thought. It is a truly interdisciplinary effort and the development of its technology involves many fields of engineering, operations research, and other fields of science. To start with, the pointed end of the threat (so to speak) was not anymore a conventional high-explosive bomb but potentially a chemical, biological, or even nuclear warhead. While the world lived under the nuclear threat for several decades, the situation after 1991 was markedly different. For one (and unlike the conditions during the Cold War) the potential adversaries were not necessarily responsible and careful governments. Second, several regimes with access to ballistic missiles had a previous history of using chemical weapons both against their foes and against their own populations. So the technical (engineering if you will) problems of ways and means of totally destroying such warheads, both unitary and bomblet carrying ones, had to be solved.

This led to a constantly increasing sophistication of the interceptor warhead. But the relatively high price-tag of the various interceptors precluded expenditure of too many weapons against each target. This in turn led to the question of "warhead kill assessment," which became much more important and furthermore, had to be answered in real time (during an actual engagement) and not later at the projected impact point.

Since this effort could not be kept under wraps it had to be assumed that the potential adversaries (whoever they might be) would do their best to overcome the defenses. This brought up the much-involved problems of decoys and their effects, both on the incoming warhead's capabilities (weight and volume) and the defense's effort, and the questions of the adversary's technical (indigenous or purchased) capabilities in advancing and further developing such concepts. This question was compounded by the fact that several other countries (some of them technologically more advanced) actively engaged in long-range missiles, occasionally selling their wares to whomever was willing to pay. This in turn brings up the question of a reliable threat assessment. On the one hand correctly appreciating the real threat, but without sliding into a panicky, knee-jerk response of preparing for doubtful threats. Although such a course of action may seem prudent, it should be remembered that in today's cash-strapped defense budgets, too prodigious an expenditure of resources undoubtedly will affect other defense requirements, which may be no less critical. (The development of the atomic bomb was initiated because of erroneous information and misinterpretation of German activity.)

The technical questions of the interception itself pose other problems. While a large body of research and literature exists about the interception of various airborne targets, from sea-skimming missiles to supersonic aircraft, all of it deals with basically slow targets, up to approximately Mach 2. The problems involved in the interception of small targets, travelling at Mach 6 and more, were not just a question of extending the scale (the velocities of the target and the interceptor). In essence these were new problems of different substance, pushing on occasion the performance envelopes of the various disciplines such as aerodynamics and maneuverability, materials, sensors, electronics, and computing. Furthermore, with the new interception systems, which are to perform above most of the Earth's atmosphere, this is akin to space operations, with their technological challenges.

III. Defense of Assets

Up to now we discussed essentially technological questions, but the defense of a country against ballistic missiles also involves less tangible questions (some of them concerning ethics and public opinions) which are harder to test in the laboratory or even in a simulation. These questions, and the needed research to answer them, grew out of the requirement to defend the maximum of assets, both of population and of war fighting capabilities, and involving questions of technical capabilities vs geographical distribution of the various assets. Furthermore, it should be remembered that even now there is more than one antimissile system, with various capabilities. A successful and efficient integration of the various systems, considering the various threats and various adversaries, can reap useful operational and economic dividends.

A corollary to this problem is the possibility of future coalition warfare or at least the support of the antimissile defense by an ally with possibly different systems and probably different doctrines. There is also the problem of multinational space assets, both for early warning and for threat trajectory computing and updates. Because of the short time constants in any missile-against-missile engagements, the smooth and quick meshing of the various components of such a combined effort is both important and elusive.

Finally there is the problem of battle management. With regard to conventional air defense this problem is not new and some of its fundamental tenets were established back in the 1930s. However, when dealing with antimissile defenses, this problem acquired several new twists, never before encountered. The first grew up from the very high speeds of the threats and the fact that the interceptors are rocket propelled with no loiter capability. This means that interceptor launch windows are extremely narrow and thus the timing of the launch has to be exact, with little margins. Furthermore, in contrast to traditional air defense, each interceptor (and sometimes more than one) has to be assigned specifically to a particular threat. All this in an environment (possibly) cluttered with decoys and various other counter measures that must be quickly resolved by long range sensors. Furthermore, because there are no humans at the point of actual combat who can contribute their input as the battle is evolving, all decisions and control are performed on the ground, sometimes scores of kilometers away. Although human control and the ability to intervene are retained, the overall physical aspects of the engagement have to be managed by powerful computers.

In traditional air defense, numerical odds can be manipulated and affected (to some extent) by training and quality of the defending pilots and their equipment (consider the Battle of Britain experience). In antimissile defense, however, and even assuming a perfect, up-to-specs operation, to a large extent this is a straight, quantitative, one-to-one exchange. This poses an additional burden on the defense because, at least for the time being, and disregarding potential damage on the ground, defensive assets are costlier than many of the threats. On the other hand, in contrast to traditional air threats, most, if not all, current missile threats fly in fixed trajectories during the reentry phase that, once determined, will also point at the potential targets. An efficient battle management system will be able to grade threats according to their potential danger and use defensive assets so as to maximize their effect. Finally, the fast pace of such an engagement will have a decisive effect on the degree of centralization or decentralization of the battle management structure, which in turn will decide the required assets, amount of redundancy, communication networks, and sophistication of the computing systems.

IV. Role of this Book

This book was written by professionals whose job it is to look at the different problems posed by this new battle environment, analyze them, and attempt to find suitable answers. For two reasons this is a continuously ongoing effort. First, the threat itself is constantly evolving because of the widening proliferation of offensive weapon systems and the growing technological sophistication of the weapons themselves. Second, the continuous development of the various defense technologies requires a constant readjustment of the various components of the defensive system so that the overall system will be well balanced and be able to utilize its capabilities to maximum effects. The book itself is intended for both the technical community and for decision makers. In the new environment of high-tech warfare, no single person is capable of mastering all of the myriad technologies involved in a major weapon system. Thus the aim of the book is to present some of the technical questions in such a manner that workers from different scientific disciplines can understand the problems (and solutions) of their coworkers. Without exception this will contribute to a more efficient product. The decision makers will benefit by understanding some of the more esoteric problems in a critical battlefield, the complex solutions involved, and by inference, some of the political and economic complexities involved.

No comprehensive single text, giving an overall view of all aspects of the problem, and dealing both with technicalities of high-speed interception and some of the intangibles of such combat scenarios, was published before. Much of the work that eventually led to the current state of the art in missile defense, presented in this book, was previously presented at the annual AIAA International Conferences on Theater Missile Defense. The various authors of this volume acknowledge their debt to this solid foundation laid down by many years of patient work. It should be realized that while this book represents the most recent work on the subject, this is not the final word in this field. As pointed out before, the threat is constantly evolving both in scope and in magnitude, and consequently the thinking and technologies intended to thwart this threat have to keep up.

V. Final Comments

No book can cover all aspects of such a complex problem. Consequently the material presented here constitutes only a sample of the store of knowledge in this field. Furthermore, for obvious reasons not all of the material can be openly discussed. We trust that this initial sample will in turn lead to more publications, both contemporary and archival, on the various aspects of this important field. We believe that by itself the wider dissemination of this knowledge contributes to the deterrence effect, and so all this know-how will never have to be utilized in practice.

Appendix A

Extant Systems for Theater Ballistic Missile Defense

Eitan Yariv* and Azriel Lorber†
WALES Ltd., Ramat-Gan, Israel

FROM essentially a science fiction concept ("hitting a bullet with a bullet") and through an ambitious research program (the Strategic Defense Initiative), which became a political football, the idea that a ballistic missile can, and should, be intercepted and destroyed by less than a nuclear warhead slowly gained ground. The failures (or almost successes) of missile interceptions during the 1991 Persian Gulf War finally brought two facts home to the decision makers. Tactical ballistic missiles are a growing menace, but one that can be countered with a reasonable amount of technological investment.

The last 10 years saw a tremendous growth both in the political will to discuss the necessity of such systems and to commit the required resources to this purpose. Consequently, during this period several systems, and the thinking about their employment, matured to the point where they are either actually operational, like the American Patriot, the Russian SA-300, and the Israeli Arrow, are on the verge of being operational or are at an advanced state of development.

This appendix lists these systems, the general thinking behind their design and concepts of operation, and their important technical and operational characteristics. As already described, only operational, near-operational, and systems that are under development, but that are technologically mature, are included. We may add that if the current pace of technological advancement will continue, the number of such systems, in all categories, will increase dramatically.

Copyright © 2000 by the American Institute of Aeronautics and Astronautics, Inc. All rights reserved.

*Team Leader, Interoperability, External Cueing, and Concept of Operations. Member AIAA.
†Senior Consultant. Senior Member AIAA.

Table A1 ATBM weapon systems

Missile system	Tier	Deployment	ATBM interceptor types	Radar/sensor	BMC	Guidance	W/H	Seeker
Patriot PAC III	Air defense and lower tier missile defense	Land based colocated remote launchers point defense sector of 120-deg	**GEM** against SRBM **Erint** against MRBM	**MPQ-53** C-band Detection Tracking FCR	**ECS** for FU **ICC** for battalion	TVM Active	HTK + Lethality enhancement	RF Ka-band electro-magnetic active seeker
AEGIS NAD Navy area defense	Lower tier	Sea based 360-deg	**Standard SM2 Block IVA** against SRBM, MRBM	**AN/SPY-1** S-band Detection Tracking FCR	**ACS**	**Inertial + Semiactive**	HE fragments	Imaging IR seeker
AEGIS NTW Navy theater wide	Upper tier outside the atmosphere	Sea based 360-deg ascend/descend phase	**Standard SM-3 LEAP** kinetic kill vehicle against MRBM LRBM	**AN/SPY-1** (improved) S-band Detection Tracking FCR	**ACS** AEGIS combat system	Active with uplink corrections from the FCR	HTK with kinetic kill vehicle	IR + RF seeker

THAAD theater high-altitude area defense	Upper tier outside and inside the atmosphere	Land based	**THAAD** against SRBM MRBM LRBM	**GBR** 120-deg X-band detection tracking FCR	**TOC**	Inertial with FCR directions via uplink + self IR homing	HTK with kinetic kill vehicle	IR
AWS Arrow weapon system	Medium tier outside and inside the atmosphere	Land based	**ARROW II** against SRBM MRBM LRBM	**Green Pine** L-band detection tracking FCR	**Citron Tree**	Inertial + FCR updates via uplink + self IR homing	HE directed fragments	IR + RF
FSAF SAMP-T Aster	Lower-tier	Land + sea based	**Aster 30** SRBM air defense	**ARABEL MFR 360-deg** I.X.KU-band detection tracking FCR	**EM**	Inertial + FCR updates	HE Blast fragments	Active RF J-band
ABL airborne laser	Boost-phase	Airborne onboard 747/400	Direct energy against MRBM LRBM	**IRST**	**Airborne FCR** and director	Direct energy	N/A	N/A

(*Cont.*)

Table A1 ATBM weapon systems (Continued)

Missile system	Tier	Deployment	ATBM interceptor types	Radar/ sensor	BMC	Guidance	W/H	Seeker
S-300 V PMU SA-10/12	Lower tier	Land based	**Grumble** against SREM MRBM	**36N85** I-J band 9S19 search **9S32-1** detection tracking FCR	**Baikal NPO 83M6E2**	Inertial + command uplink updateds TVM	Directed fragments	Semiactive RF Possible active RF seeker
MEADS	Lower tier	Land based	**ERINT** against SRBM Air defense	**APAR C-band**	**BM3**	Inertial + TVM + Active	HTK + leathality enhancement	RF Ka-band electro-magnetic Active seeker
HAWK	Lower tier	Land based	**PIP III** against SRBM air defense	**TPS-59** L-band **IHPI MPQ46** illuminator for tracking	**PCP FDC ICC**	Semiactive	Fragments	RF Semiactive

Table A2 ATBM early warning and cueing systems

Warning system	Deployment	Accuracy	Sensor	Notes
DSP defense support program	GEO stationary spaced based + ground segment 360-deg	Low; track only boost phase prediction of trajectory after end of boost	IRST	In use
SBIRS Low	LEO 20–30 cross linked constellation of satellites + ground segment 360-deg	High; with tracking updates from boost phase and during all trajectory	IRST	Development
SBIRS High	GEO Synchronous orbit satellites + Ground segment 360-deg	High	IRST	Development
GBR	Land based 120-deg	Very high	Radar X-band	In use
Pave-Paws AN/FPS-115	Fixed land based 360-deg	Very high	Radar UHF	In use
Cobra-Dane AN/FPS-80	Fixed land based 120-deg	Very high	Radar UHF	In use

Appendix B

Persian Gulf War—Intelligence, Early Warning, and the Home Front

Benny Michelsohn*
WALES Ltd., Ramat-Gan, Israel

I. Introduction

THE Al-Hussein is a road-mobile descendant of the Soviet SCUD-B, the first modern tactical ballistic missile that dates from the 1950s. The Al-Hussein is a single-warhead, Iraqi-constructed missile that is made from the parts of several Soviet-supplied SCUD-B missiles. The missile's inaccuracy and limited payload restricted Iraqi use of the Al-Hussein in both the Iran–Iraq and Gulf Wars to striking large urban targets and population centers.

The Iraqi Al-Hussein—or SCUD—medium-range ballistic missile was a key coalition target during the Persian Gulf War. The United States used a large number and variety of national and tactical intelligence assets to support the coalition targeting effort against the Iraqi missile force. U.S. reconnaissance satellite reporting provided extensive support to military operations and bomb damage assessments. One important asset used to detect Iraqi missile launches was the defense support program (DSP) satellite, a missile warning vehicle equipped with infrared sensors to detect launch ignition or the rocket plume of a missile during flight.

The DSP satellite monitored missile launches from its 35,000 km geostationary perch by means of a scanning infrared (IR) telescope, capable of 3-km resolution. The satellite relayed the SCUD missile's IR plume signature to a ground controller who undertook target discrimination, a process occupying some 2 min of the SCUD's 7-min flight time.

The missile's trajectory, timing, and expected impact area were then relayed via communications satellite to alert Patriot batteries in Saudi Arabia and Israel, and provided early warning to the entire Israeli population.

In addition to satellite systems, a high percentage of quality coalition aircraft were used to search for mobile missile units. Surveillance of suspected Al-Hussein operating and launch areas helped to appreciate missile activity and launches and passed collated information to F-111, F-15, F-16, and A-10 fighter aircraft. Key

Copyright © 2000 by the American Institute of Aeronautics and Astronautics, Inc. All rights reserved.

*Senior Consultant, Intelligence and Operations.

platforms such as the airborne warning and control system (AWACS), the TR-1 (the descendant of the U-2) and the E-8A joint surveillance target attack radar system (JSTARS) were involved in the effort to try and locate the Al-Hussein launchers. It also was reported that British and U.S. special operations forces were inserted behind enemy lines to help locate and target mobile missile units.

Despite this level of effort, the Iraqi mobile missile forces were extremely difficult targets to locate and destroy. Based on Soviet practices, the missile force is subject to some operational practices that are designed to promote its survivability. For the Al-Hussein, these included long-duration field deployments, frequent and prompt relocation following launch, reload and refire capability, and extensive deception techniques including camouflage and concealment. Iraqi operational practices successfully degraded U.S. intelligence performance during the Persian Gulf War, despite the aforementioned reconnaissance effort to locate the mobile launchers.

Furthermore, other concealment and deception techniques were used. Al-Hussein launches usually occurred at night, under the cover of darkness. Coalition reconnaissance assets missed the few launches that did take place in the early morning hours under cloud cover to minimize detection. The Iraqis also adeptly used dummy launch sites. Some sophisticated dummy sites, for example, used heat generators to simulate active missile engines. The Iraqis also constructed a network of drive-through trenches that might have served as dummy hide positions. Metal plates and a layer of camouflage netting covered these sites, most likely intended to confuse U.S. targeting efforts. The metal plates probably were intended to simulate hide positions for missiles or missile-related equipment, thereby attracting and wasting U.S. fire assets.

Iraqi use of strict communications security during missile launch procedures might also have complicated coalition-targeting efforts. The coalition expected to be able to intercept radar signals during the final stages of launch preparations, which would be tipped off by the release of weather balloons to collect meteorological data for trajectory calibration. Instead, the Iraqis evidently maintained complete radio silence. The lack of electronic signature suggests that the Iraqis might have relied on the use of previous missile launch data instead of balloons for final calibration.

Surprisingly, the desert background also complicated U.S. efforts to detect mobile missiles. A number of Gulf War commentators assumed that the Al-Hussein's desert surroundings would facilitate missile detection, especially compared with the problems posed by the forested terrain in Europe. Although the desert offers a less-canopied terrain in which to hide mobile missiles, the Iraqis successfully complicated coalition targeting efforts by making the most of their surroundings, typically by using broken ground and isolated groves of trees to provide cover. Destroyed vehicles and equipment also complicated detection by providing additional clutter. U.S. Gen. Norman Schwarzkopf and others noted that pinpointing mobile launchers in the desert was like the proverbial search for a needle in a haystack. Obviously, requirements for wartime targeting and peacetime arms control monitoring differ greatly in terms of the type, specificity, and timeliness of information required. Thus, the Al-Hussein forces managed to evade even the most sophisticated of U.S. intelligence detection and targeting capabilities.

It should be pointed out however that the use of intelligence assets to support targeting appears to have helped the coalition suppress the missile threat, although not one launcher was identified and destroyed during the entire war. An initial Iraqi average of four Al-Hussein launches per day was reduced to an average of one per day after armed reconnaissance patrols were increased in the second week of the war. The coalition's inability to halt Iraqi missile launches, however, reflects the difficulties associated with locating the mobile targets.

The hunt for Iraqi SCUDs in the Gulf War represents the first time a modern intelligence infrastructure was used to target mobile missiles in a wartime environment. The U.S. intelligence community apparently lacked familiarity with the doctrinal, organizational, technical, and operational details of the Iraqi missile systems. A Pentagon report to the U.S. Congress on the Persian Gulf War indicated that the intelligence profile on Iraqi mobile missiles and other equipment was prepared from scratch during the mobilization period for Operation Desert Shield. The intelligence community focused on collecting information about Iraqi weapons research programs, missile capabilities and characteristics, and military facilities only after August 1990.

Furthermore, during operations Desert Shield and Desert Storm, the intelligence community was unable to establish the exact number of Iraqi mobile launchers and missiles. U.S. intelligence agencies estimated that the Iraqis had 30 fixed launchers, more than 20 mobile launchers, and from 300 to 1000 missiles at the outset of the war. Estimates that during the war were proven as totally inaccurate.

Despite a focused targeting operation that used a substantial number and variety of intelligence resources to detect Iraqi mobile missile launchers, the outcome of the coalition effort was mixed. Iraq continued to launch missiles against Israel and Saudi Arabia, albeit at a diminished rate, throughout the duration of the war.

II. Threat Against the Civilian Population

While the extent of the failure of the coalition's antimissile campaign was not anticipated, the threat, based on the previous erroneous numbers, was perceived as real and imminent. Events and public statements in the Middle East during the summer of 1990 aggravated particularly the chemical warfare threat against the civilian population centers in Israel. The development, stockpiling, and use of chemical munitions by Arab countries had reached alarming proportions. Iraq, in its war against Iran, had employed a variety of chemical agents disseminated from aerial bombs and artillery shells. Intelligence reports and newspaper articles portrayed a production capability encompassing a wide range of chemical warfare agents, from relatively innocuous tear gases, through persistent mustard gas, and up to the most dangerous nerve agents such as Tabun and Sarin. All of these agents were weaponized and could be delivered by SCUD missiles against civilian targets. After the war, UN inspections in Iraq have shown that these intelligence reports were both true and understated.

Thus, the increased scope of chemical warfare capability in the Middle East, coupled with its proliferation and use during the Iran–Iraq War and threats in the summer of 1990, caused concern for the well-being of the Israeli civilian population in event of an outbreak of hostilities. The Civil Defense Organization has recognized the reality of the chemical warfare threats and this threat generated a response, based mainly on earlier preparations and coupled with short-term innovations, directed toward the protection and continued functioning of the civilian sector under chemical attack conditions. Furthermore, by negating the effects of such a threat, a good chemical warfare (CW) defense posture may serve as a deterrent to potential aggressors.

The effectiveness of chemical munitions depends to a large extent on whether the population has been warned of an imminent attack, and has taken various protective measures, including the use of personal protective equipment. The total flight time of an Al-Hussein missile from western Iraq to Tel-Aviv is less than 7 min. The alert time that we could expect was 3–4 min before the missile's impact. In fact, during the war the measured alert times were 1.5 min at the beginning and 5 min at the end of the war. For such (anticipated) short alert times, what we wanted to achieve was maximal dispersion of the population with good protection against possible chemical attack. The use of public shelters requires 15–20 min, and concentration of the population in them seemed to expose them as big targets.

Adequate alarm systems, sufficient protective equipment, and proper training of both the civilian population and dedicated emergency response teams can reduce casualties to a minimum. Accordingly, the civil defense units and emergency response organizations (police, fire brigade, and paramedics) must be equipped and trained to continue operations in the face of chemical contamination and the accompanying casualties. This assessment has guided the civil defense community in developing the doctrine and equipment necessary to combat the threat of chemical munitions.

III. Operational Concepts, Doctrine, and R&D

The operational concepts and requirements, which guided the civil defense community before Desert Storm, resulted in a vast R&D program and the subsequent decision to procure and distribute protective equipment to the entire civilian population. Consequently, Israel became the first country in the world to distribute antichemical warfare kits to the whole population.

The distribution of over five million protective kits before the start of hostilities generated additional requirements for special equipment for certain segments of the population, including those with medical and respiratory impairments (severe heart condition, emphysema, tracheotomies, etc.) Consequently, the omnipresent CW mask has "evolved" into a variety of devices intended to answer the needs of the following: 1) people with special facial feature such as severe scars, very narrow or very wide faces and bearded people (most of the orthodox religious people), 2) infants in incubators, and 3) children.

This equipment had to be developed, produced, and distributed in only a few months' time. The result was a round-the-clock R&D effort highly integrated with the production process. These efforts resulted in the design, development, and production of the following items: 1) an adult hood/blower system for individuals with tracheotomies or unusual faces, 2) a blower kit that could be attached to the CW mask thus compensating for poor fit or medical/respiratory impairments, 3) a blower kit for infant incubators with a battery operated power pack, and 4) a small portable infant protective crib (ages 0–6 months) equipped with a (battery powered) blower overpressure system.

In addition a personal medical treatment package, a "first-aid kit" concept based on an individual autoinjector, which allows the individual to save himself until professional medical personnel arrive on the scene. Admittedly, during the war, in some cases these kits were misused by individuals who did not understand their purpose.

In addition, the population was directed to seal a room in dwelling places. When the alarm was sounded, they were told to enter that room, seal the entrance, put on their masks, activate the radio or TV set in the room and follow the instructions provided via the public media.

The integrated CW defense doctrine was based on two principles: Survivability of the civilian population and continuance of mission of the relevant civil defense and emergency response personnel. Continuance of mission is an important element of the civil defense doctrine. All relevant civil defense and emergency response personnel should be able to continue to fulfill their tasks and missions while under chemical attack environment. The implementation of this doctrine imposes a number of additional "protective layers" on the personal and unit levels. For their use additional means were developed.

1) Simple, effective detection systems that determine both the existence of an agent and when the danger has abated. These included detector tickets with a miniature blower, "chase" detectors, and hand-held detectors. These systems and their operational deployment resulted in rapid and foolproof determination of the absence (or presence) of chemical agents.

2) Decontamination systems.

3) Equipment and training for medical treatment in hospitals.

The preceding capabilities, when fully integrated into the operational doctrine unique to each unit, would result in minimal casualties under missile attack conditions. In addition, deployment and utilization of specialized units (reconnaissance, bomb disposal, and decontamination), complement these elements and provide greater flexibility in coping with unexpected situations, which were encountered during the hostilities.

Preliminary thinking about the chemical threat started in the late 1960s, before the Six Days War. Over the years this approach to integrated and comprehensive civil defense doctrine has resulted in the definition of operational and technical concepts necessary for the research and development of antiballistic missiles civil defense systems and equipment.

These concepts were defined with the participation of the R&D community, relevant industries, and the civil defense and emergency response community. It was an interaction, resulting in the continual evolution of both doctrine and equipment, and providing a firm basis for rapid, short-term tailored responses in case of new threats. As a result, the equipment produced and procured for the 1991 crisis was several generations better than the original-issue equipment of the 1960s.

IV. Battle Damage Assessment

A. Israel

Missile impacts resulted from 33 Al-Hussein missiles and from five Al-Highara missiles (The Stone—an Al-Hussein missile with a concrete warhead).

Casualties were tabulated as follows. A total of 14 dead: two killed directly by missiles, five fatal heart attacks and seven deaths caused by misuse of protective equipment. A total of 450 injured: 228 wounded directly by missiles and 222 unnecessary Atropine injections (most of them on the first attack). In addition, 530 individuals required treatment for fear and anxiety.

Other damages in Israel included the evacuation of population from damaged homes (1,242 from Tel-Aviv and 697 from Ramat-Gan). Damage to buildings was tabulated as 6142 flats (of which over 200 were totally destroyed), 1302 buildings, 23 public buildings, 200 shops, and 50 private cars.

B. Saudi Arabia

Although several missiles were fired against Saudi targets, one in particular did considerable damage. A hit on a U.S. forces dormitory in Dhahran in late February 1991 resulted in 28 deaths and about 100 injuries.

Appendix C

Author Biographies

Haim Baruch*

H. Baruch obtained his B.A. in social studies in 1978 from the Bar-Ilan University, in Ramat-Gan, Israel. He is a reserve officer (Lt. Col.) with the Israeli Air Force where he is involved with work on C^3 systems, a field he also practices in WALES Ltd. as a senior expert.

Abraham Baum

A. Baum obtained his B.Sc. in mechanical engineering from the Technion, Israel Institute of Technology, in Haifa, Israel, in 1973, and in the year 2000 was awarded a B.A. at the University of Tel Aviv. He started as a designer in the IAI, was the manager of research projects in IAI/MLM, headed the Arrow–Target project, and currently is the manager of R&D for IAI/MLM.

Joseph Z. Ben-Asher*

J. Ben-Asher received his B.Sc. in aerospace engineering from the Technion in Haifa in 1978 and an M.Sc. (1986) and a Ph.D. (1988) in aerospace and ocean engineering from the Virginia Polytechnic Institute and State University. J. Ben-Asher is an associate professor at the Department of Aerospace Engineering at the Technion, Israel Institute of Technology, in Haifa, Israel, and a special consultant to WALES Ltd. His interests include systems engineering, optimization techniques, missile guidance, optimal control theory, and flight dynamics. J. Ben-Asher has published extensively, including another book published by AIAA in the Progress in Astronautics and Aeronautics Series, on missile guidance, which was coedited by I. Yaesh.

Dror Cohen*

D. Cohen holds a B.Sc. in mathematics from the Technion (1992). He is married with two children. Since 1994 he has been president of WALES Ltd. His primary fields of activity are operations research and analysis of military systems. He presented four papers at the AIAA Multinational Conferences on Theater Missile Defense.

Reuven Eyal*

R. Eyal holds a B.Sc. in aeronautical engineering from the Technion in Haifa (1966). He served as a pilot and retired from the Israeli Air Force as the head

*Lead author.

of IAF Intelligence with the rank of brigadier general. For many years he was involved in threat assessment and strategic research and evaluation. He is now senior threat and operations analyst with WALES Ltd. He has published numerous research papers (many of them classified) on these subjects, including three papers for the AIAA Multinational Conferences on Theater Missile Defense.

Nathan Farber*

N. Farber received his B.Sc. (1966), M.Sc. (1974), and Ph.D. (1981) in aeronautical engineering from the Technion in Haifa. He worked in IMI in the fields of ballistics, aerodynamics, and propulsion. During the years 1993–1996 he was employed as chief scientist of the Rocket Systems Division at IMI. N. Farber has published several AIAA papers (including for the Multinational Conferences on Missile Defense) and NASA reports on applications of differential games to the analysis of air-combat problems. His interests include flight dynamics, operations research, and guidance and control. Since 1996 he has been employed as senior systems engineer at WALES Ltd.

Moshe Guelman*

M. Guelman was educated at the Facultad de Ingenieria de Montevideo, Uruguay, and received the Diplome d'Etudes Approfondies (1967) and the Docteur en Electronique (1968) from the Faculte des Sciences, Universite de Paris. M. Guelman is a professor at the Faculty of Aerospace Engineering and head of the Asher Space Research Institute in the Technion in Haifa, Israel. He was previously with Rafael (Israeli MOD) in different capacities in the general fields of aerospace systems guidance and control. In periods of leave of absence he worked, among others, at the International Satellite Organization, Washington, D.C., and the National Aerospace Laboratory, The Netherlands. M. Guelman originated Israel's concept of boost-phase interception for missile defense. He has published extensively in the open literature, is a member of the Committee on Astrodynamics at the International Astronautical Federation, a corresponding member of the International Academy of Astronautics, and is a recipient of the prestigious Israel Defense Award. Since 1997 M. Guelman has served as a special consultant to WALES Ltd.

Ayala Gur*

A. Gur received her B.A. in physics from the Technion in Haifa (1987) and is now completing her M.E. in systems engineering. She served in the Israeli Air Force, attaining the rank of captain. Her last position in the Air Force was as test manager of the IAF test range. She is now with WALES Ltd. as senior systems analyst. She published (as principal and coauthor) seven papers at the AIAA Multinational Conferences on Theater Missile Defense.

Alik Hermetz*

A. Hermetz has a B.Sc. in industrial and management engineering (1977) and an M.A. in public policy (1988), both from the University of Tel Aviv. After a distinguished career he retired as a colonel from the IDF. He then worked (at IAI/MLM) as deputy program manager of the Arrow missile program. Since 1995 he has been president of WALES Ltd. and the program manager of the Israeli System Architecture and Integration study. A. Hermetz served on a variety of planning and consultation committees advising the IMOD, the Knesset (Israeli parliament), and various government ministries. During his military service he authored numerous papers on topics of strategy and long-term planning.

Ronia Lapid

R. Lapid ended a 29-year-long career in the IDF (final positions as the commander of the Air Defense Forces of the Israeli Air Force) with the rank of brigadier general. He holds a B.A. in economics (developing countries) and political science from the University of Tel Aviv (1968). He worked for El-Op Industries as director of corporate strategic planning and as director of marketing administration. Since 1988 he has been executive vice president of WALES Ltd. and heads the Israeli test-bed experiment and analysis team in this company.

Elie Levy

E. Levy holds a colonel's rank in the Israeli Air Force reserves (last regular assignment was an airbase commander) and now is vice president for systems engineering at WALES Ltd. He is a graduate of the Technion in aeronautical engineering (1963) and obtained there his M.Sc. in the same discipline in 1969. His areas of expertise are armaments, missiles and rockets, telecommunications, and space systems. He is a frequent lecturer at the AIAA Multinational Conferences on Theater Missile Defense.

Azriel Lorber*

After service in the IDF [last rank, major (R) armor corps], A. Lorber received a B.S. in mechanical engineering from the University of Pittsburgh (1961) and an M.S. in aerospace engineering (1963) and a Ph.D. in aerospace and ocean engineering (1974) from the Virginia Polytechnic Institute and State University. He worked in the IAI, IMI, and the private sector, and served as principal assistant to the director general of the Ministry of Science and Technology. A. Lorber is now with WALES Ltd. He published extensively (including three books) on military technology, as well as several papers at the AIAA Multinational Conferences on Theater Missile Defense.

Benny Michelsohn*

B. Michelsohn started his military career in 1968 and served as armor officer during the Attrition and Yom Kipur Wars. He later transferred to the intelligence branch, rising to the rank of full colonel and fulfilling a variety of assignments. He ended his active military service as chief of military history in the IDF. B. Michelsohn is a graduate of the IDF C&GS College, holds a B.A. in military history (1987) and an M.A. in military and diplomatic history (1994) from the University of Tel Aviv, and is a member of the board of the Israeli Society for Military History. In his civilian career he has worked as director of marketing research for the IMI, is a consultant to the IMOD, and is a visiting professor at the Japanese National Defense Academy and a lecturer at the IDF C&GS College. Now he is with WALES Ltd. as a senior consultant on intelligence and operations. B. Michelsohn publishes and lectures extensively on intelligence and national defense topics.

Aron Moss*

A. Moss obtained his B.Sc. in aeronautical engineering in 1959 from the Technion in Haifa. He received an M.S. in aerospace engineering from the

Polytechnic Institute of New York (1963) and a Ph.D. in management sciences from the University of Paris (1972). He is the director, international programs and cooperation and concurrently he is the director, ballistic missiles defense cooperation office, both in the Directorate of Defense R&D in the Israeli MOD. A. Moss is the recipient (for 1995) of the AIAA David R. Israel Award for Meritorial Achievement in the Area of TMD.

Ben-Zion Naveh*

B. Naveh obtained his B.Sc. and M.Sc. in aeronautical engineering from the Technion (1959 and 1962) and a Ph.D. in aeronautical and mechanical engineering (1975) from the University of Notre Dame, South Bend, Indiana. In 1959 B. Naveh started working in Rafael (Armament Development Authority) and in 1978 was appointed its managing director. In 1982 he was appointed head of research, development, and infrastructure in the Israeli MOD. Later he joined and managed several nonmilitary advanced technology companies and is now with WALES Ltd. as special consultant and chief systems architect. B. Naveh has published extensively and authored a book on management of high-tech companies; he is the recipient of the Israel Defense Award.

Dan Peretz

D. Peretz received a B.Sc. in civil engineering (1967), an M.Sc. in mechanical engineering (1969), both from the Technion and a D.Sc. from the School of Engineering, Washington University, St Louis, Missouri, in 1971. He worked as a researcher and consultant in the United States and Israel and taught at the Technion and at Texas A&M University. D. Peretz worked on warheads at Rafael and was director of the armor-anti-armor center there. Since 1990 he has been with IAI/MLM where he worked on the Arrow warhead and systems and currently is the director of the Arrow program. He publishes extensively on materials, warheads, and lethality and missile technology. D. Peretz is the recipient of awards for excellence in teaching from the Technion and for excellence in performance from Rafael and the IAI. In 1998 he received the *Aviation Week and Space Technology* award for Outstanding Performance in Aeronautics and Propulsion, and in 2000 he received the AIAA David R. Israel Award.

Karel A. Pick*

K. Pick holds a Ph.D. in physics/atmospheric sciences from the University of Tel Aviv (1991). He worked in weather forecasting, R&D in meteorology and climatology, operational weather prediction, meteorology for weapon systems, and test ranges and environmental risks. Current interests encompass operations research, weapon systems human-in-the-loop, test range safety and fire danger rating system development, test planning, and geodesy. K. Pick retired from the Israeli Air Force as a lieutenant colonel, and is now with WALES Ltd., doing system analysis and operations research. He is a member of the Israeli chapter of the International Test and Evaluation Association and the Israeli Meteorological Society.

Moshe Prinz

M. Prinz obtained his B.Sc. (1966) and M.Sc. (1973) in mechanical engineering from the Technion in Haifa and a Ph.D. in mechanical engineering from Stanford

University (1986). He held the positions of project manager and chief engineer of air-to-surface missile systems at Rafael (IMOD) and program manager of the Israeli boost intercept system at WALES Ltd. M. Prinz is now deputy general manager for strategic planning, marketing, and business development of the missile division at Rafael.

Yair Ramati*

Y. Ramati obtained a B.Sc. in aeronautical engineering from the Technion in 1976, completed his military service in the IDF Air Force (last rank major), and concurrently obtained an M.Sc. in aeronautical engineering (1980) from the Technion. From 1982 he has been with the IAI/MLM where he has worked in the areas of system engineering, guidance and control, and testing. He was the Arrow program manager, director of advanced programs, and currently he is the general manager of IAI/MLM. Y. Ramati is the recipient of the AIAA David R. Israel Award.

Uzi Rubin*

After serving in the Artillery Corps of the IDF, U. Rubin received his B.Sc. in aeronautical engineering (1962) from the Technion and an M.E. in aeronautical engineering (1962) from the Rensselaer Polytechnic Institute, Troy, New York. U. Rubin fulfilled a variety of engineering and management positions, including design and test engineer at the IAI, assistant director, R&D Directorate, IMOD, head of the SDIO Cooperation Office in the R&D Directorate, IMOD, codirector of a study on missile proliferation at the CISAC at the Stanford University, and head of the Israel Missile Defense Organization (IMDO). Currently he is the senior director for proliferation and technologies in the Israeli National Security Council. In 1996 U. Rubin received the Israel Defense Award and is the 2000 recipient of the AIAA David R. Israel Award. He published numerous papers on missile technology and is a frequent lecturer at the AIAA BMD conferences.

Josef Shinar*

J. Shinar received his B.Sc. (Summa Cum Laude) in aeronautical engineering from the Technion in Haifa (1959), a degree of Maître és Sciences Aéronautiques (avec nention "Trés Bien") from the École Nationale Supérieur de l'aéronautique in Paris (1963) and a D.Sc. in technology from the Technion (1973). From 1959 until 1974 he served as an R&D engineer in the Israel Air Force, retiring with the rank of lt. colonel. Since 1974 he has been with the faculty of Aerospace Engineering in the Technion where he is currently Max and Lottie Dresher Professor in aerospace performance and propulsion. In the years 1990–1993 he served as the dean of the faculty. His research interests include missile guidance and avoidance, aircraft trajectory optimization, and application of differential game models for air combat and missile guidance. Recently he has focused his research on theater missile defense.

Isaac Yaesh

I. Yaesh received his B.Sc. in electrical engineering from the Technion and an M.Sc. (EE) and a Ph.D. from the systems department at the University of Tel Aviv. He worked as a research engineer at the IDF and is currently with the advanced systems division of the Israeli Military Industries, heading the department of control simulations and aerodynamics. His interests include robust H_∞ control and estimation and differential games and their applications. I. Yaesh has published extensively and coauthored with J. Ben-Asher a book on missile guidance, also published in the AIAA Progress in Aeronautics and Astronautics Series.

Eitan Yariv

E. Yariv retired from the Israeli Air Force as chief of the Air Defense Corps with the rank of brigadier general. During the Persian Gulf War he was recalled to active duty and served as deputy commander of the A.D. Corps. He holds a B.A. in history and mid-east studies from the University of Tel-Aviv (1982) and an MBA from the University of New Haven, Connecticut (1998). At WALES Ltd. he is leading the team studying interoperability, external cueing, and concept of operations.

Joseph Zack

J. Zack obtained his B.Sc. in electrical engineering from the Technion in 1959. He worked as an electronics engineer for the IDF and the IMOD and later was deputy chief engineer of IAI/TAMAM (Precision Instruments Industry). In 1984 he moved to IAI/MLM as chief of the Directorate for Advanced Technologies and later headed the Arrow program. In 1992 he was named deputy general manager of IAI/TAMAM. In 1996 he joined WALES as senior system engineer for advanced weapons and technologies.

Author Index

Subject Index

PROGRESS IN ASTRONAUTICS AND AERONAUTICS SERIES VOLUMES

***1. Solid Propellant Rocket Research (1960)**
Martin Summerfield
Princeton University

***2. Liquid Rockets and Propellants (1960)**
Loren E. Bollinger
Ohio State University
Martin Goldsmith
The Rand Corp.
Alexis W. Lemmon Jr.
Battelle Memorial Institute

***3. Energy Conversion for Space Power (1961)**
Nathan W. Snyder
Institute for Defense Analyses

***4. Space Power Systems (1961)**
Nathan W. Snyder
Institute for Defense Analyses

***5. Electrostatic Propulsion (1961)**
David B. Langmuir
Space Technology Laboratories, Inc.
Ernst Stuhlinger
NASA George C. Marshall Space Flight Center
J. M. Sellen Jr.
Space Technology Laboratories, Inc.

***6. Detonation and Two-Phase Flow (1962)**
S. S. Penner
California Institute of Technology
F. A. Williams
Harvard University

***7. Hypersonic Flow Research (1962)**
Frederick R. Riddell
AVCO Corp.

***8. Guidance and Control (1962)**
Robert E. Roberson
Consultant
James S. Farrior
Lockheed Missiles and Space Co.

***9. Electric Propulsion Development (1963)**
Ernst Stuhlinger
NASA George C. Marshall Space Flight Center

***10. Technology of Lunar Exploration (1963)**
Clifford I. Cumming
Harold R. Lawrence
Jet Propulsion Laboratory

***11. Power Systems for Space Flight (1963)**
Morris A. Zipkin
Russell N. Edwards
General Electric Co.

***12. Ionization in High-Temperature Gases (1963)**
Kurt E. Shuler, Editor
National Bureau of Standards
John B. Fenn, Associate Editor
Princeton University

***13. Guidance and Control–II (1964)**
Robert C. Langford
General Precision Inc.
Charles J. Mundo
Institute of Naval Studies

***14. Celestial Mechanics and Astrodynamics (1964)**
Victor G. Szebehely
Yale University Observatory

***15. Heterogeneous Combustion (1964)**
Hans G. Wolfhard
Institute for Defense Analyses
Irvin Glassman
Princeton University
Leon Green Jr.
Air Force Systems Command

***16. Space Power Systems Engineering (1966)**
George C. Szego
Institute for Defense Analyses
J. Edward Taylor
TRW Inc.

***17. Methods in Astrodynamics and Celestial Mechanics (1966)**
Raynor L. Duncombe
U.S. Naval Observatory
Victor G. Szebehely
Yale University Observatory

***18. Thermophysics and Temperature Control of Spacecraft and Entry Vehicles (1966)**
Gerhard B. Heller
NASA George C. Marshall Space Flight Center

***19. Communication Satellite Systems Technology (1966)**
Richard B. Marsten
Radio Corporation of America

---

*Out of print.

***20. Thermophysics of Spacecraft and Planetary Bodies: Radiation Properties of Solids and the Electromagnetic Radiation Environment in Space (1967)**
Gerhard B. Heller
NASA George C. Marshall Space Flight Center

***21. Thermal Design Principles of Spacecraft and Entry Bodies (1969)**
Jerry T. Bevans
TRW Systems

***22. Stratospheric Circulation (1969)**
Willis L. Webb
Atmospheric Sciences Laboratory, White Sands, and University of Texas at El Paso

***23. Thermophysics: Applications to Thermal Design of Spacecraft (1970)**
Jerry T. Bevans
TRW Systems

***24. Heat Transfer and Spacecraft Thermal Control (1971)**
John W. Lucas
Jet Propulsion Laboratory

25. Communication Satellites for the 70's: Technology (1971)
Nathaniel E. Feldman
The Rand Corp.
Charles M. Kelly
The Aerospace Corp.

26. Communication Satellites for the 70's: Systems (1971)
Nathaniel E. Feldman
The Rand Corp.
Charles M. Kelly
The Aerospace Corp.

27. Thermospheric Circulation (1972)
Willis L. Webb
Atmospheric Sciences Laboratory, White Sands, and University of Texas at El Paso

28. Thermal Characteristics of the Moon (1972)
John W. Lucas
Jet Propulsion Laboratory

***29. Fundamentals of Spacecraft Thermal Design (1972)**
John W. Lucas
Jet Propulsion Laboratory

***30. Solar Activity Observations and Predictions (1972)**
Patrick S. McIntosh
Murray Dryer
Environmental Research Laboratories, National Oceanic and Atmospheric Administration

***31. Thermal Control and Radiation (1973)**
Chang-Lin Tien
University of California at Berkeley

***32. Communications Satellite Systems (1974)**
P. L. Bargellini
COMSAT Laboratories

***33. Communications Satellite Technology (1974)**
P. L. Bargellini
COMSAT Laboratories

***34. Instrumentation for Airbreathing Propulsion (1974)**
Allen E. Fuhs
Naval Postgraduate School
Marshall Kingery
Arnold Engineering Development Center

***35. Thermophysics and Spacecraft Thermal Control (1974)**
Robert G. Hering
University of Iowa

36. Thermal Pollution Analysis (1975)
Joseph A. Schetz
Virginia Polytechnic Institute
ISBN 0-915928-00-0

***37. Aeroacoustics: Jet and Combustion Noise; Duct Acoustics (1975)**
Henry T. Nagamatsu, Editor
General Electric Research and Development Center
Jack V. O'Keefe, Associate Editor
The Boeing Co.
Ira R. Schwartz, Associate Editor
NASA Ames Research Center
ISBN 0-915928-01-9

***38. Aeroacoustics: Fan, STOL, and Boundary Layer Noise; Sonic Boom; Aeroacoustics Instrumentation (1975)**
Henry T. Nagamatsu, Editor
General Electric Research and Development Center
Jack V. O'Keefe, Associate Editor
The Boeing Co.
Ira R. Schwartz, Associate Editor
NASA Ames Research Center
ISBN 0-915928-02-7

***39. Heat Transfer with Thermal Control Applications (1975)**
M. Michael Yovanovich
University of Waterloo
ISBN 0-915928-03-5

*Out of print.

***40. Aerodynamics of Base Combustion (1976)**
S. N. B. Murthy, Editor
J. R. Osborn, Associate Editor
Purdue University
A. W. Barrows
J. R. Ward, Associate Editors
Ballistics Research Laboratories
ISBN 0-915928-04-3

***41. Communications Satellite Developments: Systems (1976)**
Gilbert E. LaVean
Defense Communications Agency
William G. Schmidt
CML Satellite Corp.
ISBN 0-915928-05-1

***42. Communications Satellite Developments: Technology (1976)**
William G. Schmidt
CML Satellite Corp.
Gilbert E. LaVean
Defense Communications Agency
ISBN 0-915928-06-X

***43. Aeroacoustics: Jet Noise, Combustion and Core Engine Noise (1976)**
Ira R. Schwartz, Editor
NASA Ames Research Center
Henry T. Nagamatsu, Associate Editor
General Electric Research and Development Center
Warren C. Strahle, Associate Editor
Georgia Institute of Technology
ISBN 0-915928-07-8

***44. Aeroacoustics: Fan Noise and Control; Duct Acoustics; Rotor Noise (1976)**
Ira R. Schwartz, Editor
NASA Ames Research Center
Henry T. Nagamatsu, Associate Editor
General Electric Research and Development Center
Warren C. Strahle, Associate Editor
Georgia Institute of Technology
ISBN 0-915928-08-6

***45. Aeroacoustics: STOL Noise; Airframe and Airfoil Noise (1976)**
Ira R. Schwartz, Editor
NASA Ames Research Center
Henry T. Nagamatsu, Associate Editor
General Electric Research and Development Center
Warren C. Strahle, Associate Editor
Georgia Institute of Technology
ISBN 0-915928-09-4

***46. Aeroacoustics: Acoustic Wave Propagation; Aircraft Noise Prediction; Aeroacoustic Instrumentation (1976)**
Ira R. Schwartz, Editor
NASA Ames Research Center
Henry T. Nagamatsu, Associate Editor
General Electric Research and Development Center
Warren C. Strahle, Associate Editor
Georgia Institute of Technology
ISBN 0-915928-10-8

***47. Spacecraft Charging by Magnetospheric Plasmas (1976)**
Alan Rosen
TRW Inc.
ISBN 0-915928-11-6

***48. Scientific Investigations on the Skylab Satellite (1976)**
Marion I. Kent
Ernst Stuhlinger
NASA George C. Marshall Space Flight Center
Shi-Tsan Wu
University of Alabama
ISBN 0-915928-12-4

***49. Radiative Transfer and Thermal Control (1976)**
Allie M. Smith
ARO Inc.
ISBN 0-915928-13-2

***50. Exploration of the Outer Solar System (1976)**
Eugene W. Greenstadt
TRW Inc.
Murray Dryer
National Oceanic and Atmospheric Administration
Devrie S. Intriligator
University of Southern California
ISBN 0-915928-14-0

***51. Rarefied Gas Dynamics, Parts I and II (two volumes) (1977)**
J. Leith Potter
ARO Inc.
ISBN 0-915928-15-9

***52. Materials Sciences in Space with Application to Space Processing (1977)**
Leo Steg
General Electric Co.
ISBN 0-915928-16-7

---

*Out of print.

***53. Experimental Diagnostics in Gas Phase Combustion Systems (1977)**
Ben T. Zinn, Editor
Georgia Institute of Technology
Craig T. Bowman, Associate Editor
Stanford University
Daniel L. Hartley, Associate Editor
Sandia Laboratories
Edward W. Price, Associate Editor
Georgia Institute of Technology
James G. Skifstad, Associate Editor
Purdue University
ISBN 0-915928-18-3

***54. Satellite Communication: Future Systems (1977)**
David Jarett
TRW Inc.
ISBN 0-915928-18-3

***55. Satellite Communications: Advanced Technologies (1977)**
David Jarett
TRW Inc.
ISBN 0-915928-19-1

***56. Thermophysics of Spacecraft and Outer Planet Entry Probes (1977)**
Allie M. Smith
ARO Inc.
ISBN 0-915928-20-5

***57. Space-Based Manufacturing from Nonterrestrial Materials (1977)**
Gerald K. O'Neill, Editor
Brian O'Leary, Assistant Editor
Princeton University
ISBN 0-915928-21-3

***58. Turbulent Combustion (1978)**
Lawrence A. Kennedy
State University of New York at Buffalo
ISBN 0-915928-22-1

***59. Aerodynamic Heating and Thermal Protection Systems (1978)**
Leroy S. Fletcher
University of Virginia
ISBN 0-915928-23-X

***60. Heat Transfer and Thermal Control Systems (1978)**
Leroy S. Fletcher
University of Virginia
ISBN 0-915928-24-8

***61. Radiation Energy Conversion in Space (1978)**
Kenneth W. Billman
NASA Ames Research Center
ISBN 0-915928-26-4

***62. Alternative Hydrocarbon Fuels: Combustion and Chemical Kinetics (1978)**
Craig T. Bowman
Stanford University
Jorgen Birkeland
Department of Energy
ISBN 0-915928-25-6

***63. Experimental Diagnostics in Combustion of Solids (1978)**
Thomas L. Boggs
Naval Weapons Center
Ben T. Zinn
Georgia Institute of Technology
ISBN 0-915928-28-0

***64. Outer Planet Entry Heating and Thermal Protection (1979)**
Raymond Viskanta
Purdue University
ISBN 0-915928-29-9

***65. Thermophysics and Thermal Control (1979)**
Raymond Viskanta
Purdue University
ISBN 0-915928-30-2

***66. Interior Ballistics of Guns (1979)**
Herman Krier
University of Illinois at Urbana–Champaign
Martin Summerfield
New York University
ISBN 0-915928-32-9

***67. Remote Sensing of Earth from Space: Role of "Smart Sensors" (1979)**
Roger A. Breckenridge
NASA Langley Research Center
ISBN 0-915928-33-7

***68. Injection and Mixing in Turbulent Flow (1980)**
Joseph A. Schetz
Virginia Polytechnic Institute and State University
ISBN 0-915928-35-3

---

*Out of print.

***69. Entry Heating and Thermal Protection (1980)**
Walter B. Olstad
NASA Headquarters
ISBN 0-915928-38-8

***70. Heat Transfer, Thermal Control, and Heat Pipes (1980)**
Walter B. Olstad
NASA Headquarters
ISBN 0-915928-39-6

***71. Space Systems and Their Interactions with Earth's Space Environment (1980)**
Henry B. Garrett
Charles P. Pike
Hanscom Air Force Base
ISBN 0-915928-41-8

***72. Viscous Flow Drag Reduction (1980)**
Gary R. Hough
Vought Advanced Technology Center
ISBN 0-915928-44-2

***73. Combustion Experiments in a Zero-Gravity Laboratory (1981)**
Thomas H. Cochran
NASA Lewis Research Center
ISBN 0-915928-48-5

***74. Rarefied Gas Dynamics, Parts I and II (two volumes) (1981)**
Sam S. Fisher
University of Virginia
ISBN 0-915928-51-5

***75. Gasdynamics of Detonations and Explosions (1981)**
J. R. Bowen
University of Wisconsin at Madison
N. Manson
Universite de Poitiers
A. K. Oppenheim
University of California at Berkeley
R. I. Soloukhin
Institute of Heat and Mass Transfer, BSSR Academy of Sciences
ISBN 0-915928-46-9

***76. Combustion in Reactive Systems (1981)**
J. R. Bowen
University of Wisconsin at Madison
N. Manson
Universite de Poitiers
A. K. Oppenheim
University of California at Berkeley
R. I. Soloukhin
Institute of Heat and Mass Transfer, BSSR Academy of Sciences
ISBN 0-915928-47-7

***77. Aerothermodynamics and Planetary Entry (1981)**
A. L. Crosbie
University of Missouri-Rolla
ISBN 0-915928-52-3

***78. Heat Transfer and Thermal Control (1981)**
A. L. Crosbie
University of Missouri-Rolla
ISBN 0-915928-53-1

***79. Electric Propulsion and Its Applications to Space Missions (1981)**
Robert C. Finke
NASA Lewis Research Center
ISBN 0-915928-55-8

***80. Aero-Optical Phenomena (1982)**
Keith G. Gilbert
Leonard J. Otten
Air Force Weapons Laboratory
ISBN 0-915928-60-4

***81. Transonic Aerodynamics (1982)**
David Nixon
Nielsen Engineering & Research, Inc.
ISBN 0-915928-65-5

***82. Thermophysics of Atmospheric Entry (1982)**
T. E. Horton
University of Mississippi
ISBN 0-915928-66-3

***83. Spacecraft Radiative Transfer and Temperature Control (1982)**
T. E. Horton
University of Mississippi
ISBN 0-915928-67-1

***84. Liquid-Metal Flows and Magneto-hydrodynamics (1983)**
H. Branover
Ben-Gurion University of the Negev
P. S. Lykoudis
Purdue University
A. Yakhot
Ben-Gurion University of the Negev
ISBN 0-915928-70-1

*Out of print.

***85. Entry Vehicle Heating and Thermal Protection Systems: Space Shuttle, Solar Starprobe, Jupiter Galileo Probe (1983)**
Paul E. Bauer
McDonnell Douglas Astronautics Co.
Howard E. Collicott
The Boeing Co.
ISBN 0-915928-74-4

***86. Spacecraft Thermal Control, Design, and Operation (1983)**
Howard E. Collicott
The Boeing Co.
Paul E. Bauer
McDonnell Douglas Astronautics Co.
ISBN 0-915928-75-2

***87. Shock Waves, Explosions, and Detonations (1983)**
J. R. Bowen
University of Washington
N. Manson
Universite de Poitiers
A. K. Oppenheim
University of California at Berkeley
R. I. Soloukhin
Institute of Heat and Mass Transfer, BSSR Academy of Sciences
ISBN 0-915928-76-0

***88. Flames, Lasers, and Reactive Systems (1983)**
J. R. Bowen
University of Washington
N. Manson
Universite de Poitiers
A. K. Oppenheim
University of California at Berkeley
R. I. Soloukhin
Institute of Heat and Mass Transfer, BSSR Academy of Sciences
ISBN 0-915928-77-9

***89. Orbit-Raising and Maneuvering Propulsion: Research Status and Needs (1984)**
Leonard H. Caveny
Air Force Office of Scientific Research
ISBN 0-915928-82-5

***90. Fundamentals of Solid-Propellant Combustion (1984)**
Kenneth K. Kuo
Pennsylvania State University
Martin Summerfield
Princeton Combustion Research Laboratories, Inc.
ISBN 0-915928-84-1

91. Spacecraft Contamination: Sources and Prevention (1984)
J. A. Roux
University of Mississippi
T. D. McCay
NASA Marshall Space Flight Center
ISBN 0-915928-85-X

92. Combustion Diagnostics by Nonintrusive Methods (1984)
T. D. McCay
NASA Marshall Space Flight Center
J. A. Roux
University of Mississippi
ISBN 0-915928-86-8

93. The INTELSAT Global Satellite System (1984)
Joel Alper
COMSAT Corp.
Joseph Pelton
INTELSAT
ISBN 0-915928-90-6

94. Dynamics of Shock Waves, Explosions, and Detonations (1984)
J. R. Bowen
University of Washington
N. Manson
Universite de Poitiers
A. K. Oppenheim
University of California at Berkeley
R. I. Soloukhin
Institute of Heat and Mass Transfer, BSSR Academy of Sciences
ISBN 0-915928-91-4

95. Dynamics of Flames and Reactive Systems (1984)
J. R. Bowen
University of Washington
N. Manson
Universite de Poitiers
A. K. Oppenheim
University of California at Berkeley
R. I. Soloukhin
Institute of Heat and Mass Transfer, BSSR Academy of Sciences
ISBN 0-915928-92-2

96. Thermal Design of Aeroassisted Orbital Transfer Vehicles (1985)
H. F. Nelson
University of Missouri-Rolla
ISBN 0-915928-94-9

97. Monitoring Earth's Ocean, Land, and Atmosphere from Space—Sensors, Systems, and Applications (1985)
Abraham Schnapf
Aerospace Systems Engineering
ISBN 0-915928-98-1

---

*Out of print.

98. Thrust and Drag: Its Prediction and Verification (1985)
Eugene E. Covert
Massachusetts Institute of Technology
C. R. James
Vought Corp.
William F. Kimzey
Sverdrup Technology AEDC Group
George K. Richey
U.S. Air Force
Eugene C. Rooney
U.S. Navy Department of Defense
ISBN 0-930403-00-2

99. Space Stations and Space Platforms—Concepts, Design, Infrastructure, and Uses (1985)
Ivan Bekey
Daniel Herman
NASA Headquarters
ISBN 0-930403-01-0

100. Single- and Multi-Phase Flows in an Electromagnetic Field: Energy, Metallurgical, and Solar Applications (1985)
Herman Branover
Ben-Gurion University of the Negev
Paul S. Lykoudis
Purdue University
Michael Mond
Ben-Gurion University of the Negev
ISBN 0-930403-04-5

101. MHD Energy Conversion: Physiotechnical Problems (1986)
V. A. Kirillin
A. E. Sheyndlin
Soviet Academy of Sciences
ISBN 0-930403-05-3

102. Numerical Methods for Engine-Airframe Integration (1986)
S. N. B. Murthy
Purdue University
Gerald C. Paynter
Boeing Airplane Co.
ISBN 0-930403-09-6

103. Thermophysical Aspects of Re-Entry Flows (1986)
James N. Moss
NASA Langley Research Center
Carl D. Scott
NASA Johnson Space Center
ISBN 0-930430-10-X

***104. Tactical Missile Aerodynamics (1986)**
M. J. Hemsch
PRC Kentron, Inc.
J. N. Nielson
NASA Ames Research Center
ISBN 0-930403-13-4

105. Dynamics of Reactive Systems Part I: Flames and Configurations; Part II: Modeling and Heterogeneous Combustion (1986)
J. R. Bowen
University of Washington
J.-C. Leyer
Universite de Poitiers
R. I. Soloukhin
Institute of Heat and Mass Transfer, BSSR Academy of Sciences
ISBN 0-930403-14-2

106. Dynamics of Explosions (1986)
J. R. Bowen
University of Washington
J.-C. Leyer
Universite de Poitiers
R. I. Soloukhin
Institute of Heat and Mass Transfer, BSSR Academy of Sciences
ISBN 0-930403-15-0

***107. Spacecraft Dielectric Material Properties and Spacecraft Charging (1986)**
A. R. Frederickson
U.S. Air Force Rome Air Development Center
D. B. Cotts
SRI International
J. A. Wall
U.S. Air Force Rome Air Development Center
F. L. Bouquet
Jet Propulsion Laboratory, California Institute of Technology
ISBN 0-930403-17-7

***108. Opportunities for Academic Research in a Low-Gravity Environment (1986)**
George A. Hazelrigg
National Science Foundation
Joseph M. Reynolds
Louisiana State University
ISBN 0-930403-18-5

109. Gun Propulsion Technology (1988)
Ludwig Stiefel
U.S. Army Armament Research, Development and Engineering Center
ISBN 0-930403-20-7

*Out of print.

110. Commercial Opportunities in Space (1988)
F. Shahrokhi
K. E. Harwell
University of Tennessee Space Institute
C. C. Chao
National Cheng Kung University
ISBN 0-930403-39-8

111. Liquid-Metal Flows: Magnetohydrodynamics and Application (1988)
Herman Branover
Michael Mond
Yeshajahu Unger
Ben-Gurion University of the Negev
ISBN 0-930403-43-6

112. Current Trends in Turbulence Research (1988)
Herman Branover
Micheal Mond
Yeshajahu Unger
Ben-Gurion University of the Negev
ISBN 0-930403-44-4

113. Dynamics of Reactive Systems Part I: Flames; Part II: Heterogeneous Combustion and Applications (1988)
A. L. Kuhl
R&D Associates
J. R. Bowen
University of Washington
J.-C. Leyer
Universite de Poitiers
A. Borisov
USSR Academy of Sciences
ISBN 0-930403-46-0

114. Dynamics of Explosions (1988)
A. L. Kuhl
R & D Associates
J. R. Bowen
University of Washington
J.-C. Leyer
Universite de Poitiers
A. Borisov
USSR Academy of Sciences
ISBN 0-930403-47-9

115. Machine Intelligence and Autonomy for Aerospace (1988)
E. Heer
Heer Associates, Inc.
H. Lum
NASA Ames Research Center
ISBN 0-930403-48-7

116. Rarefied Gas Dynamics: Space Related Studies (1989)
E. P. Muntz
University of Southern California
D. P. Weaver
U.S. Air Force Astronautics Laboratory (AFSC)
D. H. Campbell
University of Dayton Research Institute
ISBN 0-930403-53-3

117. Rarefied Gas Dynamics: Physical Phenomena (1989)
E. P. Muntz
University of Southern California
D. P. Weaver
U.S. Air Force Astronautics Laboratory (AFSC)
D. H. Campbell
University of Dayton Research Institute
ISBN 0-930403-54-1

118. Rarefied Gas Dynamics: Theoretical and Computational Techniques (1989)
E. P. Muntz
University of Southern California
D. P. Weaver
U.S. Air Force Astronautics Laboratory (AFSC)
D. H. Campbell
University of Dayton Research Institute
ISBN 0-930403-55-X

119. Test and Evaluation of the Tactical Missile (1989)
Emil J. Eichblatt Jr.
Pacific Missile Test Center
ISBN 0-930403-56-8

120. Unsteady Transonic Aerodynamics (1989)
David Nixon
Nielsen Engineering & Research, Inc.
ISBN 0-930403-52-5

121. Orbital Debris from Upper-Stage Breakup (1989)
Joseph P. Loftus Jr.
NASA Johnson Space Center
ISBN 0-930403-58-4

122. Thermal-Hydraulics for Space Power, Propulsion and Thermal Management System Design (1990)
William J. Krotiuk
General Electric Co.
ISBN 0-930403-64-9

*Out of print.

123. Viscous Drag Reduction in Boundary Layers (1990)
Dennis M. Bushnell
Jerry N. Hefner
NASA Langley Research Center
ISBN 0-930403-66-5

***124. Tactical and Strategic Missile Guidance (1990)**
Paul Zarchan
Charles Stark Draper Laboratory, Inc.
ISBN 0-930403-68-1

125. Applied Computational Aerodynamics (1990)
P. A. Henne
Douglas Aircraft Company
ISBN 0-930403-69-X

126. Space Commercialization: Launch Vehicles and Programs (1990)
F. Shahrokhi
University of Tennessee Space Institute
J. S. Greenberg
Princeton Synergetics Inc.
T. Al-Saud
Ministry of Defense and Aviation Kingdom of Saudi Arabia
ISBN 0-930403-75-4

127. Space Commercialization: Platforms and Processing (1990)
F. Shahrokhi
University of Tennessee Space Institute
G. Hazelrigg
National Science Foundation
R. Bayuzick
Vanderbilt University
ISBN 0-930403-76-2

128. Space Commercialization: Satellite Technology (1990)
F. Shahrokhi
University of Tennessee Space Institute
N. Jasentuliyana
United Nations
N. Tarabzouni
King Abulaziz City for Science and Technology
ISBN 0-930403-77-0

***129. Mechanics and Control of Large Flexible Structures (1990)**
John L. Junkins
Texas A&M University
ISBN 0-930403-73-8

130. Low-Gravity Fluid Dynamics and Transport Phenomena (1990)
Jean N. Koster
Robert L. Sani
University of Colorado at Boulder
ISBN 0-930403-74-6

131. Dynamics of Deflagrations and Reactive Systems: Flames (1991)
A. L. Kuhl
Lawrence Livermore National Laboratory
J.-C. Leyer
Universite de Poitiers
A. A. Borisov
USSR Academy of Sciences
W. A. Sirignano
University of California
ISBN 0-930403-95-9

132. Dynamics of Deflagrations and Reactive Systems: Heterogeneous Combustion (1991)
A. L. Kuhl
Lawrence Livermore National Laboratory
J.-C. Leyer
Universite de Poitiers
A. A. Borisov
USSR Academy of Sciences
W. A. Sirignano
University of California
ISBN 0-930403-96-7

133. Dynamics of Detonations and Explosions: Detonations (1991)
A. L. Kuhl
Lawrence Livermore National Laboratory
J.-C. Leyer
Universite de Poitiers
A. A. Borisov
USSR Academy of Sciences
W. A. Sirignano
University of California
ISBN 0-930403-97-5

134. Dynamics of Detonations and Explosions: Explosion Phenomena (1991)
A. L. Kuhl
Lawrence Livermore National Laboratory
J.-C. Leyer
Universite de Poitiers
A. A. Borisov
USSR Academy of Sciences
W. A. Sirignano
University of California
ISBN 0-930403-98-3

---

*Out of print.

135. Numerical Approaches to Combustion Modeling (1991)
Elaine S. Oran
Jay P. Boris
Naval Research Laboratory
ISBN 1-56347-004-7

136. Aerospace Software Engineering (1991)
Christine Anderson
U.S. Air Force Wright Laboratory
Merlin Dorfman
Lockheed Missiles & Space Company, Inc.
ISBN 1-56347-005-0

137. High-Speed Flight Propulsion Systems (1991)
S. N. B. Murthy
Purdue University
E. T. Curran
Wright Laboratory
ISBN 1-56347-011-X

138. Propagation of Intensive Laser Radiation in Clouds (1992)
O. A. Volkovitsky
Yu. S. Sedenov
L. P. Semenov
Institute of Experimental Meteorology
ISBN 1-56347-020-9

139. Gun Muzzle Blast and Flash (1992)
Günter Klingenberg
Fraunhofer-Institut für Kurzzeitdynamik, Ernst-Mach-Institut
Joseph M. Heimerl
U.S. Army Ballistic Research Laboratory
ISBN 1-56347-012-8

140. Thermal Structures and Materials for High-Speed Flight (1992)
Earl. A. Thornton
University of Virginia
ISBN 1-56347-017-9

141. Tactical Missile Aerodynamics: General Topics (1992)
Michael J. Hemsch
Lockheed Engineering & Sciences Company
ISBN 1-56347-015-2

142. Tactical Missile Aerodynamics: Prediction Methodology (1992)
Michael R. Mendenhall
Nielsen Engineering & Research, Inc.
ISBN 1-56347-016-0

143. Nonsteady Burning and Combustion Stability of Solid Propellants (1992)
Luigi De Luca
Politecnico di Milano
Edward W. Price
Georgia Institute of Technology
Martin Summerfield
Princeton Combustion Research Laboratories, Inc.
ISBN 1-56347-014-4

144. Space Economics (1992)
Joel S. Greenberg
Princeton Synergetics, Inc.
Henry R. Hertzfeld
HRH Associates
ISBN 1-56347-042-X

145. Mars: Past, Present, and Future (1992)
E. Brian Pritchard
NASA Langley Research Center
ISBN 1-56347-043-8

146. Computational Nonlinear Mechanics in Aerospace Engineering (1992)
Satya N. Atluri
Georgia Institute of Technology
ISBN 1-56347-044-6

147. Modern Engineering for Design of Liquid-Propellant Rocket Engines (1992)
Dieter K. Huzel
David H. Huang
Rocketdyne Division of Rockwell International
ISBN 1-56347-013-6

148. Metallurgical Technologies, Energy Conversion, and Magnetohydrodynamic Flows (1993)
Herman Branover
Yeshajahu Unger
Ben-Gurion University of the Negev
ISBN 1-56347-019-5

149. Advances in Turbulence Studies (1993)
Herman Branover
Yeshajahu Unger
Ben-Gurion University of the Negev
ISBN 1-56347-018-7

150. Structural Optimization: Status and Promise (1993)
Manohar P. Kamat
Georgia Institute of Technology
ISBN 1-56347-056-X

*Out of print.

151. Dynamics of Gaseous Combustion (1993)
A. L. Kuhl
Lawrence Livermore National Laboratory
J.-C. Leyer
Universite de Poitiers
A. A. Borisov
USSR Academy of Sciences
W. A. Sirignano
University of California
ISBN 1-56347-060-8

152. Dynamics of Heterogeneous Gaseous Combustion and Reacting Systems (1993)
A. L. Kuhl
Lawrence Livermore National Laboratory
J.-C. Leyer
Universite de Poitiers
A. A. Borisov
USSR Academy of Sciences
W. A. Sirignano
University of California
ISBN 1-56347-058-6

153. Dynamic Aspects of Detonations (1993)
A. L. Kuhl
Lawrence Livermore National Laboratory
J.-C. Leyer
Universite de Poitiers
A. A. Borisov
USSR Academy of Sciences
W. A. Sirignano
University of California
ISBN 1-56347-057-8

154. Dynamic Aspects of Explosion Phenomena (1993)
A. L. Kuhl
Lawrence Livermore National Laboratory
J.-C. Leyer
Universite de Poitiers
A. A. Borisov
USSR Academy of Sciences
W. A. Sirignano
University of California
ISBN 1-56347-059-4

155. Tactical Missile Warheads (1993)
Joseph Carleone
Aerojet General Corporation
ISBN 1-56347-067-5

156. Toward a Science of Command, Control, and Communications (1993)
Carl R. Jones
Naval Postgraduate School
ISBN 1-56347-068-3

***157. Tactical and Strategic Missile Guidance Second Edition (1994)**
Paul Zarchan
Charles Stark Draper Laboratory, Inc.
ISBN 1-56347-077-2

158. Rarefied Gas Dynamics: Experimental Techniques and Physical Systems (1994)
Bernie D. Shizgal
University of British Columbia
David P. Weaver
Phillips Laboratory
ISBN 1-56347-079-9

159. Rarefied Gas Dynamics: Theory and Simulations (1994)
Bernie D. Shizgal
University of British Columbia
David P. Weaver
Phillips Laboratory
ISBN 1-56347-080-2

160. Rarefied Gas Dynamics: Space Sciences and Engineering (1994)
Bernie D. Shizgal
University of British Columbia
David P. Weaver
Phillips Laboratory
ISBN 1-56347-081-0

161. Teleoperation and Robotics in Space (1994)
Steven B. Skaar
University of Notre Dame
Carl F. Ruoff
Jet Propulsion Laboratory, California Institute of Technology
ISBN 1-56347-095-0

162. Progress in Turbulence Research (1994)
Herman Branover
Yeshajahu Unger
Ben-Gurion University of the Negev
ISBN 1-56347-099-3

163. Global Positioning System: Theory and Applications, Volume I (1996)
Bradford W. Parkinson
Stanford University
James J. Spilker Jr.
Stanford Telecom
Penina Axelrad,
Associate Editor
University of Colorado
Per Enge,
Associate Editor
Stanford University
ISBN 1-56347-107-8

164. Global Positioning System: Theory and Applications, Volume II (1996)
Bradford W. Parkinson
Stanford University
James J. Spilker Jr.
Stanford Telecom
Penina Axelrad,
Associate Editor
University of Colorado
Per Enge,
Associate Editor
Stanford University
ISBN 1-56347-106-X

---

*Out of print.

165. Developments in High-Speed Vehicle Propulsion Systems (1996)
S. N. B. Murthy
Purdue University
E. T. Curran
Wright Laboratory
ISBN 1-56347-176-0

166. Recent Advances in Spray Combustion: Spray Atomization and Drop Burning Phenomena, Volume I (1996)
Kenneth K. Kuo
Pennsylvania State University
ISBN 1-56347-175-2

167. Fusion Energy in Space Propulsion (1995)
Terry Kammash
University of Michigan
ISBN 1-56347-184-1

168. Aerospace Thermal Structures and Materials for a New Era (1995)
Earl A. Thornton
University of Virginia
ISBN 1-56347-182-5

169. Liquid Rocket Engine Combustion Instability (1995)
Vigor Yang
William E. Anderson
Pennsylvania State University
ISBN 1-56347-183-3

170. Tactical Missile Propulsion (1996)
G. E. Jensen
United Technologies Corporation
David W. Netzer
Naval Postgraduate School
ISBN 1-56347-118-3

171. Recent Advances in Spray Combustion: Spray Combustion Measurements and Model Simulation, Volume II (1996)
Kenneth K. Kuo
Pennsylvania State University
ISBN 1-56347-181-7

172. Future Aeronautical and Space Systems (1997)
Ahmed K. Noor
NASA Langley Research Center
Samuel L. Venneri
NASA Headquarters
ISBN 1-56347-188-4

173. Advances in Combustion Science: In Honor of Ya. B. Zel'dovich (1997)
William A. Sirignano
University of California
Alexander G. Merzhanov
Russian Academy of Sciences
Luigi De Luca
Politecnico di Milano
ISBN 1-56347-178-7

174. Fundamentals of High Accuracy Inertial Navigation (1997)
Averil B. Chatfield
ISBN 1-56347-243-0

175. Liquid Propellant Gun Technology (1997)
Günter Klingenberg
Fraunhofer-Institut für Kurzzeitdynamik, Ernst-Mach-Institut
John D. Knapton
Walter F. Morrison
Gloria P. Wren
U.S. Army Research Laboratory
ISBN 1-56347-196-5

176. Tactical and Strategic Missile Guidance Third Edition (1998)
Paul Zarchan
Charles Stark Draper Laboratory, Inc.
ISBN 1-56347-279-1

177. Orbital and Celestial Mechanics (1998)
John P. Vinti
Gim J. Der, Editor
TRW
Nino L. Bonavito, Editor
NASA Goddard Space Flight Center
ISBN 1-56347-256-2

178. Some Engineering Applications in Random Vibrations and Random Structures (1998)
Giora Maymon
RAFAEL
ISBN 1-56347-258-9

179. Conventional Warhead Systems Physics and Engineering Design (1998)
Richard M. Lloyd
Raytheon Systems Company
ISBN 1-56347-255-4

180. Advances in Missile Guidance Theory (1998)
Joseph Z. Ben-Asher
Isaac Yaesh
Israel Military Industries—Advanced Systems Division
ISBN 1-56347-275-9

181. Satellite Thermal Control for Systems Engineers (1998)
Robert D. Karam
ISBN 1-56347-276-7

---

*Out of print.

182. Progress in Fluid Flow Research: Turbulence and Applied MHD (1998)
Yeshajahu Unger
Herman Branover
Ben-Gurion University of the Negev
ISBN 1-56347-284-8

183. Aviation Weather Surveillance Systems (1999)
Pravas R. Mahapatra
Indian Institute of Science
ISBN 1-56347-340-2

184. Flight Control Systems (2000)
Rodger W. Pratt
Loughborough University
ISBN 1-56347-404-2

185. Solid Propellant Chemistry, Combustion, and Motor Interior Ballistics (2000)
Vigor Yang
Pennsylvania State University
Thomas B. Brill
University of Delaware
Wu-Zhen Ren
China Ordnance Society
ISBN 1-56347-442-5

186. Approximate Methods for Weapons Aerodynamics (2000)
Frank G. Moore
ISBN 1-56347-399-2

187. Micropropulsion for Small Spacecraft (2000)
Michael M. Micci
Pennsylvania State University
Andrew D. Ketsdever
Air Force Research Laboratory, Edwards Air Force Base
ISBN 1-56347-448-4

188. Structures Technology for Future Aerospace Systems (2000)
Ahmed K. Noor
NASA Langley Research Center
ISBN 1-56347-384-4

189. Scramjet Propulsion (2000)
E. T. Curran
Department of the Air Force
S. N. B. Murthy
Purdue University
ISBN 1-56347-322-4

190. Fundamentals of Kalman Filtering: A Practical Approach (2000)
Paul Zarchan
Howard Musoff
Charles Stark Draper Laboratory, Inc.
ISBN 1-56347-455-7

191. Gossamer Spacecraft: Membrane and Inflatable Structures Technology for Space Applications (2001)
Christopher H.M. Jenkins
South Dakota School of Mines
ISBN 1-56347-403-4

192. Theater Ballistic Missile Defense (2001)
Ben-Zion Naveh
Azriel Lorber
WALES Ltd.
ISBN 1-56347-385-2

---

*Out of print.